Lasers in Maxillofacial Surgery and Dentistry

Lasers in Maxillofacial Surgery and Dentistry

Edited by

Lewis Clayman, D.M.D., M.D.
Chairman
Department of Dentistry/Oral and Maxillofacial Surgery
Sinai Hospital
Detroit, Michigan

Clinical Professor
Department of Oral and Maxillofacial Surgery
University of Detroit-Mercy School of Dentistry
Detroit, Michigan

Paul Kuo, D.M.D., M.D.
Visiting Associate Professor
Head and Neck/Plastic Reconstructive Surgery Unit
Department of Surgery
Chinese University of Hong Kong
Shatin, Hong Kong

1997

Thieme
New York • Stuttgart

Thieme Medical Publishers, Inc.
381 Park Avenue South
New York, NY 10016

Lasers in Maxillofacial Surgery and Dentistry
Lewis Clayman, D.M.D, M.D.
Paul Kuo, D.M.D, M.D.

Library of Congress Cataloging-in-Publication Data
Lasers in maxillofacial surgery and dentistry / edited by Lewis Clayman, Paul Kuo
p. cm.
Includes bibliographical references and index.
ISBN 0-86577-566-4
1. Mouth—Laser surgery. 2. Jaws—Laser surgery. 3. Face—Laser surgery.
4. Lasers in dentistry. I. Clayman, Lewis. II. Kuo, Paul, D.M.D.
[DNLM: 1. Surgery, Oral—methods. 2. Laser Surgery—methods. WU 600 L3435 1995]
RK530.5.L37 1997
617.5'2059—dc20
DNLM/DLC
for Library of Congress 96-36512
CIP

Printed in the United States of America

5 4 3 2 1

TNY ISBN 0-86577-566-4
GTV ISBN 3-13-103861-6

This book is dedicated to the patients we serve and to my wife, Minoo and children, Eric and Lara whose love and support have permitted me the time to write this book. I thank my parents, Irwin and Esther, for a lifetime of encouragement. I especially acknowledge my mentors, the late Herbert J. Bloom, D.D.S., and John Helfrick, D.D.S., M.S., without whose guidance and encouragement I would not have become an oral and maxillofacial surgeon with a passionate interest in lasers.

Contents

Contributors

Steven J. Butler, D.D.S.
Private Practice
Oral & Maxillofacial Surgeon
Fort Wayne, Indiana

Dan Castro, D.D.S.
Associate Professor
UCLA School of Medicine
Los Angeles, California

Lewis Clayman, D.M.D., M.D.
Chairman, Department of Dentistry
Oral Maxillofacial Surgery
Sinai Hospital
Detroit, Michigan

Michael D. Colvard, D.M.D.
Periodontal Surgery and Oral Medicine Associates
Schaumberg, Illinois

Lawrence M. Elson, M.D.
Clinical Manager
Laser Institute
Detroit, Michigan

Terry A. Fuller, Ph.D.
Adjunct Professor of Surgery
Surgical Laser Technologies, Inc.
Oaks, Pennsylvania

Yves-Victor Kamami, M.D.
Private Practice
Paris, France

Paul Kuo, D.M.D., M.D.
Visiting Associate Professor
Plastic and Reconstructive/Head and Neck Surgery Unit
Chinese University of Hong Kong
Hong Kong

Claus R. Lange, M.D.
Pacific Center for Joint and Facial Surgery
Encinitas, California

Robert Meleca, M.D.
Clinical Assistant Professor
NIH Research Fellow
Department of Otolaryngology
Wayne State University
Detroit, Michigan

Jeffrey J. Moses, M.D.
Pacific Center for Joint and Facial Surgery
Encinitas, California

Richard Reid, M.D.
Assistant Professor
Department of Obstetrics/Gynecology
Wayne State University
Detroit, Michigan

Joseph S. Rosenshein, Ph.D.
Clear Vision Center
Farmington Hills, Michigan

Romaine Saxton, Ph.D.
Division of Surgical Oncology
UCLA School of Medicine
Los Angeles, California

Jacques Soudant, M.D.
Chairman, ENT Department
Hôpitaux de Paris
Groupe Hospitalier Pitié-Salpêtrière
France

Myron Strasser, D.D.S.
Private Practice
Oral & Maxillofacial Surgeon
Modesto, California

Harvey Wigdor, D.D.S., M.S.
Dental Section Chief
Ravenswood Hospital Medical Center
Chicago, Illinois

James Wooten, M.D.
Private Practice
Biloxi, Mississippi

Preface

Surgical lasers have been well accepted by all disciplines of the healing arts as useful adjuncts to the care of patients. The attitude toward their use has changed from one of "gee-whiz" appreciation for modern technology to that of acceptance of lasers as standard surgical instruments. Since the initial application of laser technology by ophthalmologists and otolaryngologists, which permitted access to relatively inaccessible body parts with a "no-touch" technique, lasers have become recognized as standard delivery systems for treatment in dermatology, oral and maxillofacial surgery, plastic surgery, general surgery, urology, gynecology, and neurosurgery. Hard tissue applications have been more difficult to develop. However, a role has been defined for intra-articular surgery, and the search for a satisfactory alternative to the high-speed dental drill continues. Definite advantages for the application of laser technology to other aspects of dentistry have been well delineated. By the diligent application of basic scientific study, which has enabled us to understand how to match target chromophores to specific laser wavelengths, consistently reproducible results have established new standards of care which reduce the suffering of patients who require surgery.

Now that the applications of laser technology to medicine and dentistry have entered the age of sophisticated and rational treatment, we have attempted to distill our experience both in the laboratory and with patients over the past twenty years into a form which we hope will help disseminate this knowledge, thereby stimulating our colleagues in surgery and dentistry to use and improve upon the information presented in this book to better the lives of their patients.

This book is particularly useful for those who are involved in the care of patients with oral precancer and cancer. The techniques and results of therapy are presented both in principle and by illustrative cases. Dentists, oral and maxillofacial surgeons, plastic surgeons, and otolaryngologists will also find models for laser-assisted therapy of most common oral and facial conditions as well as some of the less common ones. Research scientists in both the "basic" and clinical sciences will find much useful information relating to low-level photobiostimulation, fusion of biologic surfaces, and future studies conducted in the weightless medium of space.

It is our hope that this book will serve as an instructional guide and reference for solving problems of daily practice which are best treated by lasers, while stimulating our colleagues to learn and apply the methods detailed in this book.

Lewis Clayman
Paul Kuo

Foreword

In this book, the editors, Drs. Clayman and Kuo, have woven a well-focused text, discussing the use of lasers in the maxillofacial and dental fields. Dr. Clayman is himself a pioneer in the use of surgical lasers in these fields, having produced seminal research in the seventies as an early member of the Sinai Hospital of Detroit Laser and Photobiology Institute. The authors have drawn extensively on the experience of many other members of this pioneering group and, with the addition of other experts in this field, have created a definitive and comprehensive volume.

After a conventional introduction to laser physics, laser safety, and laser use, the book thoroughly discusses such issues as: the laser treatment of preneoplasias, transoral resection of oral cancers, facial rejuvenation by wrinkle removal, gingival hypertrophy, and LAUP for snoring and sleep apnea. Photodynamic therapy is thoroughly discussed, as are new applications and future uses of photo therapy, such as photobiostimulation and tissue fusion. Significant attention is paid to the rational use of lasers in dentistry.

Since many of the authors are used to collaborating with one another, an easy flow of material is achieved. This book is comprehensive, readable and not-to-be-missed reading for those practitioners of both maxillofacial surgery and dentistry who wish to understand the importance of lasers in their present practice and view the future use of lasers in the treatment of their patients.

Hugh Beckman

Lasers in Maxillofacial Surgery and Dentistry

1 Physical Considerations of Surgical Lasers

Terry A. Fuller

HISTORY

A laser, an acronym for light amplification by stimulated emission of radiation, is a device for generating a high-intensity, ostensibly parallel beam of monochromatic (single wavelength) electromagnetic radiation. The possibility of stimulated emission was predicted by Einstein in 1917; based on the work of Gordon in 1955 and Schawlow and Townes in 1958, Maiman created the first operational laser in 1960, a ruby laser emitting a brilliant red beam of light. This was followed within 3 years by the development of the argon, carbon dioxide (CO_2), and neodymium:yttrium-aluminum-garnet (Nd:YAG) lasers, which remain the most widely used lasers in medicine.

In 1963 the ruby laser was employed in the treatment of pigmented dermatologic lesions and for photocoagulation of the retina. Early applications of lasers in oral and maxillofacial surgery began to appear in the mid- to late 1970s. Potential advantages of surgical lasers were clear from the beginning, but the cost, unreliability, and operational complexity of the early machines greatly limited the actual use of lasers, except in the fields of ophthalmology and dermatology, until the past 15 to 18 years. In recent years improved understanding of light-tissue interactions and, of greatest importance to the surgeon, new technologies for delivering laser light to the tissue, has transformed lasers into versatile and valuable surgical instruments. This chapter presents the fundamentals of laser physics and introduces the reader to the interactions between light and tissue.

Full appreciation of the uses, limitations, benefits, and risks of surgical lasers requires a basic understanding of laser physics and the biologic action of light.

LIGHT

Electromagnetic radiation is energy transmitted through space. It can be viewed either as propagated waves of characteristic energies, or as discrete (and the smallest) parcels of energy called *photons*. Electromagnetic radiation is quantified in terms of two reciprocal forms of measurement: *frequency* (ν), expressed in Hertz (Hz) or cycles per second, and *wavelength* (λ), expressed in metric units of length. Which units are employed in any particular application is largely a matter of convention. The wavelength of the radiation in the visible region of the spectrum (Fig. 1–1) defines the color of the light.

Atoms (ions or molecules) at their lowest energy or *ground state* possess an intrinsic amount of energy. When excited through the process of *absorption* by the input of thermal, electromagnetic, or other forms of energy, they are raised to one of several distinct higher energy levels. The absorbed energy is subsequently and spontaneously released *(spontaneous emission)* in the form of a quantum of energy corresponding to the difference between the ground and excited states ($E_1 - E_2 = E_\Delta$). All particles making the transition between the same two energy levels will emit light of identical energy and wavelength (Fig. 1–2).

Ordinary sunlight or lamplight consists of many wavelengths; even light, colored from passing through a filter, represents a broad spectrum of many wavelengths. Such light emanates in all directions from its source. The intensity diminishes as the inverse square of the distance from the source. As discussed below, a laser uses the principle of stimulated emission to produce light of a markedly different quality.

The spontaneous emission of photons from an excited atom may occur at any time and in any direction. If, however, a photon of E_Δ strikes an atom already in an upper energy state E_2, it stimulates the emission of a second photon of light. This second photon has precisely the same energy or wavelength and is spatially and temporally synchronous with and traveling in exactly the same direction as the initial photon. If these two photons strike additional atoms in the excited state E_2, they will yield an amplifying cascade of photons—laser light—that is monochromatic (a single wavelength), coherent (synchronous waves), and collimated (parallel rays).

THE LASER

Lasers consist of a small number of basic components as shown in Figure 1–3. An *active lasing medium,* which can be a solid, liquid, or gas, is enclosed within a *laser cavity* bounded by two perfectly parallel reflectors (mirrors). High-energy radiation is pumped into the active medium by means of a *pump source.* The pump source is energy generally provided by an intense optical or electrical discharge. The energy from the pump source is absorbed by the active

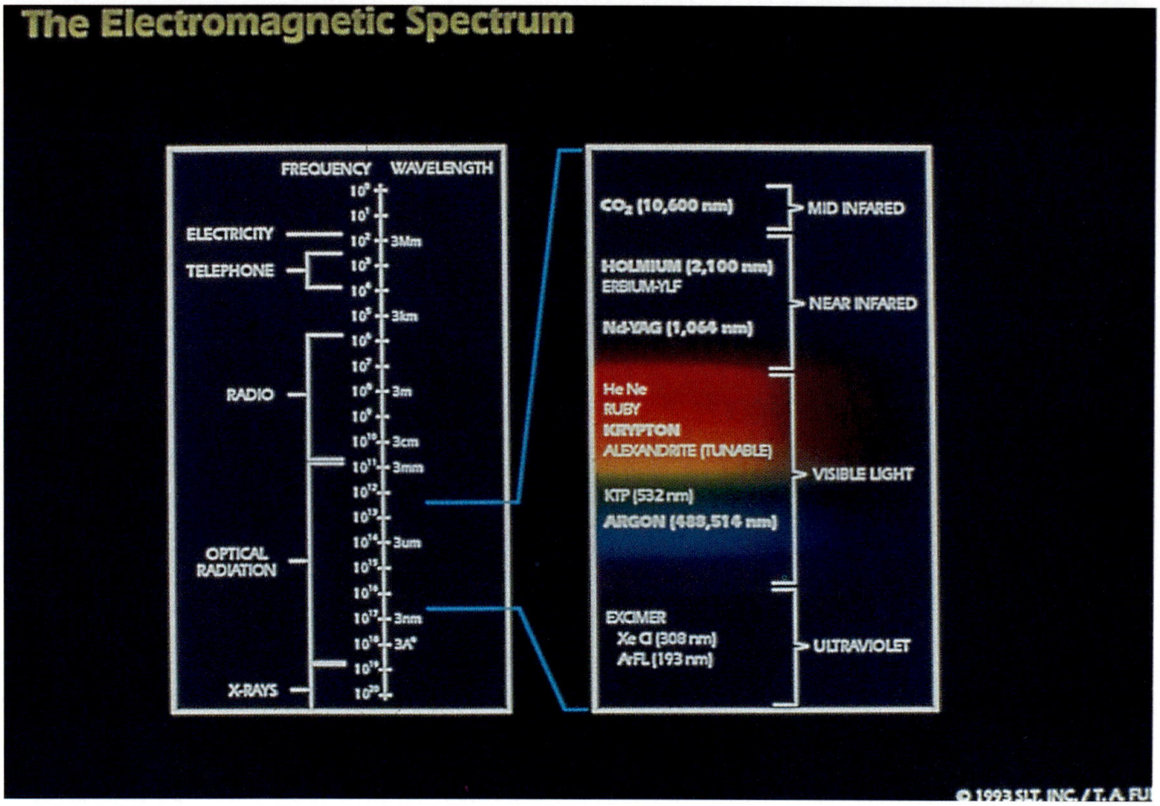

Figure 1–1. Electromagnetic spectrum.

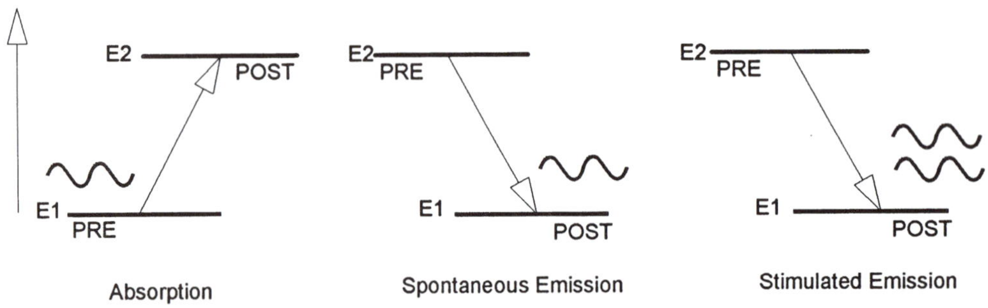

Figure 1–2. Energy state diagram.

medium until the majority of atoms, ions, or molecules are raised to their upper energy state. This is a condition known as a *population inversion* and is a necessary condition to generate laser light. The two parallel reflectors are situated at the ends of the laser cavity and act to constrain the light along and within the axis of the cavity. Thus, the light is repeatedly bounced between the reflectors. This will stimulate the emission of even more photons (amplification) in that axial direction. Light traveling in other directions escapes the cavity and is lost as heat. One of the mirrors is only partially reflective, enabling some of the light to escape the cavity as a beam of laser light.

Different lasing media, because of their particular atomic, molecular, or ionic structure and energy levels, emit light of characteristic wavelengths. The properties of the most common surgical lasers are listed in Table 1–1.

CO_2 Laser

Carbon dioxide lasers employ carbon dioxide gas (in addition to other gases required for sustained stimulated emission of radiation) as a lasing or active medium. The gases are either sealed in a tube or are circulated from a tank. When excited by direct current (DC) or radio-frequency (RF) voltage, the carbon dioxide absorbs a portion of this energy and raises the CO_2 molecule to an upper energy state. The excited CO_2 molecule spontaneously decays and emits *mid-infrared* photons at a wavelength of 10,600 nm

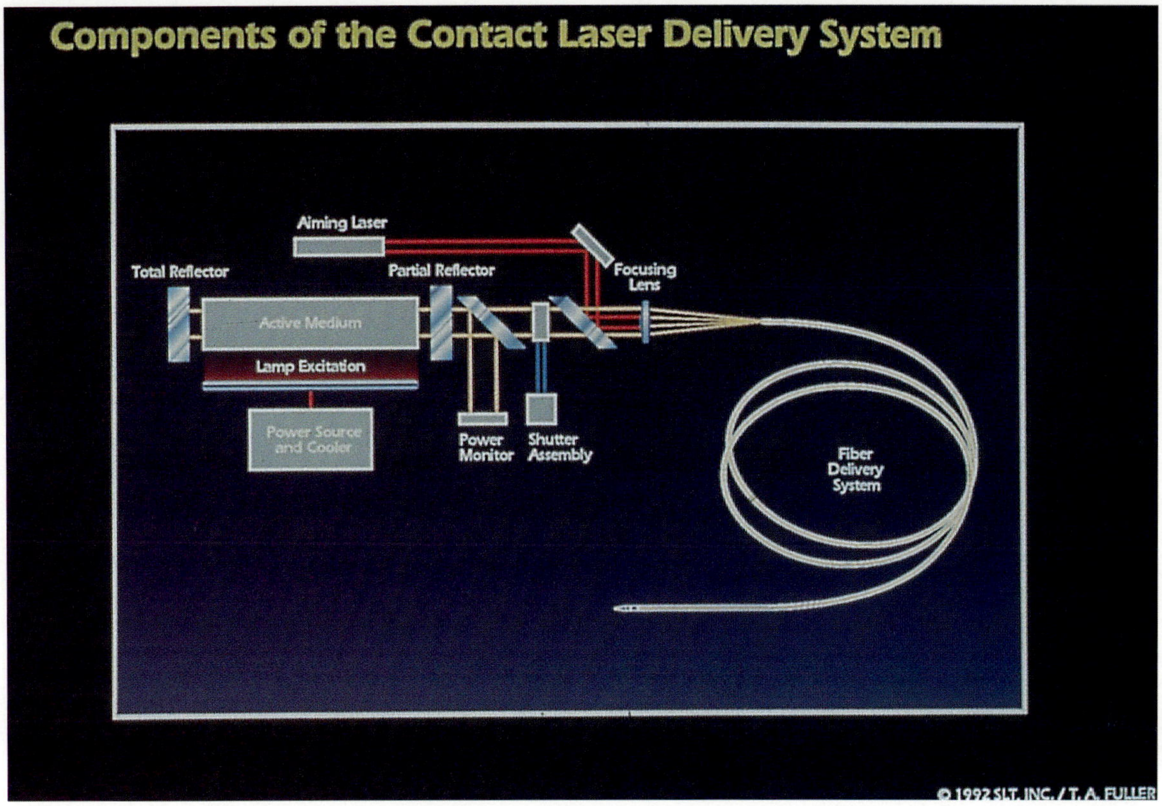

Figure 1–3. Basic laser components.

Table 1–1. Characteristics of Surgical Lasers

LASER TYPE	WAVELENGTH	SPECTRAL REGION	MODE	TYPICAL MAX POWER
CO_2	10,600 nm	Mid-Infrared	CW & Gated & Superpulsed	100W CW
Holmium	2,100 nm	Near Infrared	Pulsed	15Wavg.
Nd:YAG	1,064 nm	Near Infrared	CW & Pulsed	100W CW
Diode	800–890 nm	Near Infrared	CW	> 50W
KTP/KDP	532 nm	Visible	Pulsed	25Wavg.
Argon	488/514 nm	Visible	CW	20W
Excimer ArF	190 nm	Ultraviolet	Pulsed	550mJ
-XeCl	308 nm	Ultraviolet	Pulsed	250mJ
Erbium:YAG(Er:YAG)				

Reproduced with permission of T.A.F., modified from Fuller TA. Thermal Surgical Lasers. Philadelphia: Surgical Laser Technologies, Inc., 1992.

(10.6 μm). *Power* (measured in units of *watts,* W) is the time function of energy (measured in *joules,* J) and can be delivered either continuously (continuous wave, CW) or in a train of pulses. The carbon dioxide laser can be pulsed in a manner that results in high energy, rapidly repeating pulses typically referred to as *superpulses.* In contrast to CW surgical lasers, which generate power up to 100 W, the superpulsed CO_2 laser generates power up to 10,000 W in a repeating train of pulses. There are substantial differences in clinical effect between CW, conventional pulsing, and superpulsed modes of operation (see Chapter 3).

Infrared light is in a region of the electromagnetic spectrum that is not visible to the human eye. Therefore, a second low-power visible laser [typically a red beam from a helium-neon (HeNe) laser or visible diode laser] beam is precisely aligned and coaxial with the CO_2 laser beam for aiming purposes. The *delivery system* used to carry the laser light to the tissue is of critical importance to the surgeon. The CO_2 laser generally uses an *articulated arm* as its principal delivery system. An articulated arm is a series of hollow tubes connected together through a series of six to eight articulating mirrors. This is in contrast to very thin, continuously flexible, glass (fused silica) fiber optics generally used for near infrared and visible lasers. Glass is opaque to 10,600 nm light and thus is not suitable for CO_2 laser transmission. The CO_2 laser is primarily used for cutting and vaporizing tissue in open procedures or in procedures where rigid endoscopy is acceptable.

Argon and Frequency-Doubled Nd:YAG Lasers

Argon and frequency-doubled Nd:YAG laser (also referred to as a KTP laser), although technologically very different from each other, are devices that generate laser energy in the green region of the electromagnetic spectrum. The argon laser employs an electrically excited ionized argon gas as a lasing medium. The high heat transfer requires a water-jacketed cooling system, which permits power outputs of up to 25 W. More portable, air-cooled units are limited to power outputs of 5 to 10 W. This laser emits blue-green light at 488 and 514 nm. The KTP laser uses a Nd:YAG laser in combination with a potassium titanyl sulfate (KTP) crystal. The Nd:YAG portion of this laser system generates a wavelength of 1064-nm energy whose frequency is doubled (wavelength is halved) on passing through the KTP crystal. The result is a beam of green light at 530 nm. The emission from both the argon and KTP lasers can be transmitted through flexible glass fiber optics that can carry the light to the surgical site. Since the light is visible, no secondary aiming beam is required. Safety glasses are required to protect the patient and operating room personnel from the therapeutic beam of all surgical lasers. However, glasses used for the green lasers necessarily block green light and thus tend to obscure the overall visualization of the surgical field.

Nd:YAG Laser

The neodymium:yttrium-aluminum-garnet (Nd:YAG) laser is a solid-state device that generates light in the *near infrared* region of the spectrum at 1064 nm. The active medium of this laser is the neodymium atoms doped into a matrix of yttrium, aluminum, and garnet. The neodymium atoms are optically excited by way of a bright arc lamp. This relatively efficient laser generates a wavelength of 1064 nm and is outside the visible region of the spectrum. Therefore, the Nd:YAG laser requires an aiming beam similar to that used by CO_2 lasers. Safety glasses for this laser are transparent to visible light and do not obscure the surgeon's surgical view. The surgical Nd:YAG lasers commonly deliver continuous (CW) power up to 100 W and can be passed easily through inexpensive flexible fiber optics. In addition to the CW mode of operation, the Nd:YAG laser can be configured to operate in a special pulsed mode referred to as Q-switched. The Q-switched laser emits pulses of pico- to nanoseconds in duration. This mode is often used in ophthalmology to disrupt the posterior capsule in secondary cataracts or in shock-wave lithotripsy.

Holmium:YAG

The holmium:YAG laser is technologically associated with the Nd:YAG laser. This solid-state laser uses holmium as its active medium doped into a matrix of yttrium, aluminum, and garnet. Due to its inherently inefficient operation and certain thermal design considerations, this laser is pulsed. It emits rapid pulses of energy at 2100 nm in the mid-infrared part of the spectrum. Like the Nd:YAG laser, this laser requires an aiming beam. The holmium:YAG beam can be delivered through fiber optics. However, such fibers must be made of low OH^- (hydroxyl radical) glass due to the high absorption of this wavelength to water.

Diode Laser

In contrast to the gas and solid-state lasers discussed thus far, diode lasers are in a category of devices that emit light from semiconductor materials. They are operated in a manner similar to a transistor in which an electric potential is applied to dissimilar semiconductor materials. In contrast to gas, solid state, and liquid lasers, semiconductor lasers require no high voltages or currents, no arc lamps or optical pump sources, and have no required moving parts. They are very efficient (typically >30–35%), but are capable of generating only relatively low power levels. Individual "high-power" laser diodes typically generate only 1 to $1\frac{1}{2}$ W per diode. To gain useful power from the laser, multiple devices must be used in concert. Linear (one-dimensional) arrays or two-dimensional arrays are being developed to gain sufficient power for surgery. Additionally, ganging individual diodes in various optical configurations are being explored; each approach carries its own benefits and drawbacks. Both commercial and prototype surgical diode laser systems are able to deliver 20 to 50 W. There are currently severe fiber optic size and maximum power limitations as well as diode and system warranty and lifetime issues. Currently, the most popular diode lasers emit light in the 800- to 890-nm range. Lasers in the shorter wavelength range provide biologic effects similar to those of the Nd:YAG lasers. Longer wavelengths have higher tissue absorption characteristics.

The technological specifications of a given laser type and model indicate how much power (or in the case of a pulsed laser, energy) can be practically delivered to tissue and the means by which the power can be conveyed to tissue. When laser energy interacts with tissue its output power is distributed over the area of an illuminated spot. This distribution or *power density* or *fluence* (power/area, W/cm^2) is intimately related to the tissue effect. The power density can be altered by changing either the power of the laser or spot size of the laser beam. The effect that a particular laser emission has on tissue, and thus the surgeon's ability to effectively utilize that emission, depends upon power density and other specifications as well as the characteristics of tissue. Only by matching the characteristics of the laser beam and the tissue can one begin to accurately predict the effect that the laser will have in surgery.

THERMAL LASER—TISSUE EFFECTS

The focus of this book is on the interactions of laser energy and tissue that result in an elevation of the tissue temperature. These so-called thermal lasers represent the majority of all applications of lasers in medicine. Thus, lasers that are Q-switched or lasers that operate at low powers for biostimulation or photodynamic therapy (PDT) interactions are excluded herein from discussion. This section presents an outline of the principal variables affecting the clinical end point.

The utility of the thermal laser resides with its capability of providing the surgeon the ability to accurately predict the nature and extent of a thermally induced laser lesion in tissue. The goal of laser surgery is thus to create a *temperature gradient* (Fig. 1–4) or profile in tissue that will result in coagulation or vaporization of tissue. Coagulation provides hemostasis and, if desired, necrosis of tissue. Vaporization (the conversion of solid and liquid phase tissue components into gaseous phase components) provides the ability to cut, incise, excise, resect or ablate tissue.

Coagulation and vaporization are two different effects created by the same process: heating of tissue. Coagulation generally occurs when the temperature is elevated from 60°C to <100°C. Obvious changes occur in the tissue at these temperatures resulting from the thermal denaturation of tissue protein, and include blanching and shrinkage as well as puckering due to dehydration. When the temperature is elevated near and above the boiling point of water (100°C), vaporization of liquid and solid components occur. A frank defect is left that includes a zone of char (carbon, as a result of the combustion of tissue) surrounded by coagulated tissue. The extent of the area of vaporization, char, and coagulation (as well as a heat-affected zone surrounding the coagulation, which can cause edema) is defined by the temperature gradient. Thus, by altering the gradient, the surgical effect can be altered. There are several variables that determine the gradient. They include the laser parameters such as power density, duration of exposure, wavelength, and method of delivery of laser energy as well as tissue parameters.

Light can be absorbed, transmitted, scattered, or reflected by tissue (Fig. 1–5). Only light that has been absorbed can yield a therapeutic result. Light that is transmitted through or reflected from tissue yields no effect until and unless it is absorbed. The measure of the degree to which tissue absorbs light is the *absorption coefficient,* α (measured in units of cm^{-1}). It is a measure of the amount of energy ab-

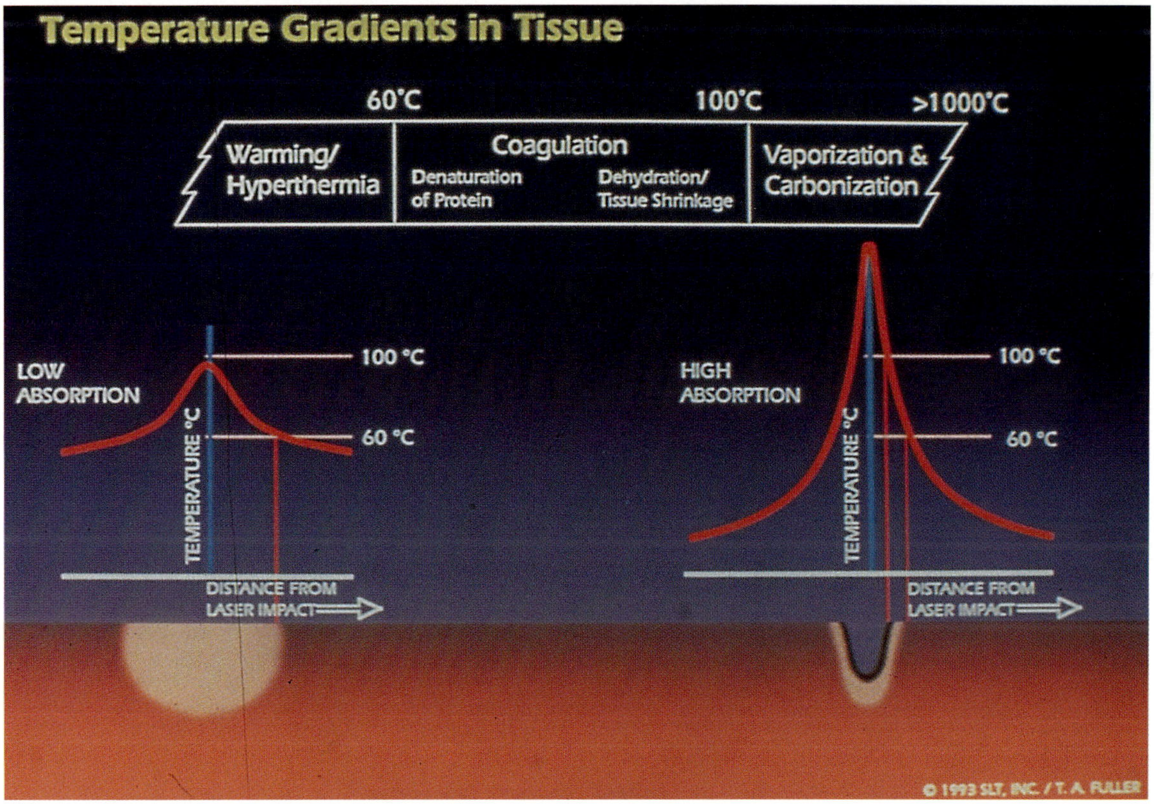

Figure 1–4. Temperature gradients in tissue.

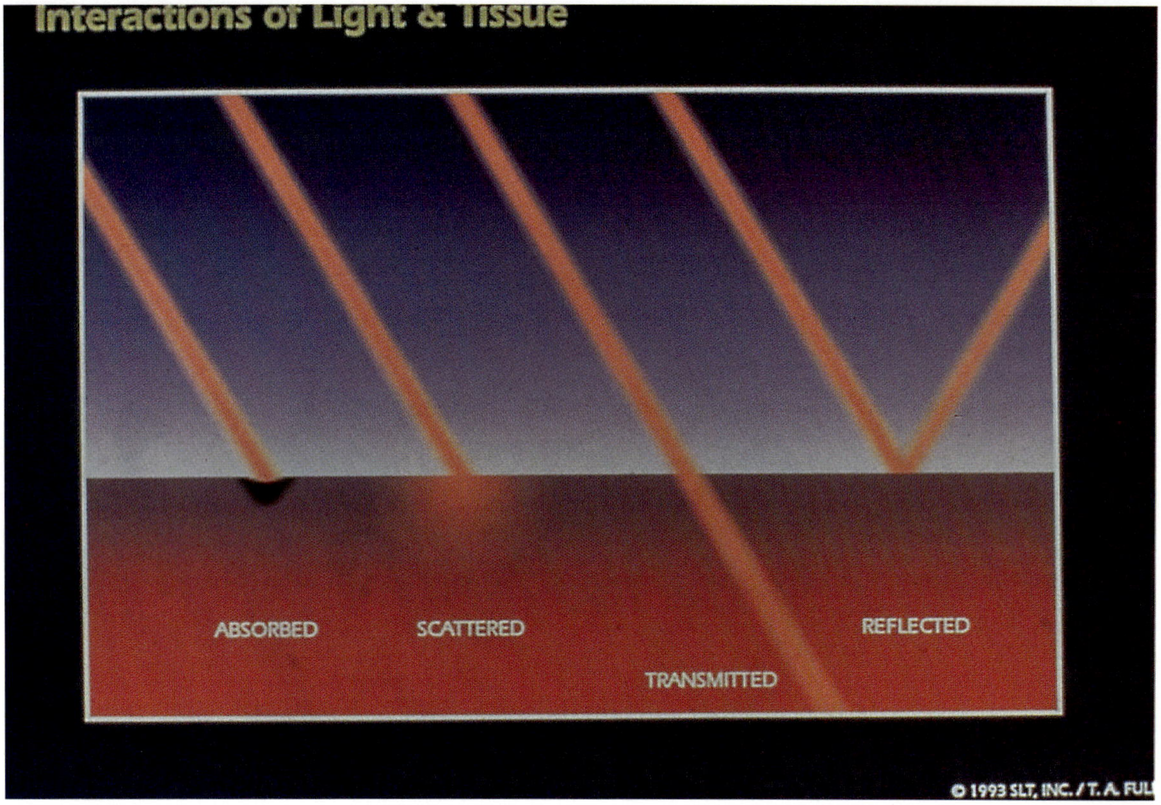

Figure 1–5. Interactions of light and tissue.

sorbed through a distance of the absorbing material. The *penetration depth* of the laser in a given tissue is proportional to the inverse of the absorption coefficient α. The more highly absorbed the light (high α), the shallower the penetration. As can be seen in Figure 1–6, this results in the light energy being converted to heat energy within a shallow layer of tissue, and therefore results in intense surface heat. A tissue with a high α will create a steep temperature gradient.

Figure 1–7 illustrates the absorption of light by tissue at different wavelengths. The y-axis indicates greater absorption (less penetration) and thus higher resulting temperatures. It can be readily seen that the CO_2 and erbium (Er):YAG lasers would create high surface temperature and very steep temperature gradients in the tissue. Both the CO_2 and Er:YAG laser beams are preferentially absorbed by water, and because water is by far the largest component of most tissue, this results in the rapid transformation of light into heat within about 0.2 to 1.0 mm of the tissue surface. The intense thermal response quickly evaporates the water and vaporizes tissue. The temperature gradient is so steep that it has relatively poor coagulation properties. The duration of exposure is another key variable in determining the extent of a laser-induced lesion. Long exposure times result in conduction of heat into surrounding tissue and thus improve hemostasis and increase coagulation necrosis. In contrast, techniques exist to diminish coagulation necrosis. The superpulse CO_2 laser is one such example. This laser uses rapidly repeating, high peak power pulses with pulse energy in the range of 50 to 120 mJ/pulse. The result of application of the superpulsed laser is the reduction of coagulation necrosis by 50% over the CW laser operating at the same average power. By way of contrast, the Nd:YAG laser will penetrate deeply in tissue with a relatively low surface temperature and shallow temperature gradient.

Scatter of light by tissue spreads the laser beam in a diffuse pattern defined by the tissue's *scatter coefficient,* β. Once the light is scattered, if it is absorbed, it will affect a volume of tissue larger than the laser's optical spot size. In some instances scatter is an attribute desired by the surgeon. For example, when Nd:YAG laser energy is used to thermally destroy a tumor, the deep penetration of the laser beam coupled with the high scatter coefficient affects a deep and wide volume of tissue. In contrast, scatter can also be detrimental if one is attempting to localize the effect of the laser.

The green light from the argon and KTP lasers is both scattered and absorbed by tissue. The degree of absorption is heavily dependent on the concentration of the chromophores hemoglobin and melanin. Thus, heavily pigmented skin or vascular areas such as a hemangioma will result in high absorption (low penetration). The scatter of the green lasers are greater than that of the CO_2 laser.

The method of delivering the laser light to the tissue also acts as a variable affecting the tissue response. In general terms this delivery of energy falls into two broad classes: *free-beam lasers* and lasers for use in contact with tissue.

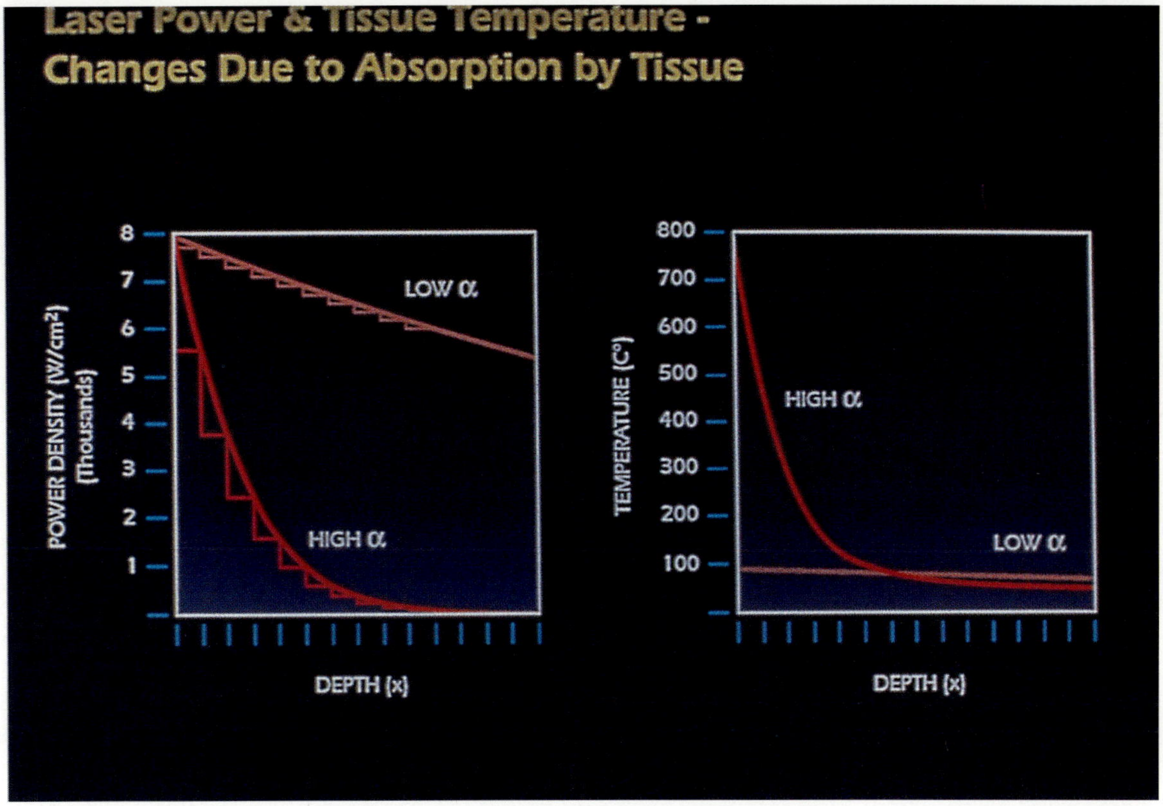

Figure 1–6. Power/depth and temperature/depth.

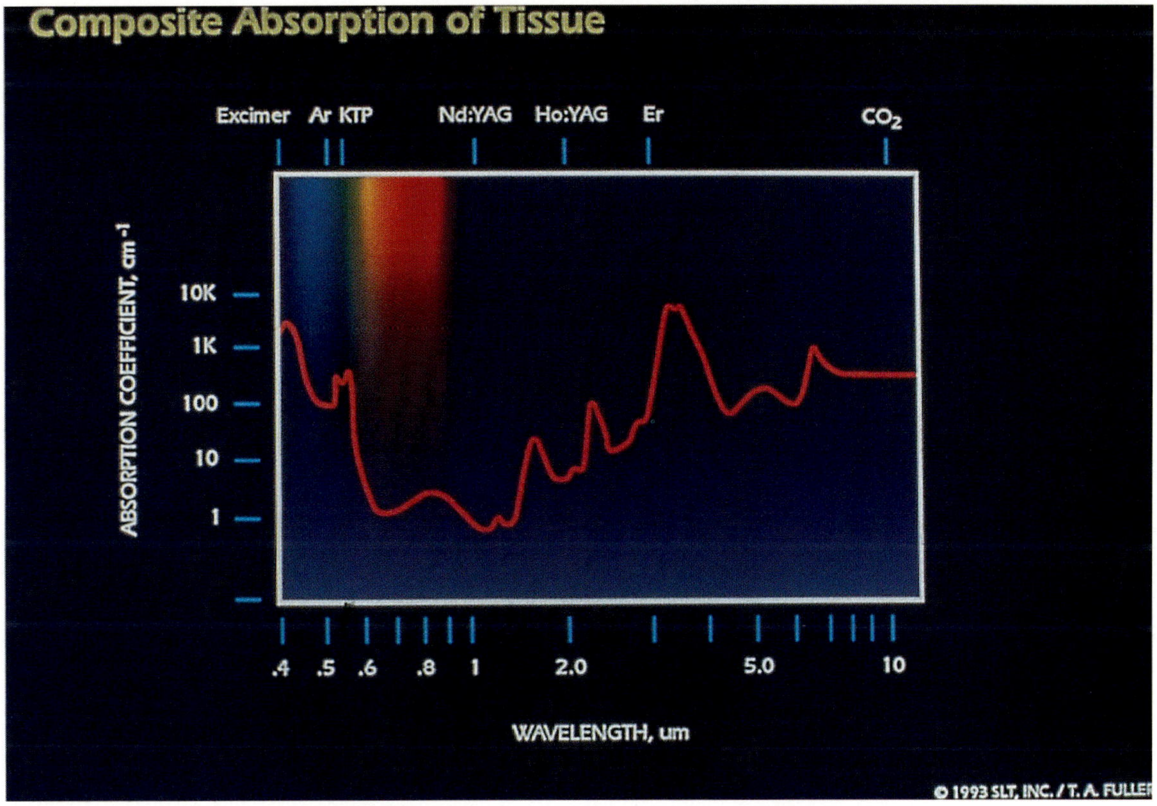

Figure 1–7. Light absorption by composite tissue.

FREE-BEAM LASERS

Free-beam (sometimes referred to as noncontact) lasers are devices that permit laser energy alone (without influence by the delivery device) to interact with tissue, causing the final clinical result. The interactions between laser light and tissue described above are specific for free-beam lasers. They result from interactions between the native laser wavelength and tissue alone. Typical free-beam delivery systems include articulating arms, micromanipulators used in conjunction with surgical microscopes, and conventional fiber optics. Characteristic of these devices is that the effect on tissue is principally that of the laser emission alone. This is typically what occurs when there is no contact between the fiber optic end of the delivery device and the target tissue. Consider the laser beam exiting a laser delivery system used in a free-beam mode (Fig. 1–8, left). The beam will converge (or diverge) as it exits the focusing lens and some portion of the energy will be reflected from the tissue on impact. Should the distance from the fiber to the tissue be altered, the power density at the tissue will change, changing the clinical effect. Substantial energy is reflected (Q_f^r) or lost as heat and in smoke (Q_v^v).

The free-beam method of delivery provides certain advantages over conventional surgery by providing a method for "non-touch" surgery, but suffers from the loss of tactile feedback. The techniques for learning and using the free-beam laser are substantially different from those of conventional instruments. Perhaps the most limiting feature of the free-beam laser is that different laser sources are required for different surgical maneuvers, e.g., Nd:YAG for coagulation and hemostasis and CO_2 for incision and excision.

Modification of Free-Beam Laser Surgery: Contact Laser Surgery

Despite the benefits of free-beam laser surgery, certain limitations and drawbacks exist. Perhaps the most significant is that to substantially change the tissue's temperature gradient (clinical effect), one must choose different laser sources, an expensive and intraoperatively difficult task. Contact Laser surgery has been developed to augment and overcome this and other fundamental deficiencies in free-beam surgery. Contact Laser surgery works by altering the tissue temperature gradient through changes in the laser delivery system, rather than by alteration in wavelength.

A decade ago researchers developed a delivery system in which an optical device is placed in direct contact with the tissue during laser surgery to increase the delivered power density and reduce changes in power density due to changes in distance to the tissue. This is accomplished by use of interchangeable contact laser probes and scalpels (tips) made from synthetic sapphire or fused silica. The tips have several different sizes and shapes and can be easily affixed to the end of fiber optics. Several benefits result from the use of these tips (Fig. 1–8, right). In addition to providing the

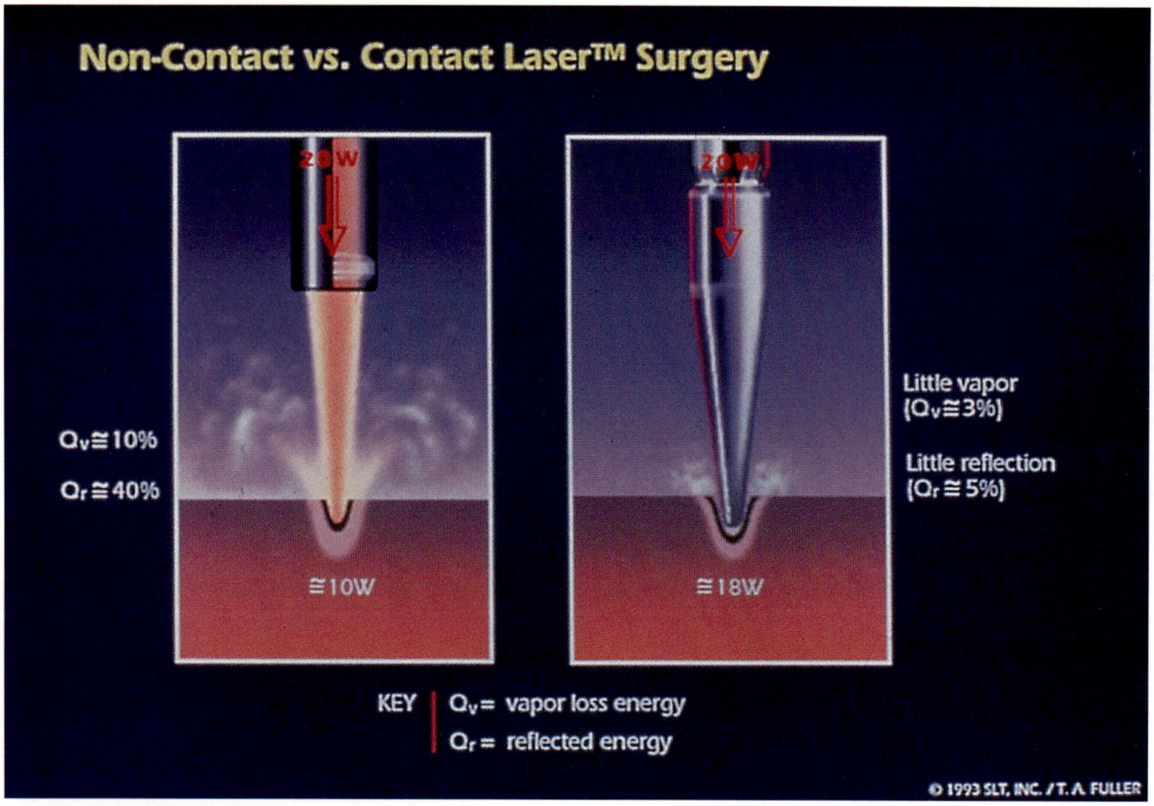

Figure 1–8. Noncontact vs. contact laser surgery.

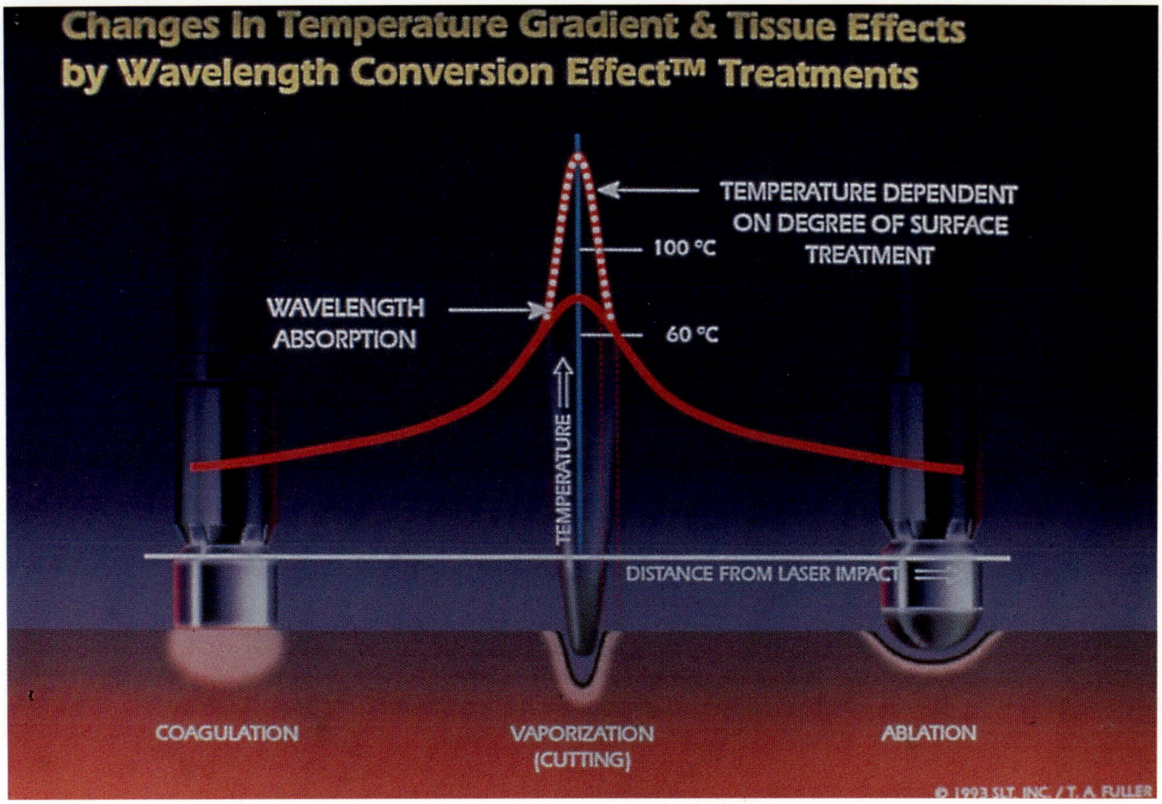

Figure 1–9. Changes in temperature gradient and tissue effect by wavelength conversion effect surface treatments.

surgeon with tactile feedback, a sense lost in free-beam surgery, and controlling power density, the reflection of light from the tissue is significantly reduced. The improved efficiency in coupling of light into the tissue results in the requirement of less power, in most cases a reduction of 40 to 50% (Fig. 1–8, right).

Altering the tip configuration of a probe and scalpel makes it possible to change not only the spot size (and thus power density), but the angle of divergence of the beam. A frustroconical tip, for example, concentrates the laser light on a small, precisely defined distal area from which light splays out at a wide angle, creating a region of high power density that drops rapidly with distance. Alterations in the tip's shape can result in a low divergence angle. In addition to placing tips onto the ends of fiber optics, the ends of fiber optics themselves can also be shaped, although they lack the mechanical strength and thermal resistance required for extended and precision use.

The Contact Laser attributes thus far described, still result in a tissue effect that is solely dependent on the absorption of the laser emission by the tissue to generate the temperature gradient. It is a major attribute of Contact Laser surgery to have the temperature gradient altered by the Contact Laser tip. By placing a small amount of light absorbing material integrally between the contact tip and the tissue, a portion of the energy will be absorbed by that material. The energy absorbed will be converted to heat and will result in a very high temperature. Since the absorbing material is in contact with the probe and the tissue, it will elevate the temperature of the tissue by thermal combustion in addition to the radiation heating caused by the native wavelength. Thus, as can be seen in Figure 1–9, by use of this absorbing material the tissue temperature gradient induced by the laser emission has been altered. Depending upon the quantity and distribution of the absorbing material the contact tip can mimic the effect of other laser wavelengths. This event is referred to as the Wavelength Conversion Effect. The wavelength conversion effect does not result in changing the wavelength of the laser; rather, it changes the effect the wavelength has in the surgical situation.

By adjusting the Wavelength Conversion Effect material on the probe tip, one can titrate the amount of laser light exiting the tip in comparison to the amount of heat generated by absorption at the tip. This means, in essence, that a single laser in combination with different interchangeable tips, can mimic the tissue temperature profile and effect of various lasers.

2 Practical Laser Safety in Oral and Maxillofacial Surgery

Lawrence M. Elson

A laser is a device that produces an intense, highly parallel beam of coherent light. It is named after the composition of the excitable medium from which the laser beam emanates [e.g., carbon dioxide (CO_2), argon (Ar), helium-neon (HeNe), etc.]. Since the late 1970s, lasers have been studied in oral and maxillofacial surgery for the treatment of soft tissue lesions and occasionally for the cutting of bone.[1] Light emitted by these surgical lasers is generally in the visible and infrared regions of the electromagnetic spectrum and is nonionizing. This radiation must be clearly differentiated from ionizing radiation exemplified by x-rays and gamma rays, which may produce deleterious effects on living tissue. Therefore, patients, medical personnel and particularly pregnant women working with or around lasers may do so without the risks[2] associated with x-rays.

Each different type of laser produces a different wavelength (color) of light that is absorbed by specific target chromophores within tissues. The biologic effect of this light on tissue is dependent upon wavelength, energy level of the beam, and absorption characteristics of the tissue receiving this energy. For example, the carbon dioxide laser (10,600 nm—middle infrared) light is absorbed heavily by water. Since human tissue is mostly water, it absorbs virtually all of the laser energy without significant reflection or backscatter from the surgical site. However, when this same light comes into contact with shiny surgical instruments, reflection will occur. In tissue, the depth of this laser's photovaporization or photocoagulation effect is directly dependent on the power density (watts/cm^2), which is determined by the intensity of the focused beam, and the energy density (joules/cm^2), which determines the rate at which energy is delivered to the tissue. The thermal damage produced adjacent to the surgical site by diffusion of heat can be reduced to a range of micrometers, depending on the energy density used. Irreversible thermal damage adjacent to the zone of photovaporization is minimized by using the highest controllable power density for the shortest amount of application time. Prior to patient use a "test spot" is made on a moistened wooden tongue blade to assess the coaxial HeNe aiming beam, spot size contour, power, and mode of operation [continuous wave (CW) or pulsed]. Hazards of the carbon dioxide laser in oral and maxillofacial surgery (OMFS) include corneal, scleral, and cutaneous injury ranging from transient pain to severe burns. Both the patient and the medical personnel are at risk for these injuries.

The argon laser emits a blue-green light of 488 and 514 nm, which is selectively absorbed by the red chromophore, oxyhemoglobin at 488 and 540/577 nm (double absorption peak). It is delivered to the target tissue by an optical fiber. This laser, depending on its spot size, power, time of application, and resulting energy density, can photovaporize or coagulate tissue with up to several millimeters of thermal damage adjacent to the zone of clinical laser treatment. The optical hazards of the argon laser include retinal and skin burns.

The neodymium:yttrium-aluminum-garnet (Nd:YAG) laser emits an invisible 1060-nm (near-infrared) light that is heavily absorbed by pigmented tissue. It can photovaporize or photocoagulate almost all biologic tissue with which it comes in contact. The zone of thermal damage of the Nd:YAG laser may extend as much as 1 cm beyond the surgical target site consequent to a deep penetrating effect that is not observable at the time of treatment. This powerful laser is delivered to the surgical site by an optical fiber or contact probe. Optical hazards of this laser are similar to that of the argon laser and include retinal and skin hazards (Fig. 2–1).

HAZARDS OF LASER SURGERY

Judgment Errors

As is the case with surgery, judgment error may be as harmful as the use of inappropriate surgical technique. Of the several types of judgment errors, the most severe is misdiagnosis or misinterpretion of the disease state being treated. After having appropriately decided to use a laser, it becomes necessary to match the wavelength, power, and energy densities to the target tissue absorptive characteristics to best eradicate the lesion. This mandates that the surgeon understand the applied laser physics and laser-tissue interactions at the selected wavelength. The technical skill to manipulate the laser delivery system safely to protect patient, surgeon, and operating room personnel must be acquired through instructional courses resulting in proper credentialing for each wavelength used. Ultimately, each surgeon should be proctored by a properly credentialed laser clinician at the hospital in which the surgeon practices for each type of procedure for which privileges are desired. In some cases, residency training may substitute for a laser

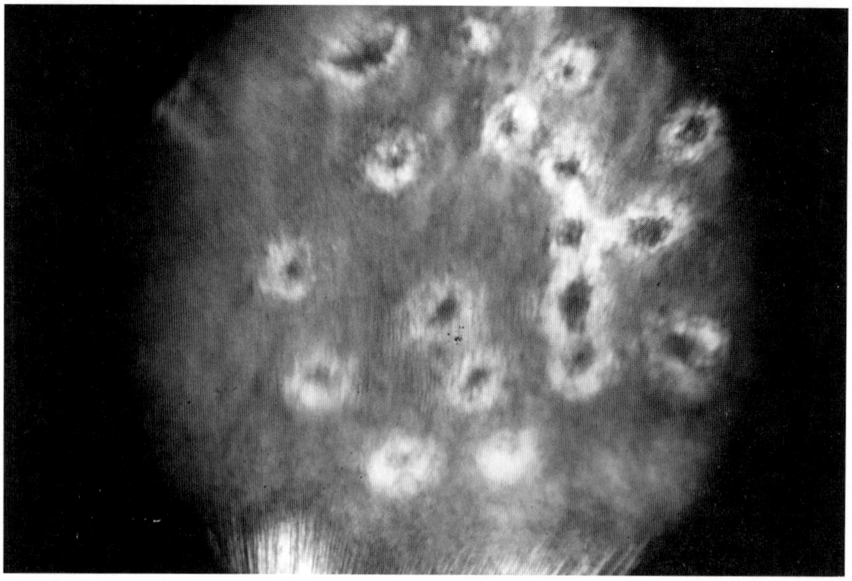

Figure 2–1. Nd:YAG-induced retinal burns in a rabbit retina.

course, but the preceptorship credentialing program is still required. It is also very important to remember that improper use converts the laser into an expensive electrocautery unit. Failing to limit the extent of the laser's lateral heat conduction by the untrained clinician may produce a conduction burn that extends well beyond the laser surgical site. This might well prove disastrous.

Optical Hazards

Since the clinical lasers utilized in oral, maxillofacial, and head and neck surgery photovaporize or photocoagulate tissue, they all have the potential to damage the eye. Depending on the laser's wavelength, different tissue effects will occur. Visible light laser radiation [argon, potassium titanyl phosphate (KTP), HeNe, gold vapor, pulsed dye, etc.], and the near-infrared Nd:YAG laser's energy will easily be transmitted through the eye directly into the retina where absorption may produce a burn (Fig. 2–2) and partial loss of vision or even blindness. Laser light that is focused through the lens of the eye will increase its effective power up to 100,000 times! The eye must *always* be protected to prevent visual field defects or blindness. Other near-infrared lasers [erbium (Er):YAG and holmium (Ho):YAG] and middle infrared lasers such as the CO_2 laser are absorbed by the water in the cornea, scleral epithelium, or eyelid and have the potential to burn or damage these areas.

Therefore, it is imperative that all individuals in the operating room, i.e., surgeons, nurses, technicians, and patients, wear adequate eye protection while the laser is being used. This will protect their eyes from direct exposure to misaimed laser light as well as from specular reflections from instruments or tissues at the surgical site. All facilities using lasers must therefore have available appropriate wavelength-specific goggles (Fig. 2–3) or glasses with side shields to be worn by all personnel whenever the laser is operating. These laser protection devices should have an optical density (OD) stamped or imprinted on them along with the wavelength and/or name of the laser for which they are to be used. The material coating the lenses of these goggles or glasses absorbs and disperses the incident laser energy, preventing damage to the eye. For protecting the patient, in addition to wavelength-specific glasses or goggles, it is also acceptable to place wet gauze or eye pads across the closed eyelids and, depending upon the procedure (i.e., Nd:YAG laser procedures), an aluminum-metal type of eye shield should be placed over the gauze or pads.

Skin Hazards

Even though, from a laser usage standpoint, skin hazards are regarded as a minor nuisance, they are painful and may be damaging. The most common mishap occurs when the laser operator's or assistant's hands pass in front of the working laser beam causing a burn. This happens when the laser is either misfired during the course of surgery or when an assistant carelessly places a hand in contact with the laser beam. The resulting injury may potentially be substantial. It is therefore most important for the clinician to keep his foot off the foot pedal until ready to fire the laser. Simultaneously, the laser technician must be ready to change the laser to the "standby" mode whenever an interruption in laser use is encountered. The clinician should also inform the support staff of the danger of laser injuries to tissue, and must warn them to keep their hands away from the surgical site when the laser is in operation. Other important locations at risk of exposure in oral and maxillofacial surgery include the patient's facial skin, teeth, and soft tissues. Wet drapes or gauze sponges should also be placed over the patient's skin and teeth outside of the surgical site. A laser impact on a tooth has the potential to damage the enamel, penetrate into the pulp chamber, and

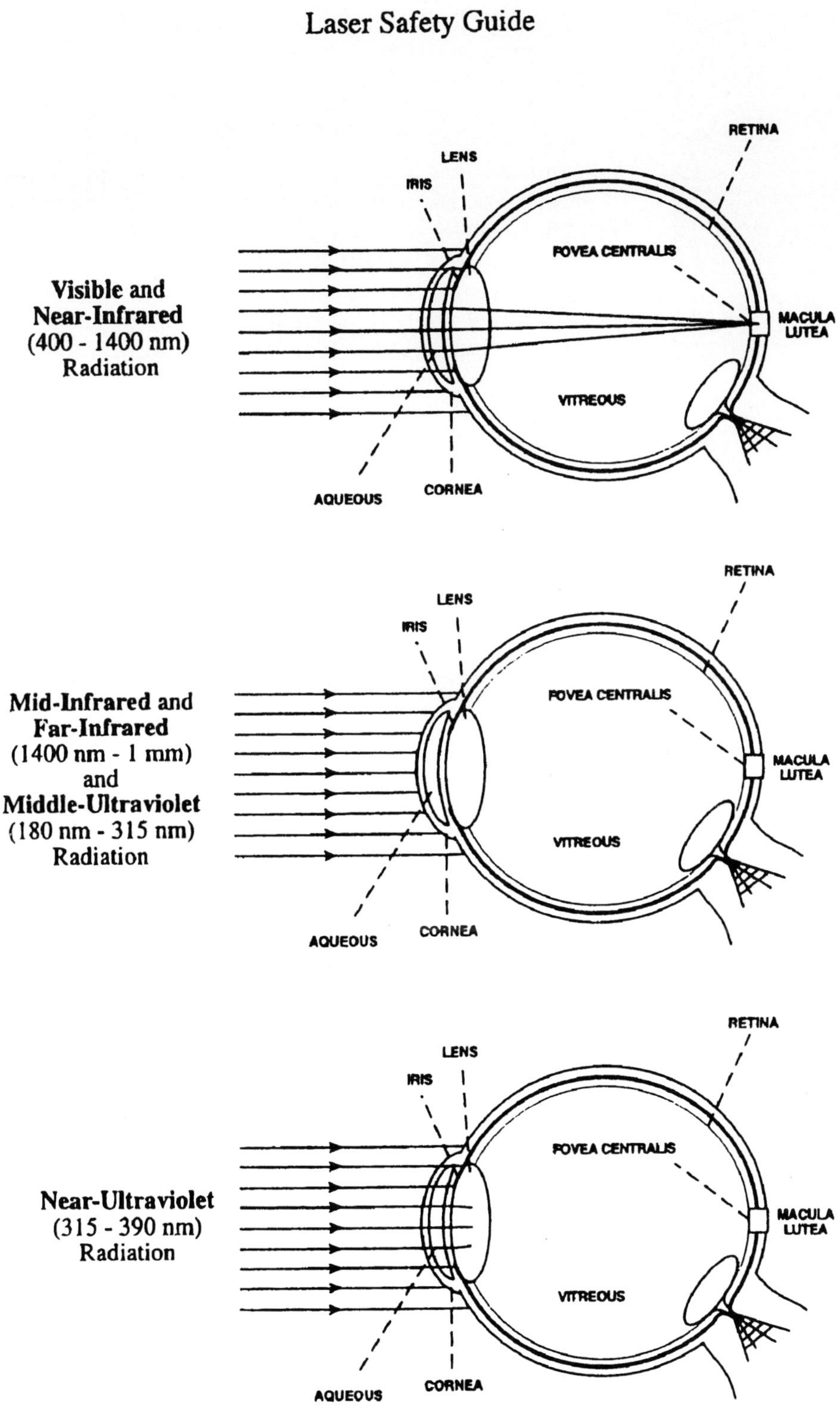

Figure 2–2. Absorption site of (**A**) visible and near-infrared radiation; (**B**) middle, far-infrared radiation and middle ultraviolet radiation; (**C**) and near-ultraviolet radiation. (Reproduced from Laser Institute of America's Laser Safety Guide.)

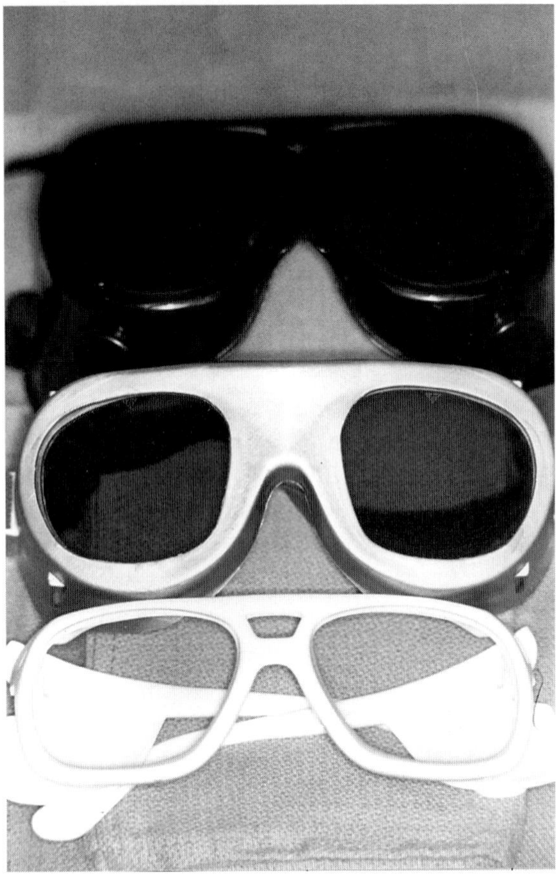

Figure 2–3. Goggles that are wavelength specific.

shatter the tooth. A tooth damaged by the laser is caries resistant but unsightly.

Fire Hazards

All lasers used in the operating suite have the potential to ignite materials on the surgical site and produce a fire hazard. Examples of these combustible materials include disposable drapes made from wood pulp, dry cotton swabs, gauze sponges, wooden tongue blades, and plastic instruments (Fig. 2–4). To reduce the potential for igniting the draping material by the laser, this author advocates the use of polypropylene surgical drapes because in my experience when hit by an incident laser beam they melt rather than burst into flame.

The greatest source of danger in surgery of the oral cavity is the endotracheal tube itself. Special care must be taken to prevent the tube from coming into contact with the laser during surgery because ignition of the endotracheal tube produces a fire with a blowtorch effect inside the patient's airway (Figs. 2–5 and 2–6). New "laser safe" endotracheal devices are available for use during laser surgery. It is important to have an airtight endotracheal tube with a metal reflective exterior. The cuff at the distal end of the tube should be filled with a saline and methylene blue dye. If the laser beam penetrates the cuff during surgery, the blue solution will spill, indicating to the surgeon and anesthesiologist that a laser-related puncture of the cuff has occurred. The stainless steel body of the armored endotracheal tubes will resist perforation by the laser. Foil-wrapped endotracheal tubes are not recommended because of the possibility that hand wrapping may leave an uncovered area that is susceptible to a laser burn, causing ignition.

Other safety-enhancing techniques to reduce fire risk include reducing the oxygen content of the anesthetic mixture

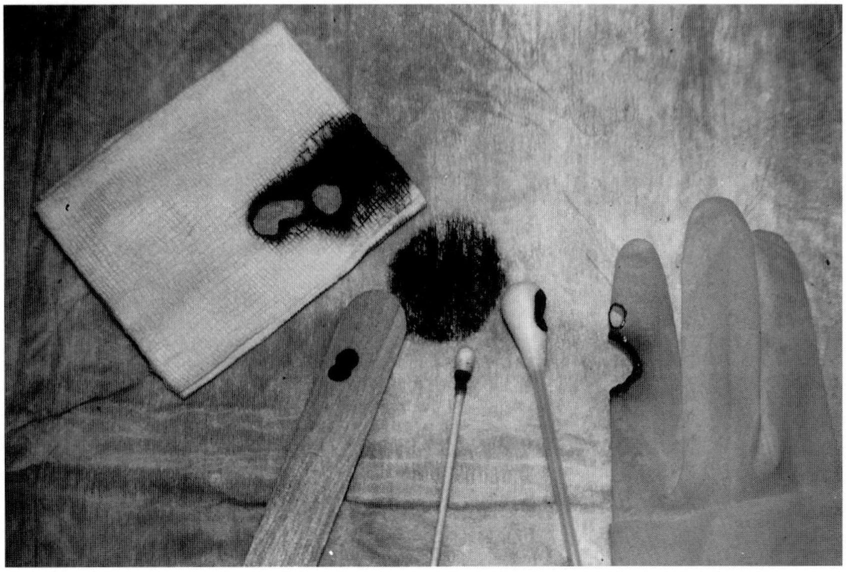

Figure 2–4. Laser burns in combustible materials present at surgery: gauze, wooden tongue blade, cotton, tipped applicators, and rubber glove.

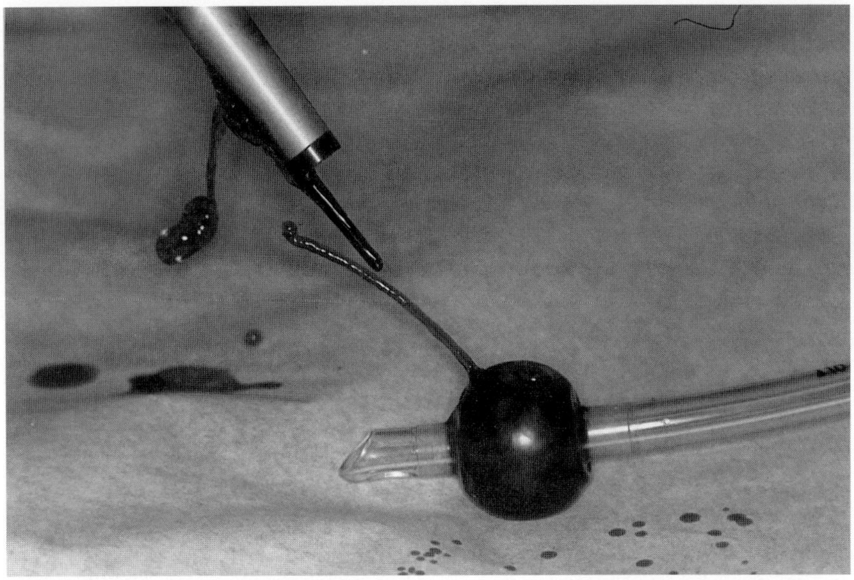

Figure 2–5. Cuff of endotracheal tube penetrated by CO_2 laser beam. Methylene blue liquid filling cuff escapes.

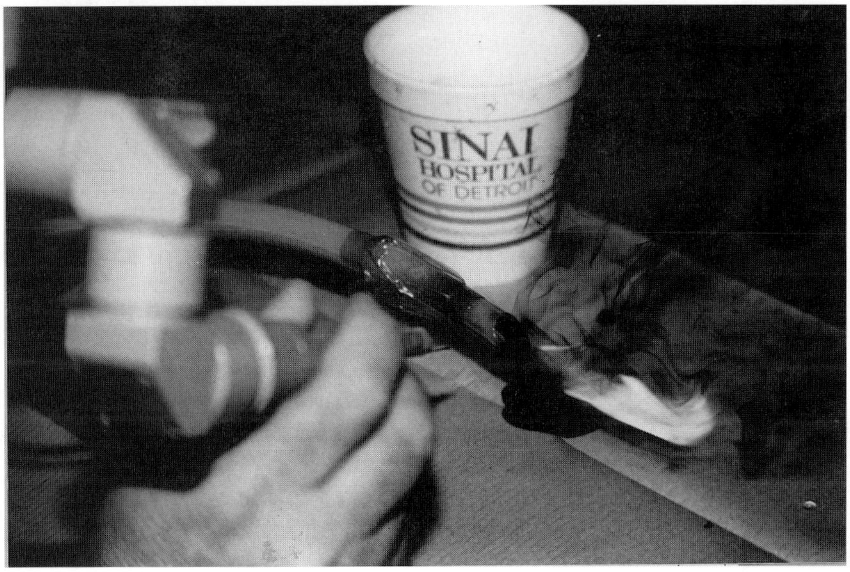

Figure 2–6. Ignition of oxygen-filled endotracheal tube results in ignition and creation of a blowtorch-like effect. Covered foot pedal.

to 30%,[3] and insertion of wet cottonoids or gauze sponges as a hypopharyngeal throat pack. These serve as additional protection for the endotracheal tube by absorbing laser light and ensuring greater protection for the patient. However, it should also be remembered that the surgeon must remove these wet packs from the patient's throat upon completion of the procedure. As for all throat packs, the anesthesiologist should record the time of placement and removal of the pack. At the end of the case, he should ask the surgeon, "Is the pack removed?" The anesthesiologist must understand the surgical procedure being performed as if he himself were performing the operation. Simultaneously, the surgeon must know of any potential anesthetic problems so that both the surgeon and anesthesiologist may foresee and avoid mishaps. As always, communication between surgeon, anesthesiologist, laser technician, and nursing staff in a safety-oriented environment is essential for successful and safe surgery.

The surgeon, anesthesiologist, and operating room staff must always be prepared and have a written plan of action should an airway fire occur. In the event of this dramatic and frightening complication, rapid planned intervention may be lifesaving. The following protocol is recommended for an airway fire: simultaneously stop lasing, cease ventilation, turn off all anesthetic gases, including oxygen, extinguish flames using saline solution from a nearby basin, deflate the cuff, and remove the endotracheal tube. Make sure the entire tube is removed. Next, ventilate the patient's lungs with 100% oxygen by bag and mask, assess the airway for burns and foreign bodies (e.g., tracheal tube and packing materials) by using a bronchoscope. If the damage is minimal, it may be possible to continue with the procedure. However, extreme caution is advised in regard to proceeding even in the case of minimal observed damage. If the damage is extensive, it may be necessary to control airway ventilation by inserting an endotracheal tube or performing a tracheostomy, ventilation proceeds using humidified gases. Antibiotics and large dose steroids[4] should also be given. Lastly, the laser safety officer and the surgeon must report the incident to the appropriate hospital quality improvement and risk management departments, as well as to the laser companies and fiber-optic manufacturers, and a report must be filed with the Food and Drug Administration.

Electrical Hazards

Of all the laser surgical-related hazards, electrical hazards have the greatest potential to be lethal, with several fatalities having been reported since the initiation of the use of lasers in surgery. These incidents have occurred as a result of either untrained and/or unauthorized individuals opening the closed laser cabinet or by technicians who did not follow prescribed electrical safety procedures. Contact with the fully charged capacitor located inside the laser cabinet may result in electrical shock or even death by electrocution.

It is mandatory that inspection, evaluation, and repair of electrical components in these specialized lasers be performed only by factory-trained technicians. Most surgical lasers use high voltage and high current electricity. The laser's direct current (DC) capacitors also have the ability to remain charged for hours after the laser has been turned off and unplugged and, therefore, remain a reservoir of lethal electrical current. Consequently, if the electrical malfunction indicator light goes on during a procedure, the laser should be turned off and a service representative should be called in immediately to evaluate the extent of the problem. If a service representative is not available, the laser aspect of the procedure must be immediately terminated (unless a standby laser is available).

Plume Hazards

One of the few negative aspects of using lasers in surgery is the resulting smoke or laser plume—a by-product of laser surgery. The laser plume is primarily composed of vaporized water (steam), carbon particles, and cellular products, which combine to produce a malodorous scent. This smoke has been found to be irritating to those operating room personnel who come in contact with it. It has also been reported that laser smoke contains many toxic substances, such as formaldehyde, hydrogen cyanide, hydrocarbons, and other airborne mutagens.[4] The particles have an average size of slightly larger than 0.3 μm.

Unfortunately, human papilloma virus DNA has been identified in the plume during the surgery for removal of papillomas.[5] The initial observers of this phenomenon cautioned against overreaction because it could not be proven that these particles could seed themselves in unsuspecting human hosts. In 1993 these researchers reported the first transmission of laser plume–related disease in cows.[6] Currently, additional research is being conducted nationally regarding this issue. As a result of the uncertainty surrounding the seeding ability of this plume material in humans, a proactive stance should be adopted. Use of a high-volume laser smoke evacuation apparatus that filters smoke particles to 0.1 μm is recommended.[7] Maintaining the suction wand within 4 cm of the surgical site to remove as much of the plume as possible is recommended. Disposable gloves and sterile technique should be used to change evacuation filters, which are treated as hazardous waste and disposed of in biohazard bags. The laser-charred material should be wiped from the surgical site and the cloth and paper products used during the laser procedure disposed of using proper biohazard handling. When working with infected patients or those at high risk for HIV/hepatitis, etc., goggles and face masks should be worn to prevent the splattering of tissue from the surgical site onto the eyes and noses of those performing or assisting during the procedure. Lastly, all surgical instruments, e.g., microscopes, operating room tables, etc., should be wiped with a hospital-approved sterilizing solution after each laser procedure.

ADDITIONAL LASER SAFETY INFORMATION

Each institution that uses lasers clinically should appoint a laser safety officer (LSO) to oversee and ensure the safe use of lasers in its facility. The LSO should attend a laser safety officer course to assist in the proper performance of his/her duties. The LSO evaluates all laser use policies and procedures, identifies potential laser-related hazards, and serves as the resource person for the education of hospital staff, medical staff, and nursing staff, and answers questions regarding laser capabilities.

It is recommended that a laser safety policy and procedure be written in each institution using laser to treat patients. Once approved by the laser committee, this information should be disseminated to the employees of the operating room staff and to all laser surgeons, dentists, physicians, podiatrists, etc., and should be followed, as written.

All lasers must have their keys removed when not in use and, if possible, they should be kept in a locked room to maintain equipment safety and security. Only LSO-approved personnel should have access to operate the laser equipment.

Laser safety warning signs should be placed on the door of any operating room using lasers prior to usage. These signs should include the type and power of the laser being used. All operating room windows should be covered with an opaque material while lasers are being used so no laser light can escape and harm an unsuspecting bystander. This is not necessary during CO_1 laser procedures because its emission is absorbed by plastic and glass. An extra pair of laser goggles should also be placed on the door handle of the operating room so that a person entering the room will have adequate eye protection.

All clinical lasers should be examined weekly and their power output should be monitored regularly with a power meter. This data should be recorded for the LSO's monthly quality assurance reports and for medical/legal record-keeping.

Remember foot pedal safety: When the laser is not in use, the clinician's foot should be removed from the pedal. If the laser is not being used for a substantial period of time, the laser should be placed in the standby mode with the approval of the clinician. The covered design of the foot pedal helps prevent accidental activation of the laser.

A basin of saline should be available to be utilized in the event of fire for each laser procedure. *Remember:* In case of fire, use the laser fire safety protocol and act quickly. *Do not use water to extinguish fires on electrical equipment.*

All operating room personnel should know where and how to use the fire extinguishers located near the operating room. *Remember:* P.A.S.S.—pull, aim, squeeze, sweep.

REFERENCES

1. Clayman L, Fuller T, Beckman H. Healing of continuous-wave rapid superpulsed, carbon dioxide, laser-induced bone defects. *J Oral Surg* 1978;36:932–937.
2. Reid R, Elson L, Absten G. A practical guide to laser safety. *Colposc Gynecol Laser Surg* 1986;2(3):121–132.
3. Rontal M, Rontal E, Wenokur M, Elson L. Anesthetic management for tracheobronchial laser surgery. *Ann Otol Rhinol Laryngol* 1986;95:556–560.
4. Sosis MB, ed. *Problems in Anesthesia: Anesthesia for Laser Surgery.* Philadelphia: J.B. Lippincott; 1993.
5. Intact viruses in CO_2 laser plume spur safety concern. *Clin Laser Month* 1987;5(9):101–103.
6. New research confirms laser plume can transmit disease. *Clin Laser Month* 1993;11(6):81–84.
7. Recommended practices for laser safety in the practice setting. *AORN J* 1989;155–158.
8. American National Standard: For the safe use of lasers in health care facilities. *ANSI Z136.3.* 1988.

3 Specific Guide to the Use of Lasers

Lewis Clayman, Richard Reid

CARBON DIOXIDE LASER

The carbon dioxide (CO_2) laser, which is the workhorse of contemporary laser surgery, is a molecular gas laser emitting in the mid-infrared (IR) range configured in either flowing gas or sealed tube form. In the former, the continuously degrading active medium is replenished with fresh gas and the laser consistently produces power outputs of up to 100 watts (W). It is noisy but reliable. The sealed tube laser is of smaller size and lower output power. Its lower maintenance requirements make it suitable for office use.

To bring the laser light to the target tissue, two basic delivery systems have been developed: an articulated arm and a waveguide. At present, there is no commercially available fiber-optic delivery system, although feasibility for one was demonstrated when a prototype was developed by Terry A. Fuller in 1982.

The articulated arm consists of a series of metal tubes, linked by freely movable joints containing precisely aligned mirrors that maintain the laser beam in the center of each segment of the arm. This prevents degradation of beam integrity within the articulated arm. The distal end of the articulated arm is attached to a handpiece containing a focusing lens, or to a micromanipulator attached to an operating microscope (Figs. 3–1 and 3–2).[1,2]

A flexible hollow waveguide, consisting of a small diameter metal tube coated with a highly reflective material applied to its interior, is available for some CO_2 lasers, generally with maximum power outputs of less than 20 W. The laser beam bounces from point to point within the waveguide to reach the handpiece. The greater flexibility of this delivery system permits increased freedom of movement, allowing the operator to reach less accessible areas of the oral cavity and oropharynx. Additional flexibility is achieved by outfitting the waveguide with curved or contra-angled tips. In contradistinction to the articulated arm system that attaches to either a handpiece containing a focusing lens or a microscope, the waveguide system does not transmit the laser beam through a lens system. The beam, as it emerges from the latter, immediately begins to diverge. Therefore, the focal point is considered to be at the tip of the waveguide. Divergence is rapid, resulting in a more rapid decrease in power density than is the case for an articulated arm-focusing handpiece system.

Why Use a CO_2 Laser?

The CO_2 laser emits a coherent light beam in the mid-IR region at 10,600 nm which is near a major spectroscopic absorption peak for water. Because the target chromophore is water and all tissues contain water, all tissues have the capability of interacting with the CO_2 beam. The extent to which this interaction will occur, and therefore the extent to which it may be controlled, is determined by the water content of the tissue and the irradiance, fluence, and geometry of the CO_2 laser beam (also see Chapter 1). This laser has unique application in the evaporative ablation (photovaporization) of superficial mucosal disease of the oral cavity. It can also function as a precise thermal knife for the excision of soft tissue lesions affecting mucosa or skin (Chapter 6). Properly used, the CO_2 laser will produce results either superior to or not achievable with a scalpel or electrocautery. The following are the advantages and disadvantages of the CO_2 laser.

Advantages

1. Improved operating conditions:
   - Rapid incision or ablation (evaporative photovaporization of tissue).
   - Minimal damage to normal tissue adjacent to the area of treatment.
   - Preservation of histologically readable "margins."
   - Good intraoperative hemostasis.
   - "Quiet field" secondary to lack of muscle contraction of the target tissue during laser surgery.
   - Sterilizing action of the beam at its point of application to the tissue.
   - No need for elaborate "prep" of the operative field.
   - "No touch" technique permits surgery in difficult to reach locations (vocal cords, esophagus, paranasal sinuses).
2. Improved patient benefits:
   - Minimal postoperative swelling.
   - Very low infection rates.
   - Minimal scar formation.
   - Elimination of the need for skin grafting in floor of mouth surgery.
   - Healed tissue is supple and maintains normal healing capability if repeat surgery is required.

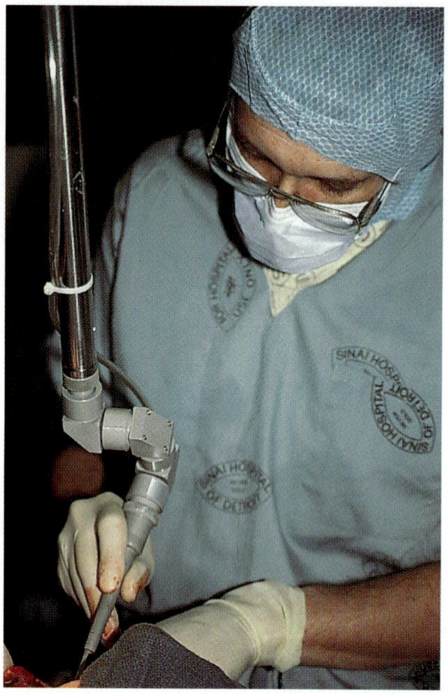

Figure 3–1. Handpiece and articulated arm.

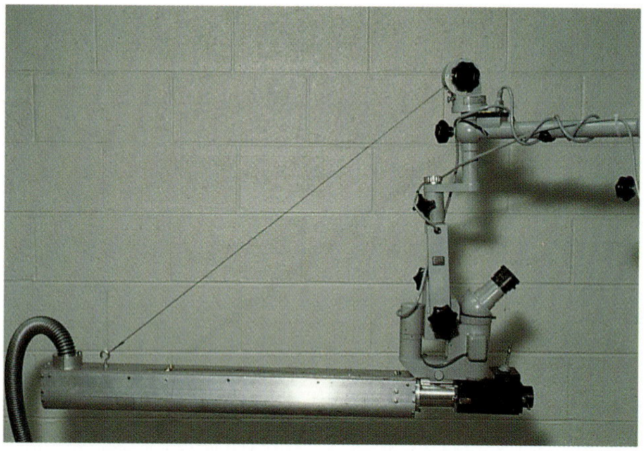

Figure 3–2. Microslad.

- Healing is more rapid than for other thermal instruments (diathermy,[1] cryoprobe[2–4]).
- Minimal tissue handling is required.

Disadvantages

Operative:

- Loss of tactile sense with which surgeon is most familiar and comfortable.
- Additional safety requirements for use in the operating theater.
- Laser safety personnel (laser technician) required in operating theater.[5]
- Anterior floor of mouth surgery is complicated by microstomia, limited mouth opening, or other anatomic abnormalities.[6]
- Special attention required to avoid contact with the endotracheal tube.
- Possible source of unexpected injury to patient, staff, or surgeon.
- Laser-specific education and credentialling required for surgeons.
- High cost of equipment.

Rational Basis for the Use of the CO_2 Laser

Electromagnetic radiation reaching the target tissue is reflected, transmitted, scattered, or absorbed. Ultimately, absorption determines the effect of the laser on the tissue. For the CO_2 laser, absorption is proportional to water content. Therefore, tissues with high aqueous content like epithelium, connective tissue, or muscle readily absorb the incident beam. This is especially true for corneal epithelium, which, because of its high water content, completely absorbs the laser energy within 50 μm of the epithelial surface. Therefore, the corneal thermal lesion is very superficial.[7] Tissues like muscle and skin, which have less water content, suffer greater thermal damage of respective depths of 0.055 mm and 0.25 mm in response to continuous wave (CW) CO_2 at low power density (PD).[8] In comparison, nonaqueous tissues like bone, tendon, or fat are poor absorbers that may sustain more heat damage. Using a rapid superpulsed (RSP) beam instead of CW will minimize the heat effects. In addition, bone will rapidly melt thereby becoming even more anhydrous, resulting in excessive heating even to the point of incandescence followed by actual flaming with continued application of the beam. For anhydrous tissue like bone, one must use a shorter wavelength laser like the erbium:yttrium-aluminum-garnet (Er:YAG) (2.92 μm) or the holmium (Ho):YAG (2.127 μm) to avoid the excessive heating occurring with CO_2. The other commonly used lasers in head and neck surgery, neodymium (Nd): YAG and argon, respectively, have pigmented chromophores for targets. Argon has affinity for the red pigment of hemoglobin,[7] whereas Nd:YAG is selective for the dark pigments of melanin and protein. Nd:YAG is usually used for excision as a contact laser with a sapphire or silica tip. Argon, on the other hand, is used for photocoagulation of vascular lesions with a fiberoptic or handpiece delivery system. The intensity of the tissue interaction also depends on the energy of the incident beam.

Beam energy is inversely proportional to wavelength. Hence, wavelength determines whether a laser beam will produce ionization (excimer lasers) or thermal interactions (dye, argon, potassium titanyl sulfate (KTP), Nd:YAG, Er:YAG, Ho:YAG, and CO_2 lasers). In addition, wavelength also determines whether absorption will be color dependent (dye and Nd:YAG) or color independent (excimer and CO_2). Thermal damage is a function of the optical properties of the incident energy as well as of effects induced by the absorbed irradiation.[7,9]

As the incident beam is absorbed, some heat is generated within the medium unless the application time is so short and the fluence is so low that there is no useful effect on the target tissue. Therefore, some heat effects must be accepted in the course of the performance of useful work by most lasers. During heating the optical properties of the target tissue do change. For water, as the temperature increases the absorption coefficient decreases. This becomes more pronounced with repeated laser "hits" particularly at the base of the vaporization crater. Recent studies have shown that even a single pulse will change the absorption coefficient of water. Therefore, as the temperature increases during the pulse, so does the depth of absorption. For mid-IR lasers, which emit near the 1940-nm absorption peak for water, the absorption peak decreases, which results in a slightly greater depth of penetration than was predicted. The effect is more pronounced for the CO_2 laser at 10,600 nm. At conditions of vaporization the absorption coefficient may change by a factor of 10^3. Therefore, as the energy from repeated laser pulses accumulates, thermal damage extends progressively deeper into the tissue.[10] This effect is further exaggerated if the tissue has become charred, which radically alters its optical and absorptive properties.

How is it possible for a thermal instrument to remove the target tissue without having excessive heating cause destruction of the surrounding normal tissue?

Tissue interaction with a laser beam is defined by the volume of absorption of the laser beam by the target tissue. This is the fraction of the incident light absorbed by the tissue. This becomes understandable by considering Beer's law according to which the incident light transmitted through the target tissue (I_t) is inversely proportional to the absorption coefficient (α) and the thickness of the irradiated tissue (X), thus:

$$I_t = I_0 \cdot 10^{-\alpha X}$$

This equation may be simplified by setting tissue thickness (X) equal to $1/\alpha$ so that

$$I_t = I_0\,(10^{-1}) \text{ or } I_t = I_0/10.$$

The incident transmission I_t now becomes reduced to 10% of its initial intensity. Therefore, the critical volume of tissue required to absorb 90% of the incident radiation is defined by the reciprocal of the absorption coefficient.[9,11,12] It is this extremely high absorption of the thermal energy of the laser beam within a small volume of tissue that permits the laser to selectively remove the target tissue while having minimal heat effects on the surrounding tissue. This extreme containment of the energy within a small volume of tissue results in instantaneous boiling of water within the tissue, which causes the formation of steam. This, in turn, results in explosive disruption of tissue at the impact site. The resultant crater consists of a vaporized area surrounded by a zone of carbonization (charring), which is in turn bordered by a zone of sublethal, and therefore potentially reversible, thermal injury[13–15] (Fig. 3–3). The damaged tissue zone adjacent to the vaporization crater represents a thickness of only 50 to 200 μm measured from the histologic tissue specimen. This is somewhat greater than the volume of absorption of water in laboratory studies.

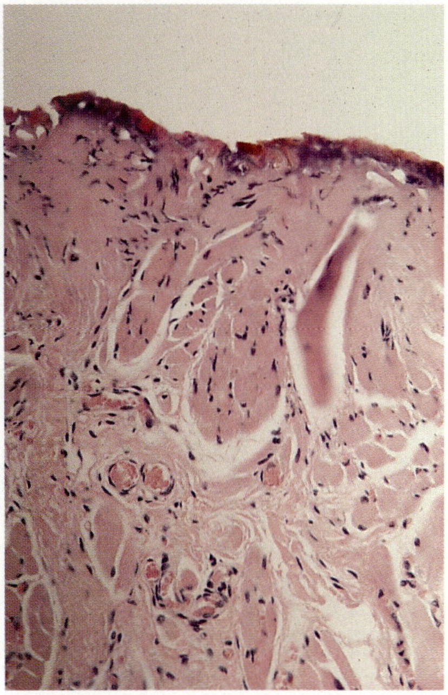

Figure 3–3. Zones of damage. H & E.

The clinical significance of the above property is that the amount of tissue removed under direct visual observation represents nearly the entire amount of vaporized and damaged tissue actually removed.

Using a superpulsed laser of adequate fluence, coagulation necrosis is limited to a narrow, sharply defined zone at the crater margin, in which energy levels do not reach the vaporization threshold (Fig. 3–4). Under these circumstances, crater depth conforms closely to the true level of thermal destruction.

With the superpulsed CO_2 laser, basically, what you see is what you get! This is its great difference compared with the Nd:YAG laser, in which, because of extensive scatter, the volume of tissue injury is approximately 40 to 50 times greater than that for CO_2.[6,9,16] In addition, with YAG there is no immediately visible change in the tissue surrounding the zone of vaporization, so it is very difficult to estimate the true extent of thermal necrosis. Studies of laser-target interactions for the CO_2 laser in water demonstrate an intense heating effect that is restricted to a small volume of water. The entire energy of the impact beam was absorbed in a depth of water of only 39 to 90 μm. To minimize lateral heat conduction, the pulse width for CO_2 must be less than approximately 1 ms. For a free-beam Nd:YAG delivered by optical fiber in the same water model the absorption depth was 4 to 6 mm.[16] This great differential in the water absorption model predicts events occurring in soft tissue.

The CO_2 beam is completely absorbed, with an intense heating effect in a small volume of water, whereas Nd:YAG is absorbed in a much larger volume of water but with less vaporization. Using a contact tip converts Nd:YAG into a predominantly thermal instrument with reduced depth of absorption compared with free-beam Nd:YAG. Argon effects are intermediate, with a depth of absorption of 0.5 to 2.0 mm.[16] However, this advantage for CO_2 may readily be lost

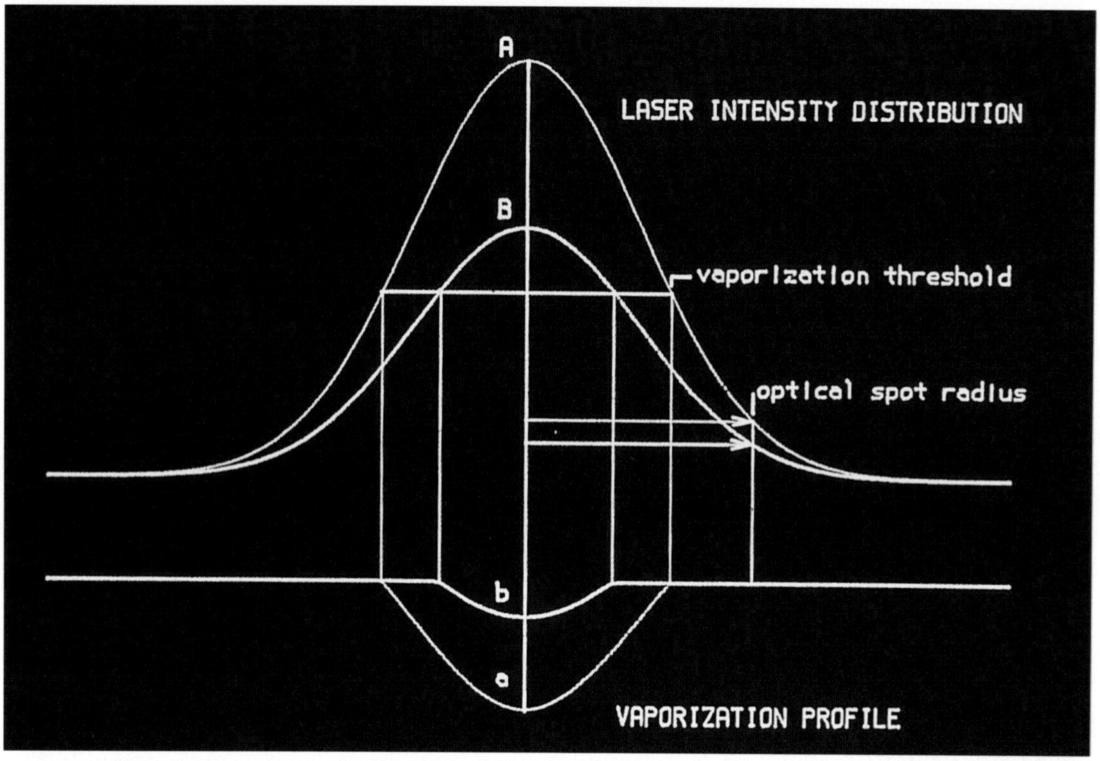

Figure 3–4. Gaussian distribution curve. Tissue removed occurs within the area defined by the "vaporization threshold." (Courtesy T.A. Fuller, Ph. D.)

if used inexpertly. Therefore, one must understand that the CO_2 laser is an instrument that works by thermal destruction (Table 3–3) as do conventional instruments like the electrocautery or the Shaw scalpel. For conventional thermal instruments to work, they must maintain contact with the tissue during a lag phase until the target tissue is heated to the necessary temperature. During this time, lateral heat conduction results in absorption of heat in a progressively larger area of tissue. In short, the tissue is burned.

Healing postoperatively will not occur until the damaged tissue is repaired, which is a slow process. On the other hand, the CO_2 laser, as previously discussed, can be administered as a series of pulses that remove tissue through explosive vaporization by the direct thermal effects of the laser radiation, but not by lateral heat conduction from the laser crater. Therefore, heat-damage adjacent to the vaporization crater is generally restricted to a zone less than 100 to 200 μm wide. The actual volume of heat necrosis is largely dependent on the application time of the laser.[17] Consequently, healing begins quickly after laser surgery and reepithelialization occurs before excessive collagen (scar) is deposited.[18,19] There are also fewer myofibroblasts in the healing laser wound than in the conventional wound, which may also contribute to reduced wound contraction and scarring.[19–21]

Irradiance (Power Density)

Once again, to achieve the desired wound characteristics listed above, optimization of tissue effects must occur. This is partly a function of the duty cycle in the pulsed mode of operation. A short pulse duration is chosen to permit photovaporization effects to predominate over photocoagulation thereby minimizing lateral heat transfer. This is accomplished by using high-power densities at pulse widths shorter than the thermal relaxation time of the target tissue. In addition, an interpulse interval at least twice as long as the pulse width permits significant, but not complete, tissue cooling between pulses. Unfortunately, rapid superpulse has one major disadvantage: the choice of a short duty cycle will reduce power output accordingly, which slows down the rate of tissue removal. Hence, in practice, rapid superpulse is generally reserved for situations in which small tissue volumes need to be treated with maximal precision.

A handy compromise between the high precision of rapid superpulse and the high power of continuous wave is obtained from the chopped mode (actually chopped CW mode; see Chapter 4, Fig. 4–15), in which the laser tube is electrically pulsed to emit broader, flatter pulses with a shortened interval between pulses. Consider, for example, the electrical pulsing of a 120-W laser tube, governed such that the ratio of on/off time (duty cycle) will never exceed 5:1. When used at the highest duty cycle, maximal output would be 100 W (i.e., $120 \times 5/6$). Conversely, selecting a 1:9 duty cycle would produce an output of only 12 W (i.e., $120 \times 1/10$). Because the peak power of each pulse is not amplified, an electronically pulsed laser tube does not have a refractory phase when used in the chopped mode. Hence, repetition rate can be increased to virtually any frequency. However, as pulse frequency approaches a duty cycle of

2:1, heat will accumulate at the impact site, and the clinical effects will resemble those of a continuous wave laser. Thus, the best compromise is a duty cycle of about 1:1 producing 60 W of power output, while preserving about half of the interpulse cooling. Physical cooling of the tissue with iced saline also helps reduce unwanted heat transfer during lasing.

Fluence (Energy Density)

In addition to power density, one must also consider the fluence (energy density), which is the rate at which energy is delivered. It must exceed the vaporization (ablation) threshold for mucosa (4 J/cm^2 per pulse) or skin (5 J/cm^2 per pulse). The fluence may be delivered in continuous or pulsed modes. The pulses themselves may be delivered in two different modes: superpulse, in which pulsing occurs within the laser tube (rapid superpulse, RSP) or "chopped" (gated) continuous wave, in which the beam is interrupted by a shutter. RSP lasers may produce peak pulse powers of individual pulses that exceed 500 W. A typical pulse duration is 150 to 300 μs at approximately 50 to 150 mJ/pulse with an interpulse interval of several milliseconds. This provides excellent control of a cool beam, which will ablate small volumes of tissue very precisely. However, the very short duration of the pulse reduces power output compared with continuous wave function. The actual average power output for a pulsed laser corresponds with the duty cycle during which the pulse is actually occurring.

Energy

Energy (joules) = Power (watts) × Time/(sec)

A given amount of energy will destroy the same volume of tissue independent of the rate at which that energy is delivered. However, the effects on the target tissue as well as on the surrounding tissue differ greatly depending upon the rate of energy delivery. With a superpulsed laser of adequate fluence emitting pulses shorter than the thermal relaxation time of the target tissue, thermal damage becomes a function of the optical properties of the incident energy. In contrast, when pulse duration exceeds thermal relaxation time, heat accumulates at the surface of the impact crater and lateral heat conduction begins. It is this technique error of prolonged time of application that causes thermal damage. This results in the loss of the major benefit of laser use: *selective* tissue removal.

The following errors most commonly lead to unwanted heat damage:

1. Use of low irradiance by excessively defocusing the beam, resulting in PD <500–600 W/cm^2 for keratinized tissue. The same applies for nonkeratinized oral mucosa at PD <350–400 W/cm^2.
2. Failure to remove carbonized debris from the wound before using the laser for its second application.
3. Irradiating a bleeding point at low PD, which heats the blood at the surface but does not coagulate the cut blood vessel. This causes cooking, not coagulation! Remember that soft tissues suffer coagulation necrosis at temperatures above 58°C[22] and bone is even more sensitive, succumbing at 47°C.[23]

Consequently, cooling the operative field with iced saline before lasing and prior to each raster is helpful in reducing unwanted heat damage.

Power Density (PD) (W/cm²)

To calculate PD, a reasonable approximation is given by

$$PD = \frac{100 \cdot W}{d^2} = 100\ W/cm^2$$

where W is power, in watts, of the exit beam, measured by the laser power meter, and d is the measured diameter in millimeters of the imprint left by a 10-W, 0.1-second pulse on a moistened wooden tongue depressor.[24] Since the inverse square law of light applies here, changing the spot size will affect PD exponentially, whereas changing the inline laser power output will affect PD only linearly. Therefore, the greatest control by the operator on laser effects will be by altering power density through changes in focus and beam geometry, not by changing power output at the beam source (Table 3–1).

Learner's Curve

Table 3–2 represents the early experience of the section of oral and maxillofacial surgery during the first year of CO_2 laser use at Sinai Hospital of Detroit in 1979–1980. There is a wide distribution of power densities used for photovaporization. As experience was gained, PD clustered around several restricted ranges, as it became apparent that there was a specific relationship between PD and clinical effect. Consequently, one may now select the appropriate PD for

Table 3–1. Power Density and Tissue Effects

POWER DENSITY	EFFECT[17,25]
<100 W/cm^2	Desiccation, denaturation, warming
>100 W/cm^2	Photovaporization, carbonization (carbon appears as target tissue temperature reaches approximately 150°C)
600–2500 W/cm^2	Photovaporization (ablation), minimal carbonization, superficial hemostasis; target tissue temperatures may reach 300°C
>10,000 W/cm^2	Ultrarapid photovaporization, thermal incision
>50,000 W/cm^2	Incision of tissue, approximately same rate of cutting as for a scalpel
>10^6 W/cm^2	Plasma formation, acoustic shock waves: tissue destruction by mechanical disruption rather than thermal denaturation

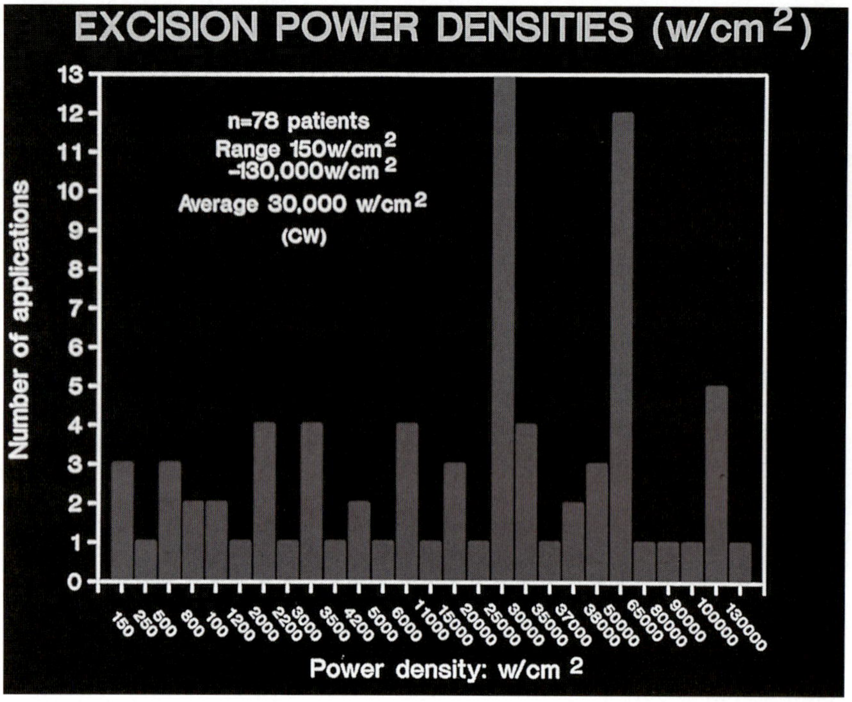

Table 3–2. Learner's curve.

ablative vaporization or incision and rapidly learn how quickly to move the beam across the target tissue to achieve the desired effect.

Beam Geometry: Gaussian Distribution of Energy

The energy within the laser beam follows a Gaussian distribution pattern with the usable component occupying the central 86% of the beam. This is the working "spot size" of the beam. However, the peripheral 14% still heats the tissue, thereby contributing to thermal conduction, denaturation and subthreshold heating. Irradiance (PD) must be kept high enough to vaporize tissue quickly because low irradiance results in desiccation. Anhydrous conditions can cause excessive heating, carbonization, and even flaming. Consequently, temperatures at the impact crater may increase

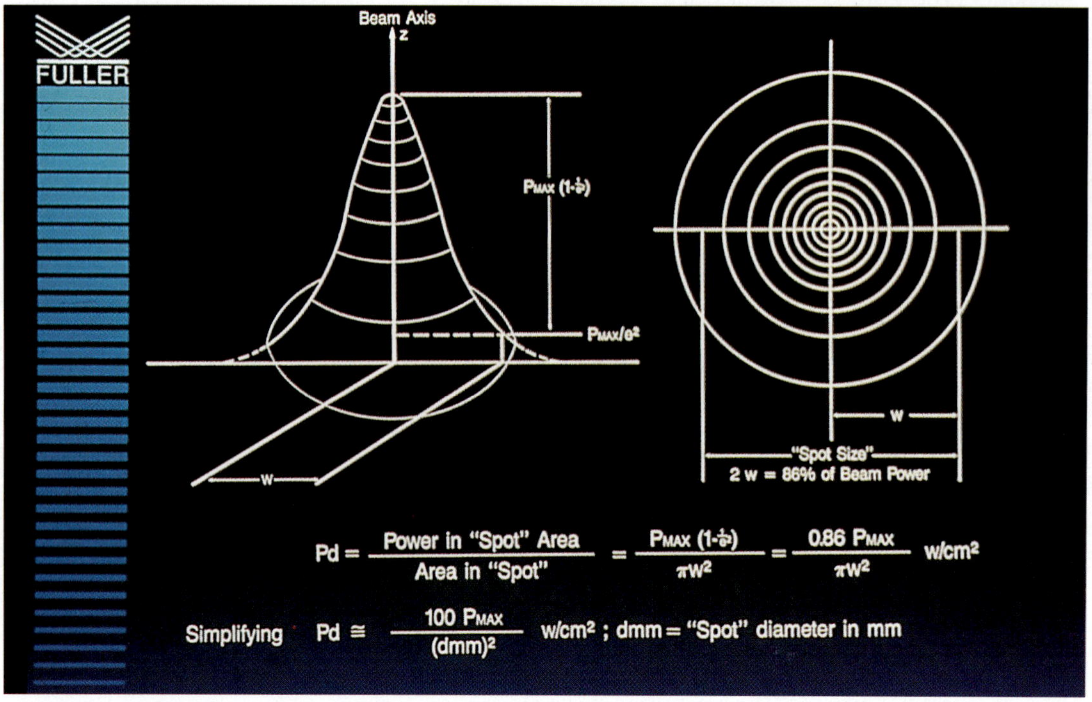

Figure 3–5. Beam profile: transverse and cross section. (Courtesy T. A. Fuller, Ph.D.)

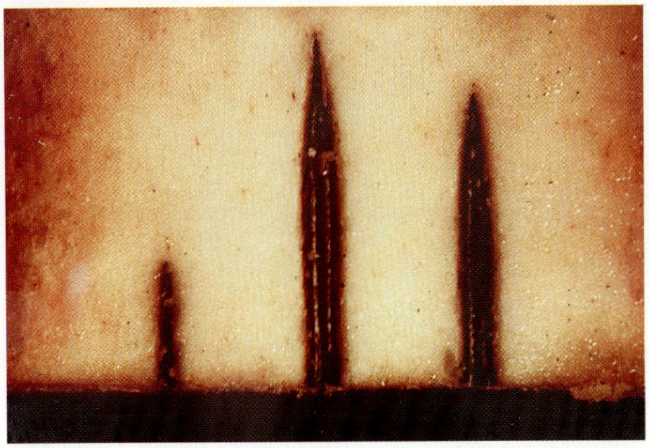

Figure 3–6. Beam profile in bone: cross section of CO_2 beam: RSP mode, in focus at high PD (left and center) and lower PD (right) (frozen ox femur). (Courtesy L. Clayman, DMD, MD and Carlo Clauser, MD.)

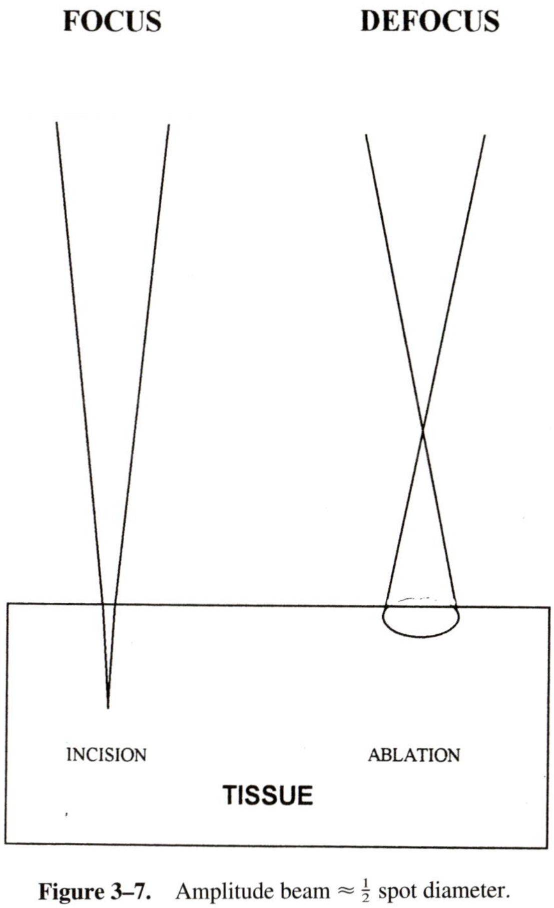

Figure 3–7. Amplitude beam ≈ $\frac{1}{2}$ spot diameter.

from 100°C to >600°C. This increased heating causes a burn, which is similar to, or even worse than, that caused by electrocautery.[9,16]

Recall that the exit beam, particularly after being modified by the lenses within a handpiece, or by the microscope's objective lenses, does not contain energy of uniform density. There is variation within the beam profile that follows a Gaussian distribution and is readily seen at the target site where the shape of the impact crater replicates the energy profile of the incident beam (Fig. 3–5). A highly focused beam, providing high PD that is suitable for incision, will produce a beam contour as seen in (Fig. 3–6). Defocusing the beam either by moving the handpiece away from the tissue or by adjusting the microslad device on the microscope by rotating its tuning dial to alter spot size will flatten out the beam. One wishes to flatten the beam profile until the amplitude of the beam is about half that of the spot diameter (Fig. 3–7).

The characteristics of the beam are also modified by the delivery system. Both systems destroy collimation, so that at the tissue the beam is slightly divergent. Both spot size and depth of field at any given wavelength will vary with the focal length of the objective lens. The operating microscope of long focal length objective (300–400 mm) produces a relatively large minimum spot size (approximately 0.6 mm) with excellent depth of field, while the handpiece objective (125 mm) produces a very small spot (0.3 mm) with a shallow depth of field. The maximum power density is higher, and the beam geometry is therefore sharper for the handpiece compared with the microscope at maximum power densities. This is the intrinsic difference that makes the handpiece the instrument of choice for rapid incision. However, the microscope is most suitable for ablation if target anatomy permits its use because it provides these advantages: (1) keeping the beam normal to the tissue maintains a circular spot size of constant PD (using the defocused handpiece in a "pencil grip" is more likely to permit obliquity and an oval spot size of nonuniform PD); (2) enhanced visual resolution increases both beam control and monitoring of direct tissue effects.

THE PLANES OF TISSUE DESTRUCTION IN ABLATION

First Plane

The objective of ablation is to selectively remove part or all of the mucosa *according to the operator's choice.* Destruction of the first plane removes only the surface epithelium. Removal stops at about the level of the basement membrane. Therefore, the vaporization crater is placed deep in the parabasal layer of mucosa or skin. To achieve proper depth, the laser spot is manipulated to describe a series of parallel lines, overlapping by about one third. Each pass of the CO_2 laser beam will cause a bubbling effect at the surface wherein the target tissue becomes opalescent, and actual bubbles occur on its surface (Fig. 3–8). This is accompanied by a crackling sound similar to that of pulmonary rales, or to the sound of Rice Krispies in milk. The presumed mechanism is that flash boiling of both intra- and extracellular water occurs, which ruptures the epithelium at the level of attachment of keratinocytes to the basement membrane. This first layer of removal is also referred to as the first raster. Either of these two distinctive signs (opalescence and bubbling) can be lost if deep penetration beyond

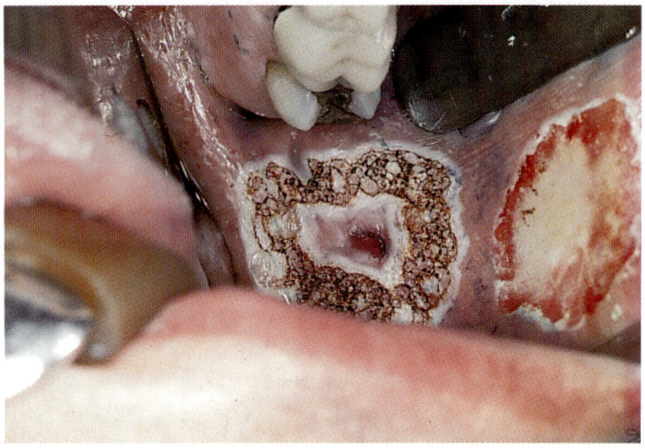

Figure 3–8. Surface bubbling and opalescence after treatment of buccal mucosa.

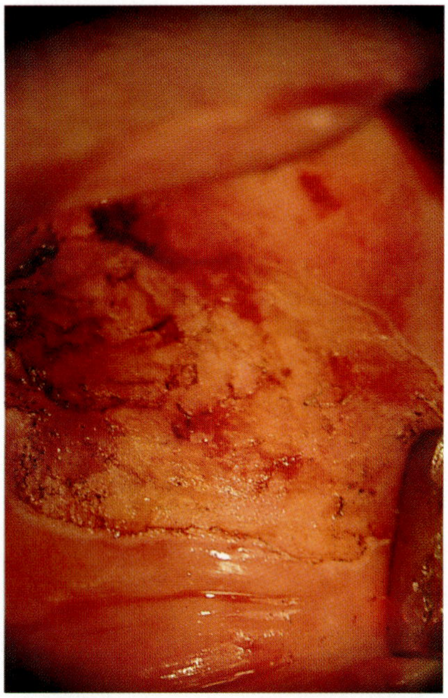

Figure 3–9. Magnified view (16×) of collagen network deep to ablated epithelium after wiping away epithelial debris.

the basement membrane occurs. Wiping away the altered tissue will expose the pink, shining, smooth intact surface of the basement membrane overlying the submucosa (Fig. 3–9). There will be no bleeding. Healing is complete by reepithelialization in less than 14 days for moderate-sized lesions and in approximately 3 weeks for large lesions. No scarring occurs.

Second Plane

Thermal destruction to the second plane removes all of the epithelium and some of the upper submucosa, or for skin the papillary dermis. This is achieved by applying a second raster, at the same PD as the first but perpendicular in direction. This time there will be no opalescence, but some bubbling will still occur (Fig. 3–10). Alternatively, a slightly

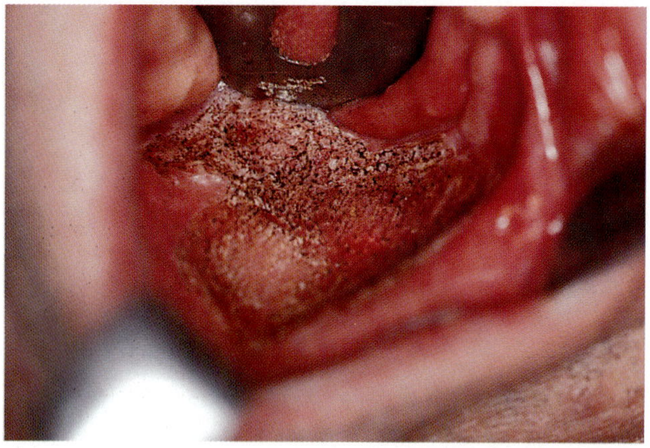

Figure 3–10. Visual end point: appearance of treatment area after second and final raster has been applied perpendicular to the initial raster.

higher PD may be used initially and the first raster will penetrate directly to plane II. After wiping away debris, the surgical site will show a roughened surface of yellow color. There is minimal heat damage to the deeper submucosa (or reticular dermis for skin). If thermal relaxation time is exceeded, then deeper transmission and wider scattering of the incident laser beam causes a larger, but predictable zone of coagulation necrosis. The extent of necrosis is directly proportional to the duration of irradiation, which elevates tissue temperature above 55°C. The sublethal zone of thermal injury remains small. Healing is rapid but slightly delayed compared with plane I, and there will be no scar contracture.

Third Plane

Plane III is rarely used for mucosa since it will obliterate the entire submucosa, following which there will be delayed healing and some scar formation. In ablative oral and maxillofacial surgery, this will be limited in use to removal or recontouring of intraoral skin grafts, for removing cutaneous scars or keloids, or for debulking nonresectable cancers.

Correct depth control is most likely obtained with use of the microscope, which allows one to recognize these landmarks in skin: (1) coarse collagen bundles appearing as gray-white fibers after epithelial ablation; and (2) a network of arterioles and venules running parallel to the epithelial surface (Fig. 3–11). There will also be drops of blood from transected blood vessels in either the reticular dermis or the deep submucosa. Good surgical technique requires slower movement of the beam guided by visual recognition of a "fibrous grain" within the crater base. Therefore, this type of lesion extends deeply enough to create a burn. Regeneration of mucosa starts from the mucosal edge and from minor salivary gland epithelium. It is somewhat delayed because the heat-damaged tissue must be removed by phagocytosis before reepithelialization begins. This delay occurs consequent to thermal damage. Excess heat may cause

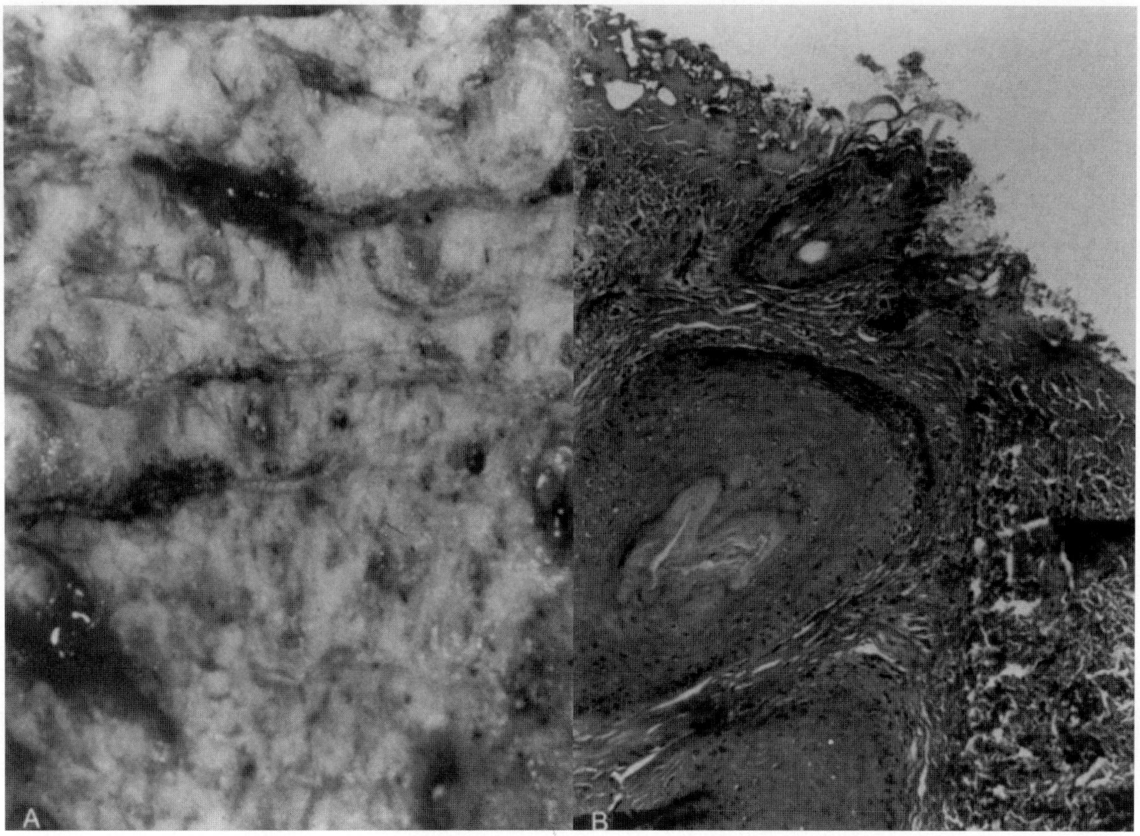

Figure 3–11. Reticular dermis: collagen fibrils exposed, blood vessels visible.

"mummification" of collagen within the submucosa (or dermis), where it further delays healing and promotes fibrosis. This is the deepest plane from which optimal healing may occur.

Postoperative Care

For oral mucosa, care is very simple. The patient uses warm dilute saline rinses four to six times per day on the first day. After that, the saline is mixed 1:1 with 3% hydrogen peroxide and used as a rinse until the mouth feels comfortable. No antibiotics are used and nonsteroidal anti-inflammatory agents are given orally to control pain.

For skin, or for postablation care of the vermilion border of the lips, an antibiotic cream or ointment is applied three times a day. Skin lesions are occluded for the first 24 to 48 hours.

Nd:YAG

Neodymium:yttrium-aluminum-garnet (Nd:YAG) lasers are solid-state devices emitting at 1060 nm in the infrared region of the electromagnetic spectrum. This is a more highly energetic beam than that of the CO_2 laser because of its shorter wavelength. (Energy is inversely proportional to wavelength.) Its target chromophores are pigmented molecules (melanin, hemoglobin, and other proteins) and it is less well absorbed by intracellular water than is the CO_2 beam. As a consequence, free-beam Nd:YAG energy causes more extensive scattering and transmission of the incident beam through the target tissue. Therefore, as expected, absorption length for water is 2 to 4 mm in a large volume of fluid[16] compared with <90 μm for Co_2. More heating of tissue occurs at lower contact temperatures than for the CO_2 laser, thereby producing a deep coagulation effect that increases with power and time of application.

The volume of tissue destruction is 40 to 50 times greater than for a similar exposure to an equal diameter incident beam from a CO_2 laser.[25] The clinical consequence of this is that the volume of tissue destruction greatly exceeds the volume of visible laser effect between the beam and the tissue.[26] Precise control of tissue effects is therefore difficult. Consequently, the YAG laser is most useful for ablation of large volumes of tissue, particularly when strict hemostasis is required (e.g., hepatic resection). On the other hand, CO_2 will be most useful for superficial ablation of surface disease or for incision where the need for hemostasis is moderate.

As mentioned above, the Nd:YAG laser is useful in situations where coagulation is essential, particularly when the underlying tissue can tolerate thermal damage, as in larger, deeply sited vascular tumors. The YAG laser's ability to seal large blood vessels greatly enhances its utility for treatment of vascular lesions. The CO_2 laser, which can be used to excise small capillary hemangiomas, is not suitable as a surgical instrument to treat these larger lesions, nor is scalpel excision, which may cause aesthetic and functional disabilities.

The most recent development permitting an increase in the range of applications of the Nd:YAG laser has been the development of contact probe tips (Fig. 3–12), which control and also limit thermal injury. This alters laser-tissue interactions without changing wavelength of the incident beam (see Chapter 1).

In considering treatment of cavernous hemangiomas and vascular malformations (AVMs) using the Nd:YAG laser, one must be cognizant of potential overtreatment, which may lead to rupture and hemorrhage of the lesions. A conservative approach is to employ a target spot technique using a 2-mm spot size free beam in single pulses at 20 to 25 W and 0.5 sec pulse width. The laser spots are placed 2 to 3 mm apart from one another to avoid overlapping of scattered laser energy. The resultant photocoagulation necrosis obliterates the pigmented or vascular lesion with preservation of normal tissue, leading to resolution of bleeding and swelling as well as improved function. One expects retreatment to be necessary to ablate residual tumor. Patients are usually reevaluated in 4 to 6 weeks for further treatment. Staged treatment helps to reduce overenthusiastic single-stage therapy, which might result in tissue sloughing and compromised healing.

The CO_2 laser resembles the electrocautery unit, the electrodiathermy, and the cryosurgical probe, in that all are instruments of thermal destruction. With conventional devices, lateral heat propagation declines along a slow, linear gradient. Adjacent tissues must recover from the ill effects of a diffuse conduction burn from thermal instruments or frostbite from cryoprobes before the healing response can begin. Moreover, collagen damaged by inept laser surgery can remain "mummified" in the dermis for many months, where it acts to delay healing and promote cicatrization.[27] The noncontact CO_2 laser consistently minimizes collateral heat damage when used properly. The Nd:YAG contact lasers act similarly and also provide tactile feedback through tissue contact.

Table 3–3. Typical Laser Use

CO_2 Laser (10,600nm)
Handpiece: Spot: 0.3 mm at focal point
  $\lambda = 10.6\ \mu m$
  Output power: 5–80 watts
  Ablation: PD: 475–750 w/cm^2
  Incision: PD: 10,000 to >50,000 w/cm^2
Pulsed average power: up to 25 W
  Duty cycle: up to 15%
  Fluence: 120–600 mJ/pulse
  Pulse width: 0.85–6.4 ms
  Maximum peak power: 500 w/pulse
CW: Same as output power at exit tube
For both: PD $\approx$ 100(W)/spot (cm)^2

Contact Nd:YAG (1060nm)
  Silica tips: varied
  Typical power
    (a) to mark tumor periphery: up to 10 W
    (b) to incise: 12–20 W

Argon Laser (488 to 514 nm)
Handpiece or fiber: 2–4 W CW mode.
ILP-fiber: 2–4 W CW mode.

CO_2: Scanner Handpiece
  $\lambda = 10.6\ \mu m$
  Spot size: 2–6mm. Varied by handpiece
  P: < 20 W
  E: 200–500 mJ/pulse
  Fluence = 5 – >15 J/cm^2
  Cycle = approx. 0.2 sec
    PRR set by computer with limits defined by length of cycle

Note: 2–4 "passes" are required to ablate skin wrinkles
Pulse width < 1 msec

Note: All lasers require protective eyewear and high-speed laser suction to evacuate plume particles.

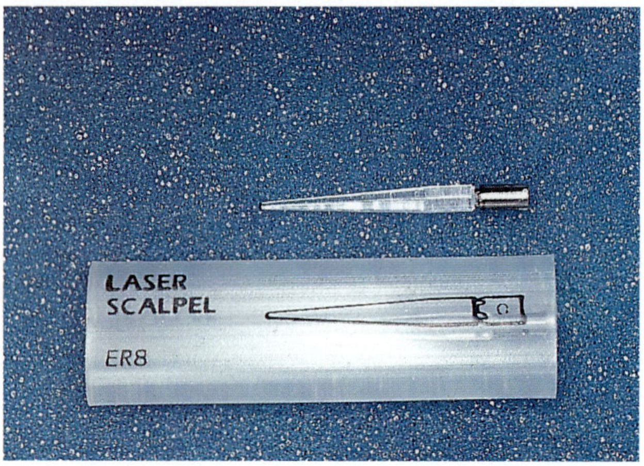

Figure 3–12. Nd:YAG contact laser probe tip.

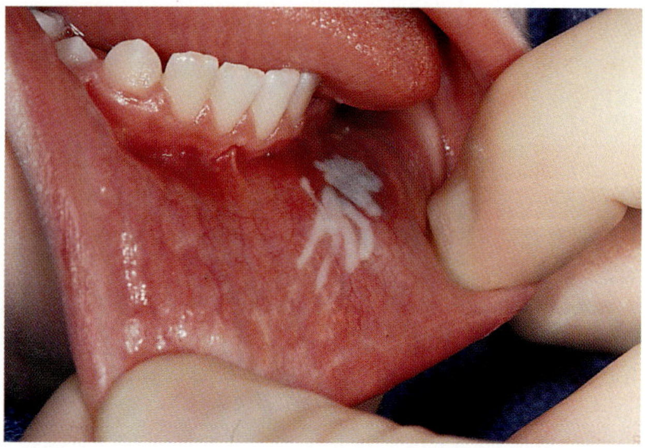

Figure 3–13. Argon laser: end point is "whitening" of lesion.

Argon Laser

The argon laser is a continuous wave laser emitting blue-green light between 488 and 514 nm (Table 3–3). Its depth of penetration is 0.5 to 2.0 mm and the energy is absorbed mainly by hemoglobin. The depth of absorption is a function both of power density and heating effects. The effect on soft tissue is to create an initial pallor (Fig. 3–13) followed by blanching (whitening). Eventually, the epithelial surface elevates, and a vesicle forms that then ruptures to reveal the effect of the laser on the subjacent deeper tissue. This vesicle itself may form from the vaporization of water into steam. This results in elevation of the epithelium away from the subepithelial plane due to dispersion and absorption of the beam within this deeper plane.[26]

For superficial coagulation a pulsed argon laser beam at 2-W output power with a 0.2-mm spot size and a 10-ms pulse width will be absorbed to a depth less than 1.0 mm. Using such a low irradiance it is possible to treat cutaneous telangiectasias without topical anesthesia by using a spot target technique of single-spot applications to the target vessels. Up to 500 vessels may be treated in a single 20-minute session this way. For extensive telangiectasias, multiple sessions, averaging between four and five in number, are required. The sessions are repeated at 3 to 4-week intervals. Slightly longer pulse duration at higher power densities will permit photocoagulation to occur to a deeper level in thicker vascular lesions. However, at higher outputs some cutaneous absorption will occur and the probability of scarring increases. Therefore, for superficial cutaneous vascular lesions like port-wine stains or telangiectasias, other lasers like flashlamp-pumped dye lasers or copper vapor lasers emitting closer to the Hb-O_2 second absorption peak of 577 nm should be used. For intramucosal vascular malformations or for those thicker malformations involving critical anatomic regions like the vermilion border of the lip, a higher dose of argon may be used either to reduce the size of the lesion and devascularize the ensuing scar prior to surgery or as definitive treatment.

TECHNIQUE

To maximize the effectiveness of the argon laser for the treatment of thicker vascular lesions (Fig. 3–14) one may employ physical adjuncts to convert a thick lesion to a thin one with a reduced rate of blood flow. This may be achieved by reducing the local blood flow by the application of ice to the lesion and by infiltration of local anesthetic containing vasoconstrictor around the lesion. At this point the argon laser is applied to the surface of a glass slide placed over the lesion to compress it (diascopy). The spot size and power is adjusted and the application time in CW is prolonged until the test target tissue turns white. The optical fiber is now used to trace a series of decreasing concentric circles from the periphery to the center of the lesion until the entire field turns white (Figs. 3–15 and 3–16). During the procedure, which takes about 1 minute, the glass slide is maintained in constant position under finger pres-

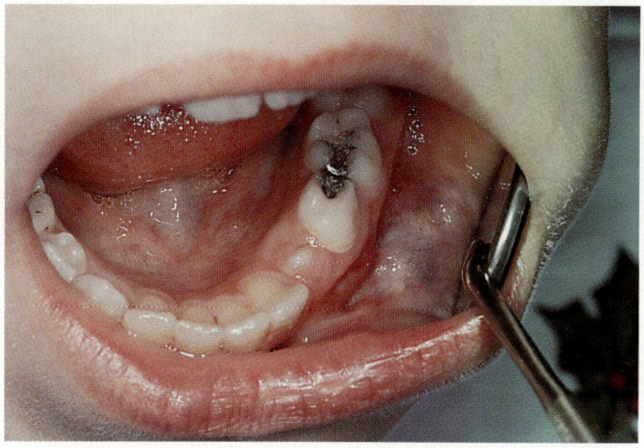

Figure 3–14. Vascular malformation of labiobuccal vestibule.

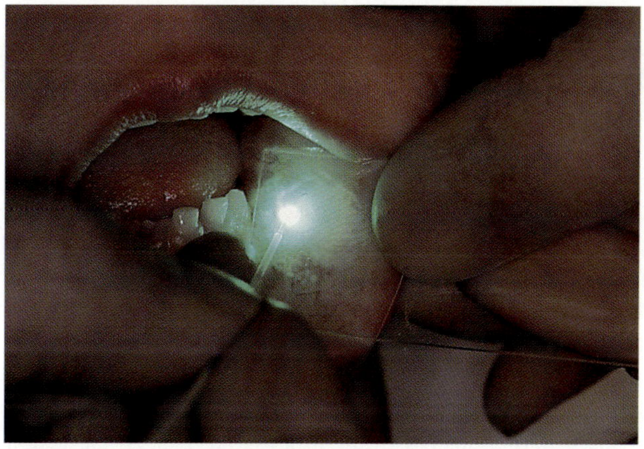

Figure 3–15. Argon laser applied by fiber to glass slide compressing the lesion. Laser beam may be used at its focal point or defocused.

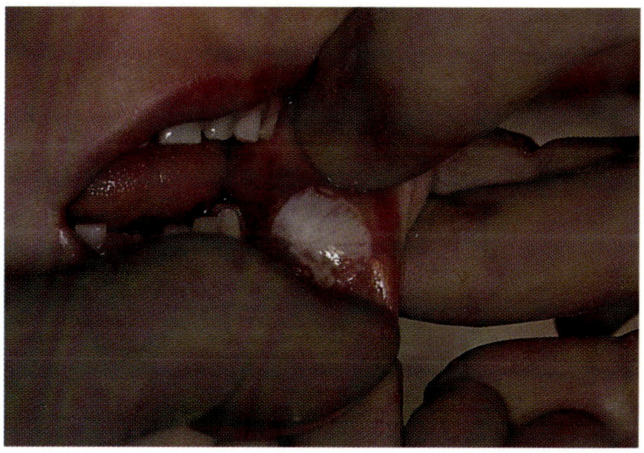

Figure 3–16. Completion of treatment: entire lesion is white.

sure. At the conclusion of the initial treatment, the slide is removed and blood flow through the lesion is visually assessed. If the lesion is still quite red, ice is reapplied and the treatment is repeated. Antibiotic ointment is applied and the patient is given wound care instructions. Swelling and discoloration at the operative site are to be anticipated.

The size of the acute lesion increases over 48 to 72 hours. Edema peaks at 72 hours and persists for several days. Wound healing, which is delayed initially, is apparent at the end of the first week.[26] Analgesics, usually in the form of nonsteroidal anti-inflammatory agents, are prescribed. The patient is seen at 5 to 7 days to monitor wound healing followed by monthly reevaluations. The healed wound is generally 20 to 30% larger than is the vascular lesion. If resolution is incomplete, the lesion is retreated after 2 months. Two or three treatment sessions may be required until the lesion is eradicated (Fig. 3–17).

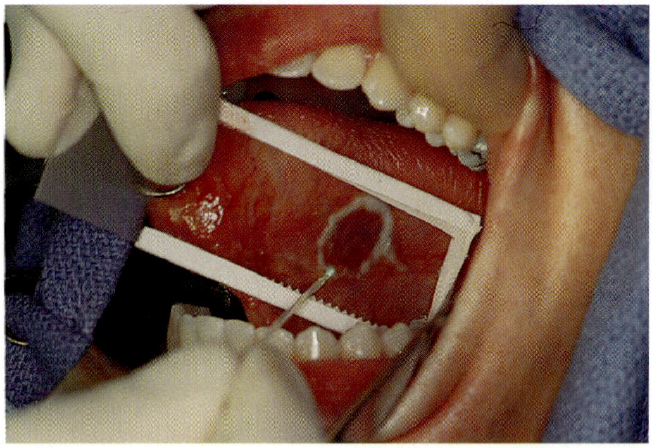

Figure 3–18. Diascopy: mucosa compressed. Lesion outlined with argon in CW mode.

ALTERNATE TECHNIQUE: INTRALESIONAL PHOTOCOAGULATION

For thicker vascular lesions, particularly for intraoral hemangiomata a more aggressive technique for photocoagulation is intralesional photocoagulation (ILP). For this technique to be effective one depends on both selective photoabsorption by the Hb-O_2 chromophore and a nonspecific heat effect. After anesthetizing the lesion with local anesthetic containing vasoconstrictor, ice is applied to help reduce blood flow, thereby diminishing the capability of a well-vascularized lesion to function as a heat sink. The optical fiber is then activated usually starting at 3 W. Using diascopy technique the lesion is compressed and photocoagulated (Figs. 3–18 and 3–19). After the tip is heated it is brought into contact with the mucosal surface of the lesion (Fig. 3–20). Using only gentle pressure, the fiber is advanced into the substance of the vascular malformation. Care is taken to ensure that the tip does not enter the surrounding normal tissue.

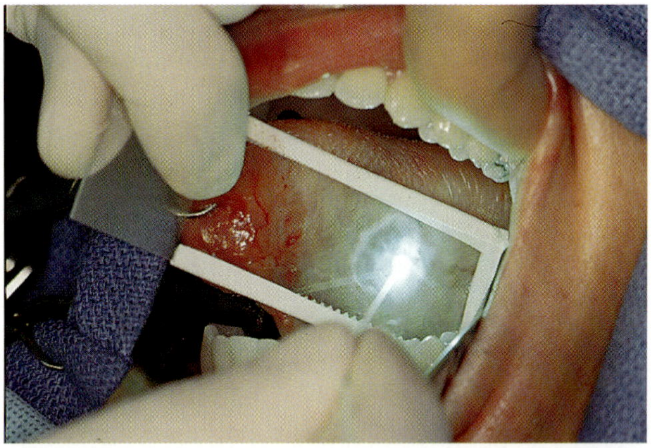

Figure 3–19. Center of lesion "filled in" with argon applied in decreasing concentric circles.

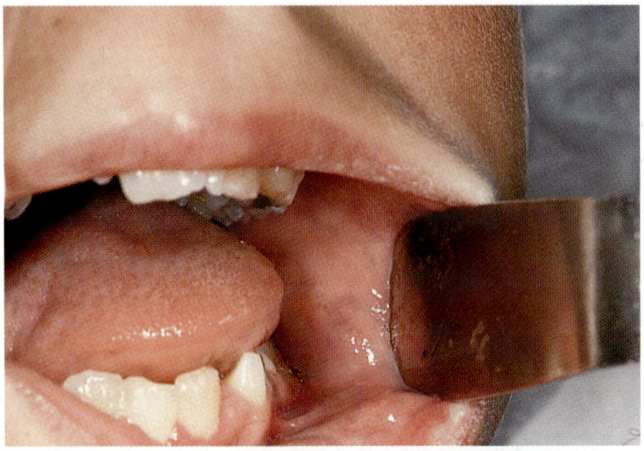

Figure 3–17. Similar case of vascular malformation of buccal mucosa eliminated. Mucosa stable at 18 months recall.

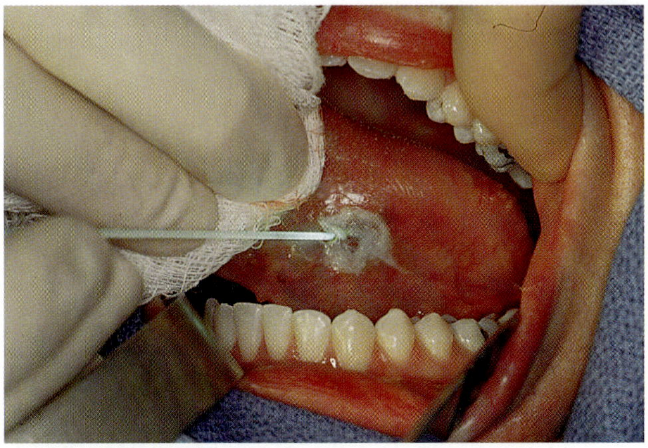

Figure 3–20. For intralesional photocoagulation the fiber tip is introduced into the lesion. First, the laser is activated and then using very gentle finger pressure so that the fiber is introduced "on its own weight," the lesion is entered. Note that entry is almost completely bloodless.

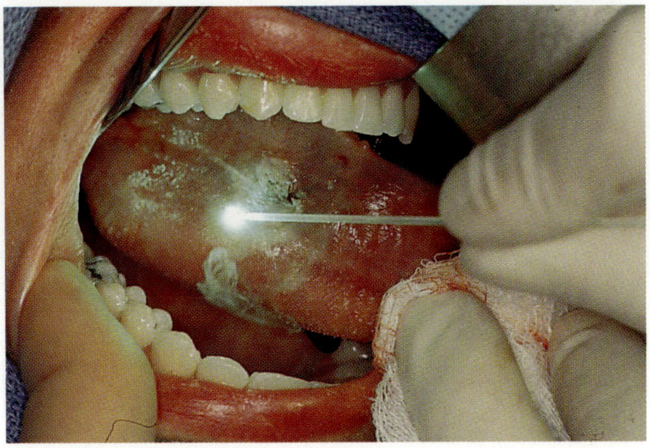

Figure 3–21. With the laser activated the fiber is brought back and forth across the lesion in a series of passes in the same manner as performance of a fine needle aspiration biopsy.

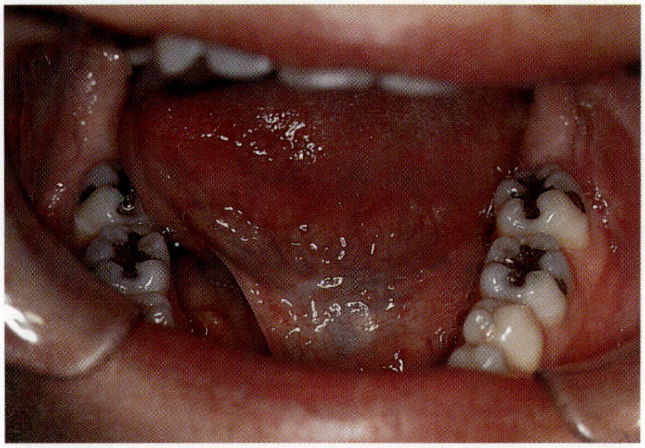

Figure 3–22. Thirty-four days after surgery healing has been complete. There is no vascular malformation present and the tongue has a full range of motion.

With the laser in active mode the fiber tip is advanced to the periphery of the lesion opposite the point of entry and is then withdrawn to a point just deep to the mucosa but still within the lesion. It is then redirected and the same action is repeated. It is the same technique used for fine needle aspiration technique to sample a mass for cytologic assessment (Fig. 3–21). Generally, four to six such passes are required. After the last pass the lesion should have become depressed and there should be little or no venous oozing from the lesion. If gentle pressure is not adequate to control bleeding, another series of ILP passes will be required. The power should be adjusted so that with each pass one hears a gentle crackling sound, indicating that absorption and some heating is occurring. If a second ILP is required, the lesion should be iced for 3 to 5 minutes between ILPs. Postoperatively a nonsteroidal analgesic is given for pain, and the patient is instructed to rinse with dilute warm saline four to six times per day. Moderate edema is expected but the amount of postoperative pain is unpredictable. The patient is recalled in 5 to 7 days for interim reexamination and then at monthly intervals to assess regression. If regression is incomplete or progression occurs at the monthly recalls, then retreatment is suggested. If more than three treatments are required, then another treatment option should be chosen. Patient acceptance is generally quite high and significant improvement is usually seen within two treatment sessions (Fig. 3–22).

ARGON: NONCONTACT

For very small lesions, the handpiece may be used to provide adequate energy to photocoagulate superficial lesions. In the following case of superficial vascular malformations of the lateral tongue border the argon laser was used at a power output of 2.5 W and a spot size of 2.0 mm in continuous wave function (Figs. 3–23 to 3–26).

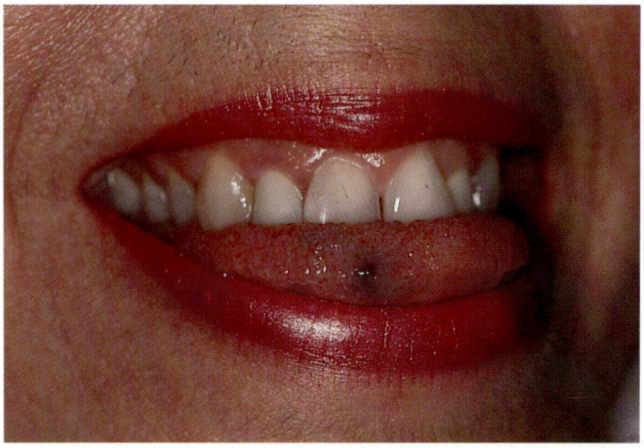

Figure 3–23. Superficial vascular malformation of free border of tongue.

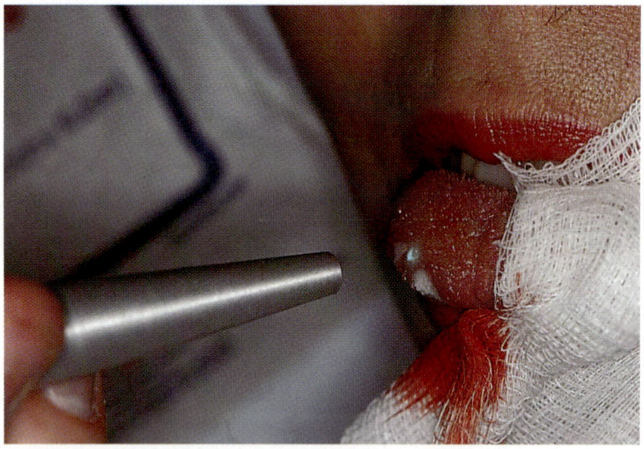

Figure 3–24. Handpiece delivery system; defocused, CW: 2.5 W.

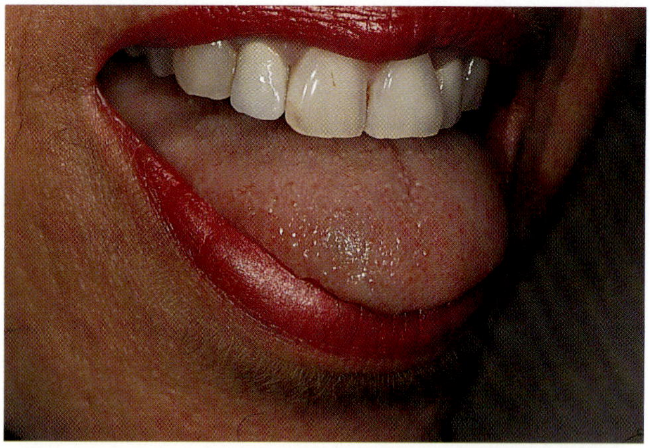

Figure 3–25. Six months postoperative. Full range of motion of tongue.

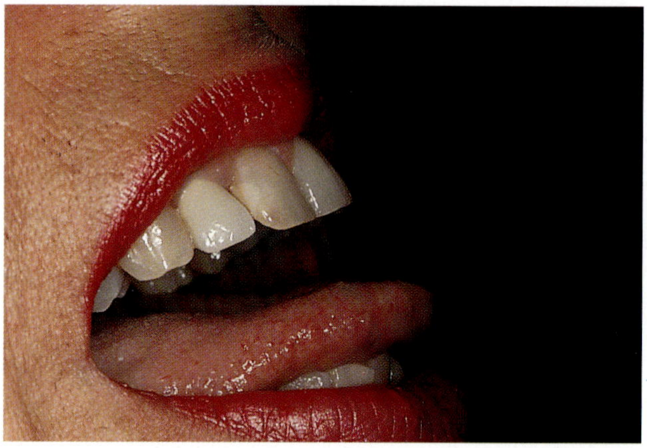

Figure 3–26. No recurrence and no scar.

ARGON: COMPLICATIONS

COMPLICATION 1: INADVERTENT SKIN PENETRATION

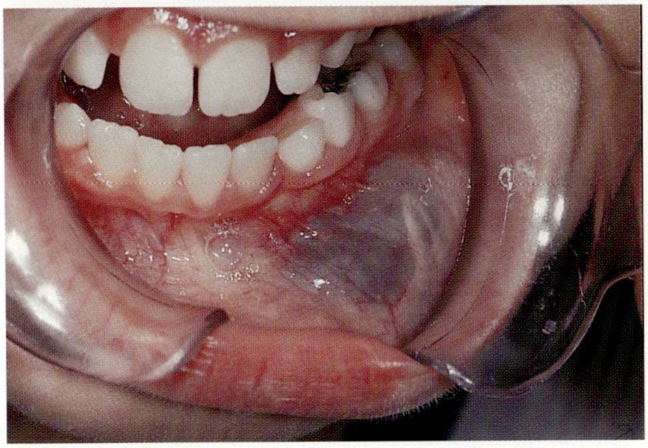

Figure 3–27. Vascular malformation of labiobuccal sulcus.

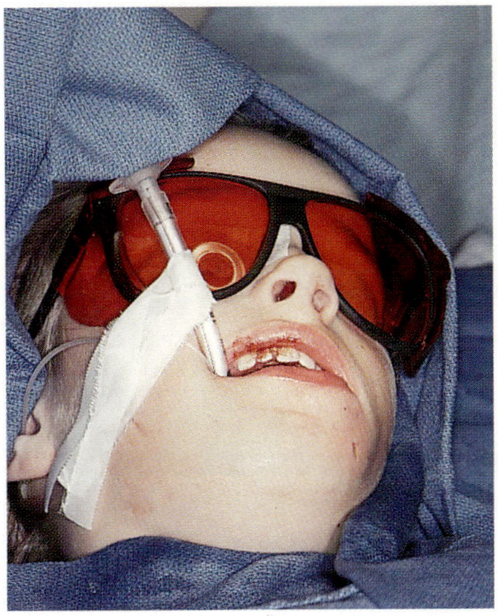

Figure 3–28. Patient properly protected with goggles.

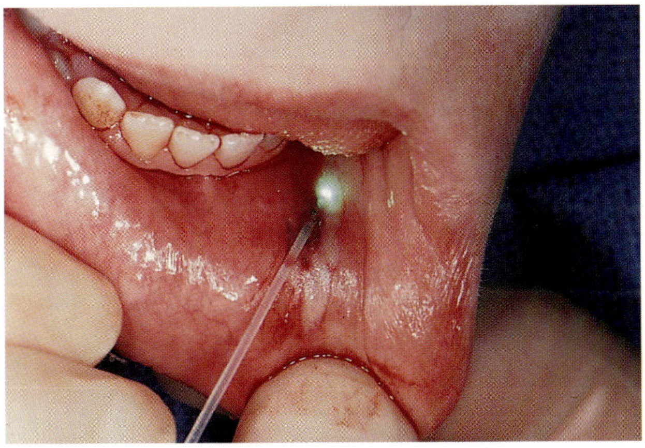

Figure 3–29. Lesion photocoagulated using intralesional photocoagulation.

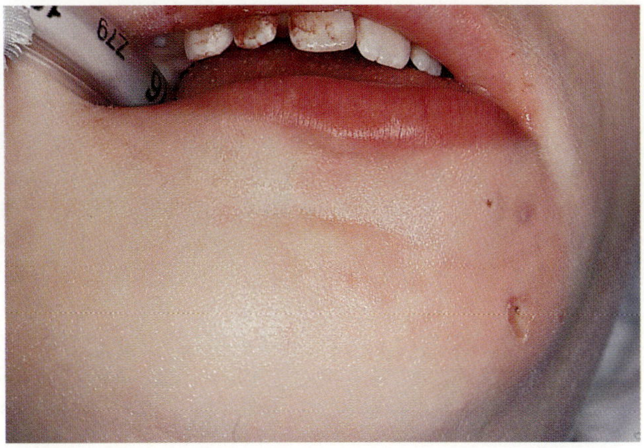

Figure 3–30. Skin damage. Fiber approached skin surface too closely during subcutaneous and submucosal photocoagulation.

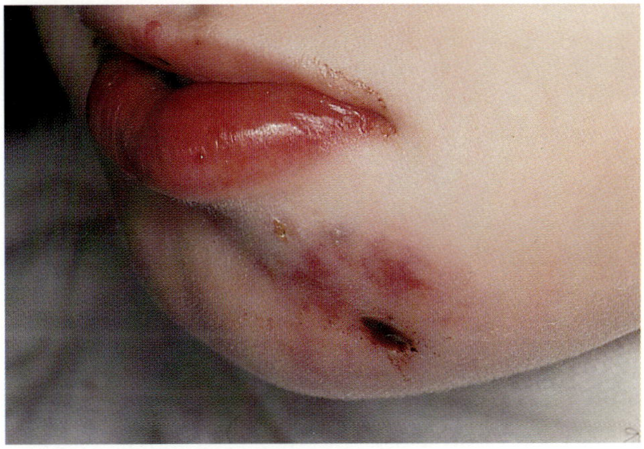

Figure 3–31. First postoperative day. Eschar forming at burn site in skin.

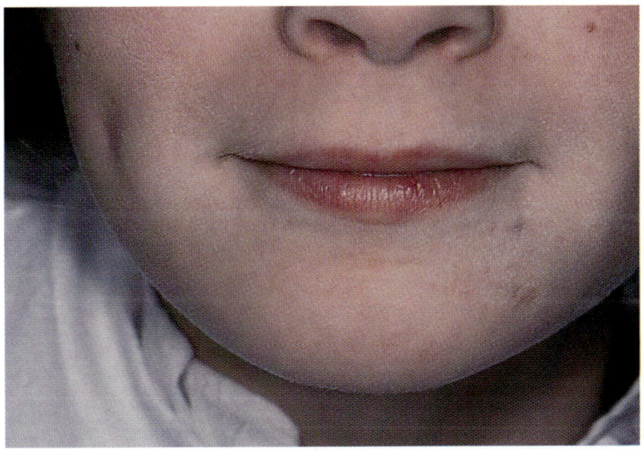

Figure 3–32. Thirteen months: depressed scar present at site of skin injury.

COMPLICATION 2: SCARRING AFTER TREATMENT OF TELANGIECTASIAS

The argon laser has been used to treat superficial telangiectasias of the skin, but because of a high rate of unfavorable scarring postoperatively, flashlamp pumped dye lasers and copper vapor lasers have largely replaced argon for this use.

In this illustrative case facial telangiectasias (Fig. 3–33) occurring along with intraoral hemangiomata in a young girl were treated by direct "tracing" by the argon fiber over the telangiectasia that was compressed by a glass slide (Fig. 3–34). Argon at 2 W CW was used at the focal point of the laser fiber. Application of energy was continued until the lesion blanched (Fig. 3–35). One year later (Fig. 3–36) there was slight skin surface scarring, although the vascularity of the telangiectasia was significantly diminished.

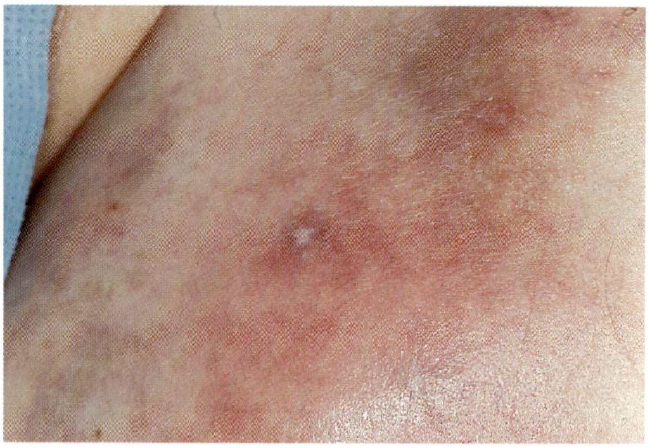

Figure 3–35. Posttreatment: feeding vessels and, especially, central part of telangiectasia has been blanched.

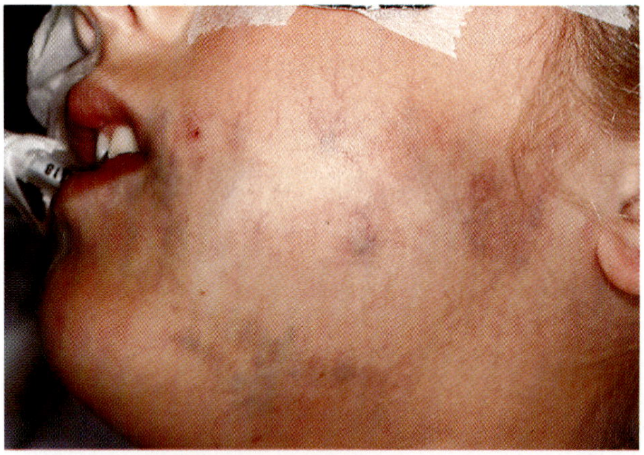

Figure 3–33. Facial telangiectasias.

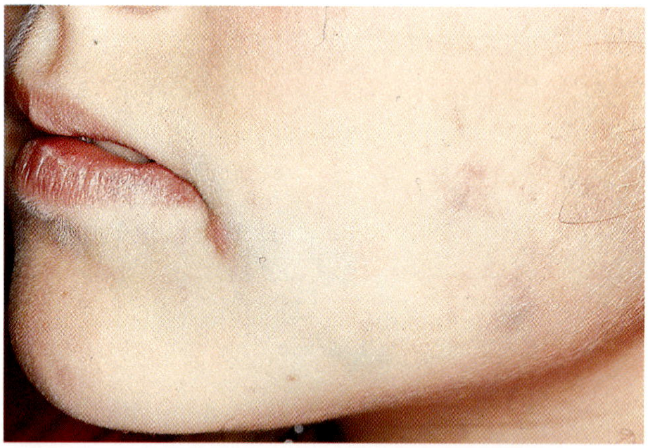

Figure 3–36. One year later, vascularity of the telangiectasia has been greatly reduced but some skin scarring has occurred.

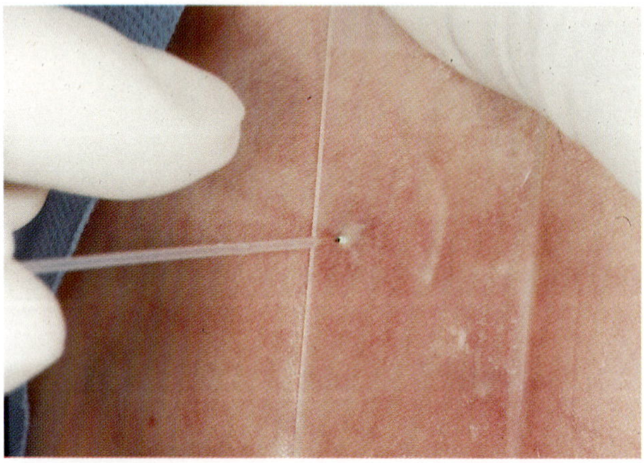

Figure 3–34. Lesion compressed (diascopy) and treated to end point of blanching.

HOLMIUM:YTRIUM-ALUMINUM-GARNETT (HO: YAG)

Holmium:YAG laser, by virtue of its ability to vaporize tissue within a fluid medium, has proven most useful for intra-articular surgery of the temporomandibular joint (TMJ). During arthroscopic surgery of the TMJ this laser is used at low power to make releasing incisions in the retro-discal tissue. At higher power it is capable of resecting fibrocartilage or bone. However, it is rare to require power greater than 10 W. In general, pulse repetition rates (PRR) of less than 10 W are sufficient. Useful characteristics of the Ho:YAG pulsed TMJ laser are listed in Table 3–1.

Table 3–4. Suitable energy levels for the Ho:YAG pulsed TMJ unit

45 WATT MODEL	60 WATT MODEL (0.5–7.0 J; 5–55 Hz; 350 μs)
2.1 μm	2.1 μm
0.5–2.8 J	0.5–2.8 J
250 μs	250 μs
45 W	60 W
2.5 mW at 650 ns up to 11 kW	2.5 mW at 650 ns

Average power—actual use in TMJ arthroscopic surgery:
Aiming Beam—0.6–1.0 J/pulse at 8–12 Hz; Avg P = 6–12 W.
Peak Power—[up to 5 J/pulse: Surgilase Ho:YAG].

ERBIUM:YTRIUM-ALUMINUM-GARNETT (ER:YAG)

The Erbium:YAG laser emits at 2.94nm and because of its shorter wavelength it is a laser of inherently higher energy than CO_2 or Nd:YAG lasers. Not only is it highly absorbed by water, being closer to the highest absorption peak than is CO_2, but it is also moderately well absorbed by hydroxyapatite, which is a major constituent of bone, dentin, and enamel. Consequently Er:YAG has potential suitability for laser-assisted surgery of hard tissues.

Er:YAG

X = 2.91nm
E = 125–625mJ/pulse
PRR = Variable, usually <20Hz
P = <ISW
chromophore: water, hydroxyapatite

REFERENCES

1. Filmar S, Jetha N, McComb P, Gomel V, et al. A comparative histologic study on the healing process after tissue transection. I. Carbon dioxide laser and electromicrosurgery. *Am J Obstet Gynecol* 1989;160(5, part 1):1063–1067.
2. Sako K, Marchetta FC, Hayes RL. Cryotherapy of intraoral leukoplakia. *Am J Surg* 1972;124:482–484.
3. Pospisil OA, MacDonald DG. The tumor potentiating effect of cryosurgery on carcinogen treated hamster cheek pouch. *Br J Oral Surg* 1981;19:96–104.
4. Poswillo DE. Cryosurgery and electrosurgery compared in the treatment of experimentally induced oral carcinomas. *Br Dent J* 1971;131(8):347–352.
5. Guerry TL, Silverman S Jr, Dedo HH. Carbon dioxide laser resection of superficial carcinoma: indications, techniques and results. *Ann Otol Rhinol Laryngol* 1986;95:547–555.
6. Catone G. Laser technology in oral and maxillofacial surgery. Part II: Applications. *Selected Readings Oral Maxillofac Surg* 1994;3(5):1–35.
7. Thomson S. Medical Lasers: How they work and how they affect tissue. *Cancer Bull* 1989;41(4):203–211.
8. Hall RR. The healing of tissues incised by a carbon dioxide laser. *Br J Surg* 1971;58(3):222–225.
9. Jacques SL. Laser tissue interaction. *Cancer Bull* 1989;41(4):211–218.
10. Jansen ED, van Leeuwen TG, Motamedi M, Borst C, Welch AJ. Temperature dependence of the absorption coefficient of water for incident infrared radiation. *Lasers Surg Med* 1994;14:258–268.
11. Polanyi TG. Laser physics: medical applications. *Otolaryngol Clin North Am* 1983;16:753–774.
12. Anderson R, Parrish K. Selective photothermolysis: precise microsurgery by selective absorption of pulsed radiation. *Science* 1983;220:524–527.
13. Beckman H, Barraco R, Sugar S, Gaynes E, Blau R. Laser iridectomies. *Am J Ophthomal* 1971;72(2):393–402.
14. Armon E, Laufer G. The response of living tissue to pulse of a surgical CO_2 laser: transections of the ASME. *J Biomech Eng* 1985;107:286–290.
15. Reid R, Elfont GA, Zirkin RM, Fuller TA. Superficial laser vulvectomy II. The anatomic and biophysical principles permitting accurate control of thermal destruction with carbon dioxide laser. *Am J Obstet Gynecol* 1985;152:261–271.
16. Absten GT. Physics of light and lasers. *Obstet Gynecol Clin North Am* 1991;18(3):407–427.
17. Walsh JT, Flotte TJ, Anderson RR, Deutsch T. Pulsed CO_2 laser tissue ablation: effect of tissue type and pulse duration on thermal damage. *Lasers Surg Med* 1988;8:108–118.
18. Dobry MM, Padilla RS, Pennino RP, Hunt WC. Carbon dioxide laser vaporization: relationship of scar formation to power density. *J Invest Dermatol* 1989;93(1):75–77.
19. Mihashi S, Jako GJ, Incze J, et al. Laser surgery in otolaryngology interactions of CO_2 laser and soft tissue. *Ann NY Acad Sci* 1976;267:263–294.
20. Gabbiani G, Ryan GB, Majno G. Presence of modified fibroblasts in granulation tissue and their possible role in wound contraction. *Experientia* 1971;27(5):549–550.
21. Loumanen M, Lehto V-P, Meurman JH. Myofibroblasts in healing laser wounds of rat tongue mucosa. *Arch Oral Biol* 1988;33(1):17–23.
22. Reid R, Dorsey JH. Physical and surgical principles of carbon dioxide laser surgery in the lower genital tract. In: Coppleson M, Monaghan JM, Morrow CP, Tattersall MHN, eds. *Gynecologic Oncology.* 2nd ed. London: Churchill-Livingstone; 1992:1087–1132.
23. Eriksson RA, Albrektsson T. Temperature threshold levels for heat-induced bone tissue injury: a vital microscopic study in the rabbit. *J Prosthet Dent* 1983;50:101–107.
24. Fuller TA. Laser tissue interaction: the influence of power density. In Baggish M, ed. *Basic and Advanced Laser Surgery and Gynecology.* New York: Appleton-Century-Crofts; 1985.
25. Reid R. Physical and surgical principles governing expertise with the carbon dioxide laser. *Obstet Gynecol Clin North Am* 1987;14:513–535.
26. Gillis TM, Strong MS. Surgical lasers and soft tissue interactions. *Otolaryngol Clin North Am* 1983;16(4):775–784.
27. Kamat BR, Carney JM, Arndt KA, et al. Cutaneous tissue repair following CO_2 laser irradiation. *J Invest Dermatol* 1986;87:268–271.

4 Preneoplasia of the Oral Cavity

Lewis Clayman

Successful treatment of superficial mucosal disease of the oral cavity mandates selective ablation of the abnormal epithelium including the parabasal layer attached to the basement membrane. The carbon dioxide laser does not impart magical properties to the tissues, but it does provide a selective therapeutic advantage for the treatment of intramucosal preneoplasia by avoiding damage to subjacent tissue, thereby eliminating scar formation and the creation of oral deformities.

Preneoplastic lesions of the oral mucosa include leukoplakia, erythroplakia, and oral submucous fibrosis, with 85% of the preneoplasias being accounted for by leukoplakia. The erosive variant of lichen planus has stimulated a great deal of debate in regard to its malignant potential; however, because this proclivity is still uncertain, erosive lichen planus will not be considered, particularly as CO_2 laser treatment of lichen planus does not alter its natural history and is therefore ineffective. High risk of malignant transformation is associated with dysplasia, multicentricity, and anatomic site of the leukoplakias.[1–6] In regard to dysplasia the risk of malignant transformation is related to its presence but not necessarily its grade.[4,7] The most recent World Health Organization (WHO) classification of leukoplakia will now include dysplasia as an indicator of risk of transformation.[8] The areas at highest risk for transformation are the floor of the mouth, buccal mucosa, soft palate/anterior tonsillar pillar, tongue, and lip vermilion.[1,3,9–11] Overall, the transformation rate ranges from 0.13 to 28% with cancer being detected on average 2.5 years after the diagnosis of the index leukoplakia.[12]

Leukoplakias are categorized as *homogeneous* (Fig. 4–1), *nodular* (Fig. 4–2), or *speckled* (Fig. 4–3). The latter occurs on the buccal mucosa adjacent to the oral commissure, which is a particularly notorious site for malignant transformation. Also worrisome are leukoplakias located on the anterior floor of the mouth covering the orifice of Wharton's duct. In this location both dysplasia and invasive carcinoma have the capability of invading directly into the lumen of the salivary ducts.[13] Different varieties of leukoplakia may also occur simultaneously in the same patient (Fig. 4–4).

The snuff dipper's lesion is usually homogeneous but may include areas of nodularity. Most commonly it is found on the area of mucosa with which the smokeless tobacco product is placed in contact. The buccal mucosa and the mandibular labiobuccal vestibule are the areas most likely to be affected (Fig. 4–5).

Erythroplakias are erythematous, are often severely dysplastic, and may include microinvasive cancer at the time of detection. Dysplasias are sharply demarcated from adjacent zones of normal mucosa and they tend to be velvety in appearance. When the oral mucosal surface is dried with a gauze sponge, the alteration in the reflective surface of the oral mucosa becomes readily apparent (Fig. 4–6).

The clinical diagnosis of the subset of lesions at high risk, the dysplastic leukoplakia, is facilitated by the application of a vital dye to the mucosal surface. The principle is similar to that supporting the use of vital staining of the uterine cervix as a method for detecting an abnormal transformation zone in cervical intraepithelial neoplasia (CIN), which is the gynecologic equivalent of leukoplakia with severe dysplasia or erythroplakia.

VITAL STAINING[14]

Toluidine blue (TN), a metachromatic vital dye, selectively stains cytoplasmic sulfated mucopolysaccharides and nuclear DNA and RNA in rapidly dividing cells. Because it is the transformed (premalignant or malignant) epithelial cell that has escaped regulation by feedback inhibition of its replication, possibly by alteration of one or more tumor suppressor genes, this rapidly dividing cell, which accepts the stain, is an abnormal cell. The specificity of vital staining with 1% toluidine blue dye ranges from 87 to 100%, and the sensitivity ranges from 96 to 100%.[15–17] False-positive rates are usually reported as being approximately 2.0% and false-negatives as 2.5%. The basic technique for vital staining requires removal of saliva from the area to be examined by washing with saline or dilute (3%) acetic acid followed by drying of the suspicious mucosa with a gauze sponge (Fig. 4–7). The TN is applied with cotton-tipped applicators and is allowed to remain in situ for 60 seconds (Fig. 4–8). The area is now rinsed with acetic acid followed by a water rinse (Fig. 4–9). Any remaining blue stain is subjectively ranked as being mildly (Fig. 4–9), moderately (Fig. 4–10), or strongly (Fig. 4–11) positive. The examiner is now guided directly to the site of most heavy staining as being representative of the "worst" area of the lesion. In this way, a directed (by the stain) biopsy of the lesion is

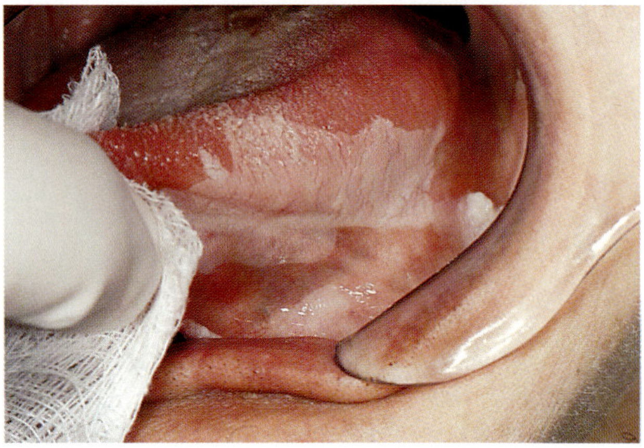

Figure 4–1. Homogeneous leukoplakia of the ventral tongue and floor of mouth.

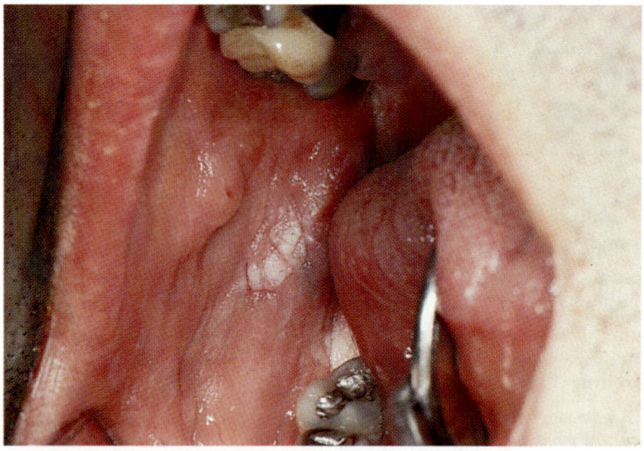

Figure 4–2. Nodular luekoplakia of the buccal mucosa.

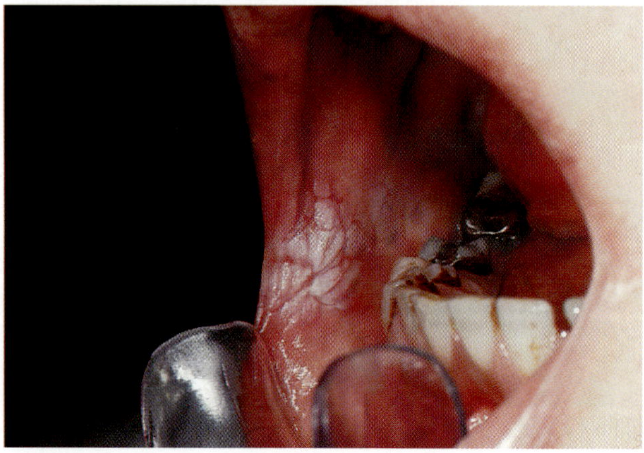

Figure 4–3. Speckled leukoplakia occurring at its most common location, the oral commissure. This is frequently accompanied by colonization with *Candida albicans.*

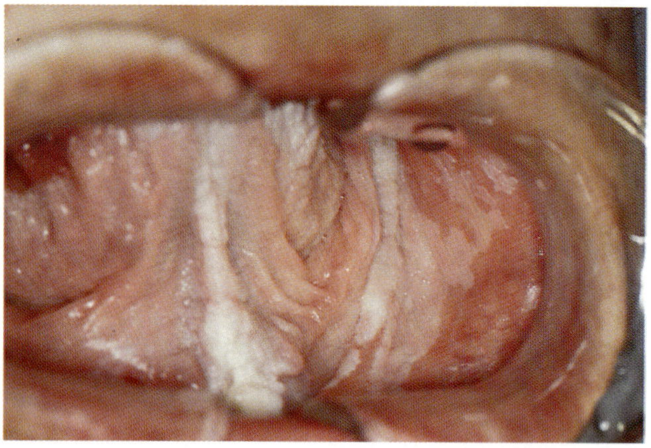

Figure 4–4. Multicentricity. Simultaneous occurrence of leukoplakia on the floor of mouth, ventral tongue and mandibular alveolar ridge. This patient also had leukoplakia of the hard and soft palate, maxillary alveolar ridge, and buccal mucosa.

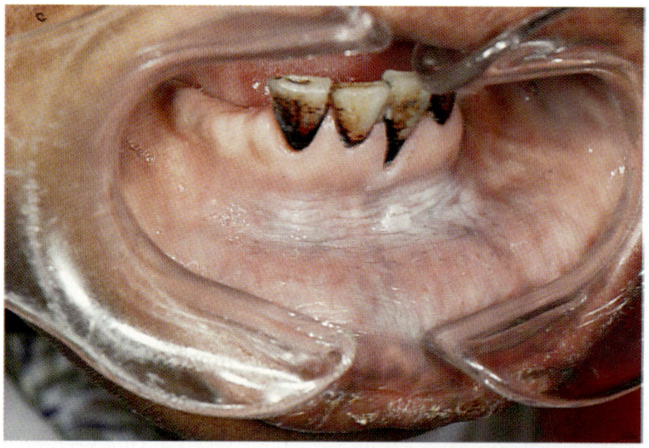

Figure 4–5. Typical snuff dippers leukoplakia at site of application of the tobacco product. Note staining of the teeth, which is also typical. In Scandinavia, these lesions rarely, if ever, progress to cancer, but in the United States, where snuff is formulated differently, they frequently do become malignant after a very long latency period.

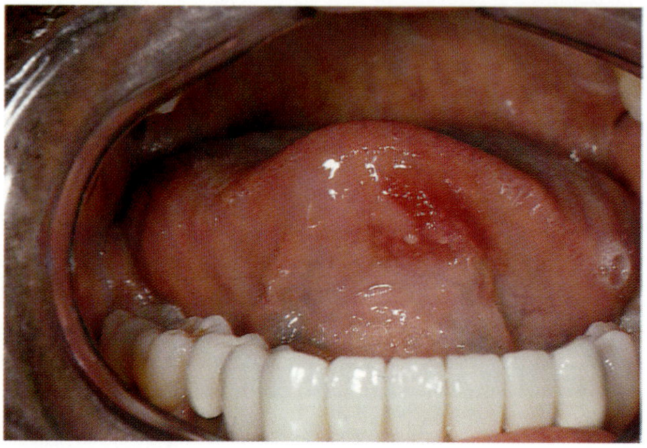

Figure 4–6. Erythroplakia of the ventral tongue. The lesion is red, slightly raised and sharply demarcated from surrounding normal mucosa.

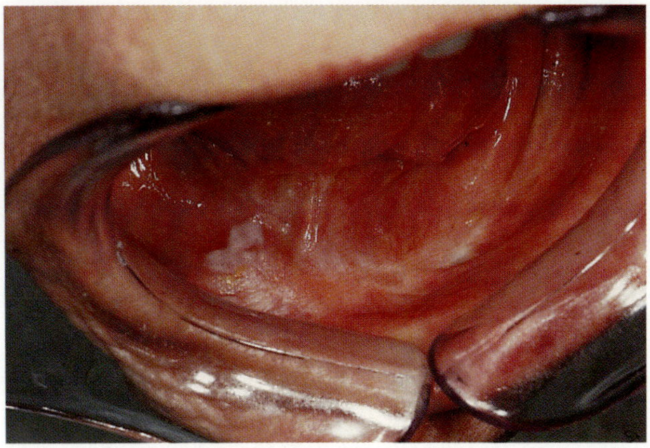

Figure 4–7. A new oral cancer of the alveolar ridge–buccal mucosa arising in a field of dysplasia 41 months after removal of a primary tumor at the same site.

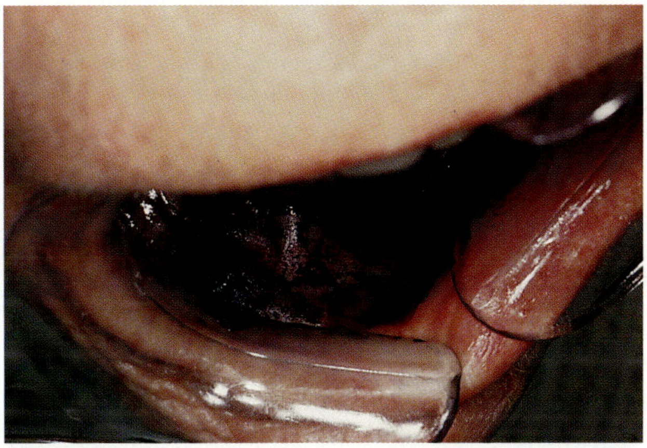

Figure 4–8. After application of 1% toluidine blue, there is dense staining of the cancer as well as the peripheral tissue.

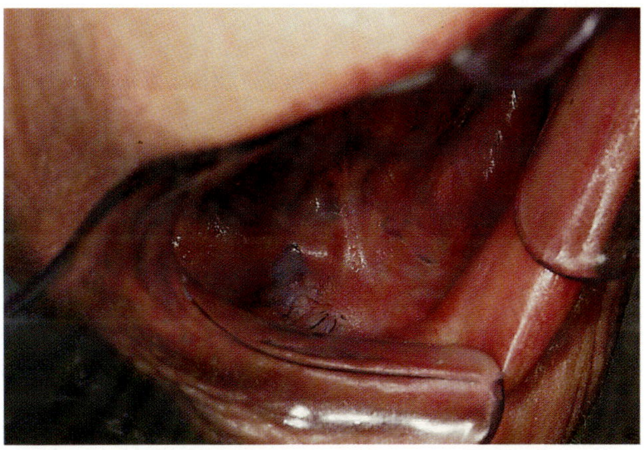

Figure 4–9. After washing with saline, the residual blue stain demarcates the area at the periphery of the lesion, which is most likely to contain areas of dysplasia. This is a mildly positive stain.

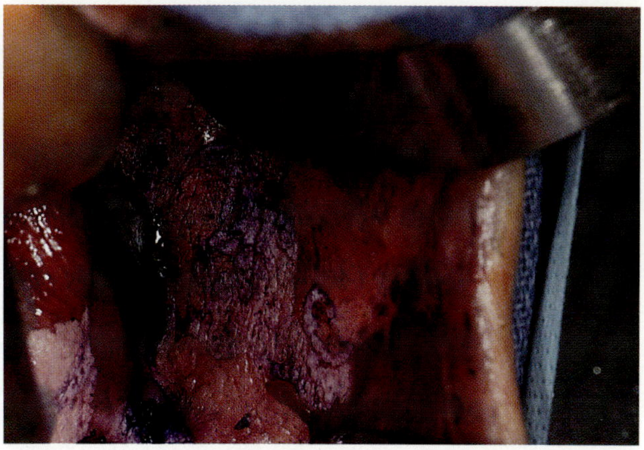

Figure 4–10. Moderately positive stain with toluidine blue: buccal mucosa, retromolar pad, and anterior tonsillar pillar.

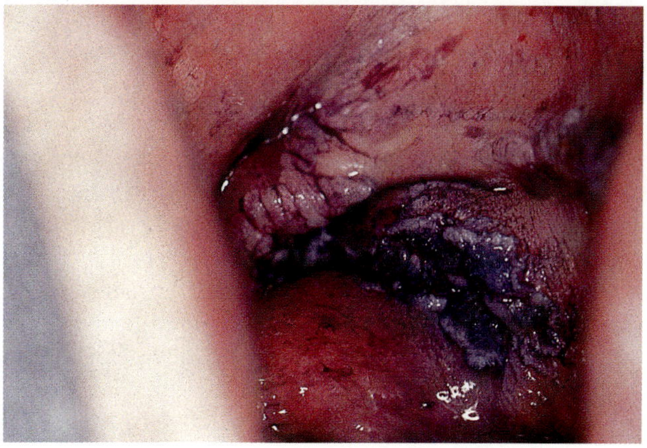

Figure 4–11. Strongly positive stain with toluidine blue.

performed, subsequent to which a definitive treatment plan is formulated. Because oral precancer and cancer is frequently multicentric, it is wisest to stain in this way all of the high-risk mucosa of the tongue, floor of mouth, soft palate–retromolar pad area, and the buccal mucosa. Staining of the more posterior area of the mouth may be carried out at the time of planned surgery of the index lesion, when the patient is sedated or anesthetized.

SURGICAL TREATMENT: CO_2 LASER

Conventional surgical treatment, which consists of excision with a scalpel, is successful and adequate for limited local disease. The literature reports control rates of around 90%.[6,18,19] Failure becomes likely when this local treatment is applied to extensive disease. Because the multicentric nature of precancer (the condemned mucosa concept) manifests itself as multifocal disease by occurring at multiple sites in the oral cavity and oropharynx, a more global treatment concept than local excision is required. Failure rates following local surgical excision are as high as 33%.[4] Multicentricity demands excision of topographically large areas of mucosa. However, the denudation of large areas of oral mucosae results in scarring and wound contraction as well as postoperative pain, edema, and nutritional depletion. Despite the greatest care, the minimum thickness of tissue removed with a scalpel results in exposure and removal of the submucosa. Both scarring and incomplete epithelial regeneration occur. The traditional solution to this problem is to replace the mucosa with a split-thickness skin graft. This, however, is an unsatisfactory solution because skin does not function as well as mucosa. The graft ultimately contracts as time passes, and the grafted skin covers remaining elements of regenerated mucosa that may be unstable. Lastly, even for local treatment, site-specific consequences may dictate against locally invasive surgery that induces scarring. For example, removal of the thinnest layer of mucosa over the opening of Wharton's or Stensen's duct may cause scarring, glandular obstruction, and infection. Excision of large lesions at the oral commissure causes deformity of the oral stoma.

The advantage of replacing traditional excisional techniques with CO_2 laser photoablation is that the laser permits removal of the damaged epithelium with as little as 0.1 to 0.2 mm of reversible thermal injury to the submucosa. Precise control of thermal damage makes it possible to remove even the epithelium directly over the salivary duct orifices without inducing sialodochitis and glandular obstruction (Figs. 4–12 and 4–13). Extensive areas of mucosa may be ablated without skin grafting because epithelium is regenerated from normal tissue at the wound periphery in no more than 5 weeks for lesions as large as 40 cm^2. After healing, the mucosa at risk is still observable by direct visual inspection during recall examination. Of equal importance, there is little postoperative swelling and patients may take oral fluids immediately after surgery. These patients may be operated upon as outpatients, and there is usually no bleeding or swelling. Pain, which is highly variable, is easily managed with oral analgesics, rarely lasts more than a few days, and only occasionally shows a secondary increase in intensity on days 3 to 5, which then abruptly terminates.[19–21]

The CO_2 laser beam itself is delivered either by a handpiece (Chapter 3, Fig. 3–1) or a microscope (Chapter 3, Fig. 3–2) delivery system. The power density is controlled by enlarging the spot size (defocusing the beam) either by direct observation of the coaxial red helium-neon (HeNe) laser aiming beam or by direct observation of the tissue effect. An estimation of the laser effect is gauged by a pretest in which a wooden tongue blade is exposed to individual pulses from the laser and then the spot size is directly measured (Fig. 4–14). In this way, the spot size, power, and application time for each of the pulses to be used during surgery are "calibrated" on a wooden tongue blade. The power density is approximately equal to the exit power of the laser (generally 15 to 40 W), divided by the square of the spot size (in cm^2). Using this rough approximation, one can achieve a power density of 500 to 1250 W/cm^2 for ablation by evaporative vaporization (ablative vaporization). Modes of application include continuous wave (CW) or variations of a pulsed mode. These latter may be gated or "chopped" CW or, preferably, rapid superpulsed (RSP) (Fig. 4–15). For ablation, RSP is most desirable because the

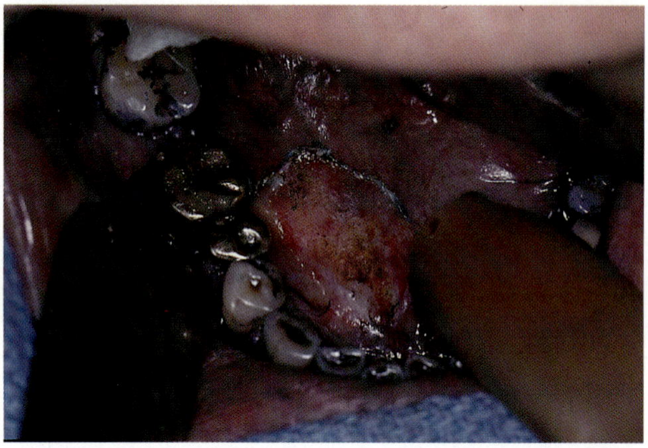

Figure 4–13. Vaporization of tissue over duct without damaging duct. No sclerosis or submandibular gland obstruction occurred postoperatively.

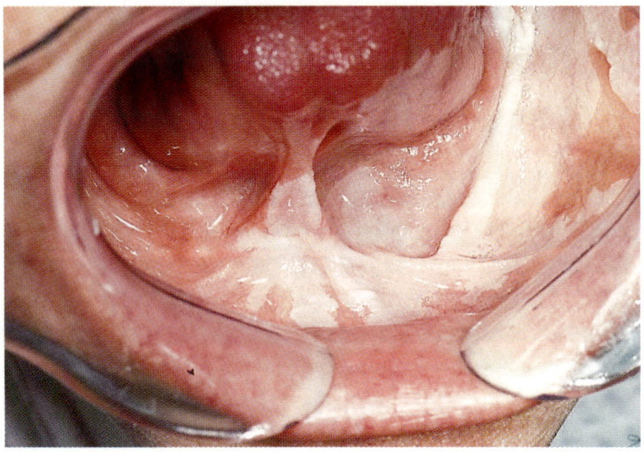

Figure 4–12. Lesion over duct.

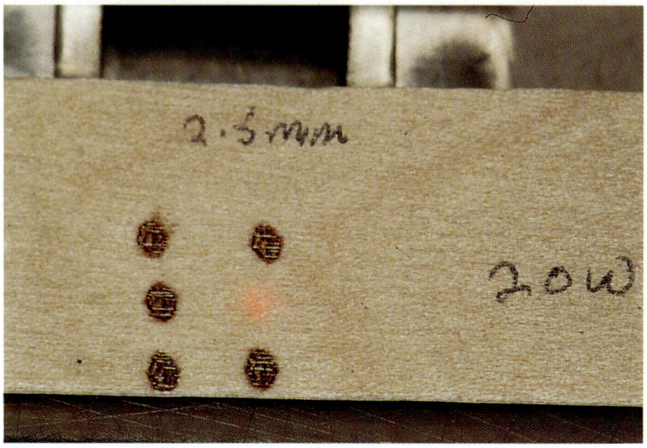

Figure 4–14. Tongue blade: spot size.

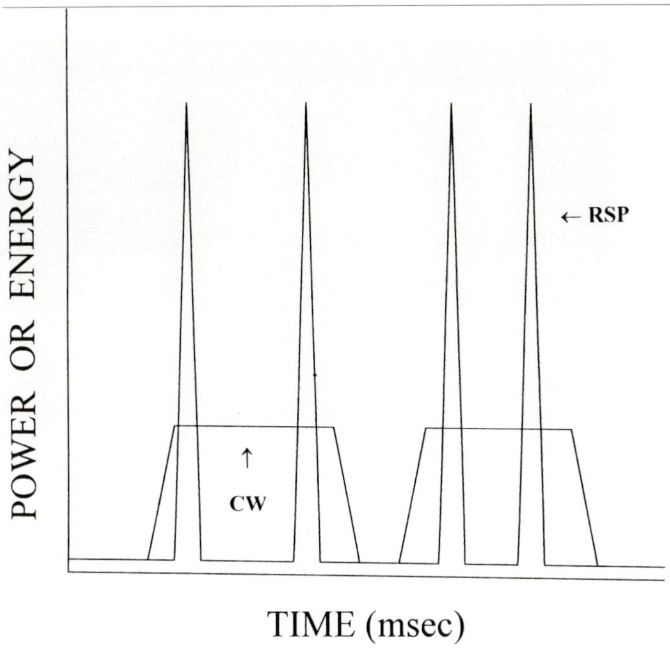

Figure 4–15. CW (chopped or gated) and RSP profiles. (Courtesy of Lara Clayman.)

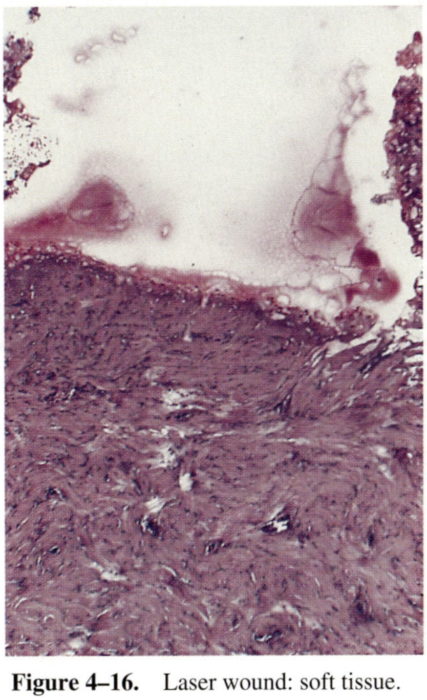

Figure 4–16. Laser wound: soft tissue.

pulse width may be designed to be as brief as 250 to 950 μs, which is shorter than the thermal relaxation time of oral soft tissues. At these power densities of 500 to 1250 W/cm^2, and using the pulsed mode at 50 to 250 pps, with a peak pulse power of 500 to 1000 W per pulse, in the range of 120 to 600 mJ/pulse the fluence actually applied to the target tissues is adequate to ablate them while limiting thermal injury to the subjacent normal tissue to less than 200 μm. As the pulse width lengthens beyond 1 msec, thereby exceeding the thermal relaxation time of the target tissue, the region of lateral thermal damage exceeds 200 μm.

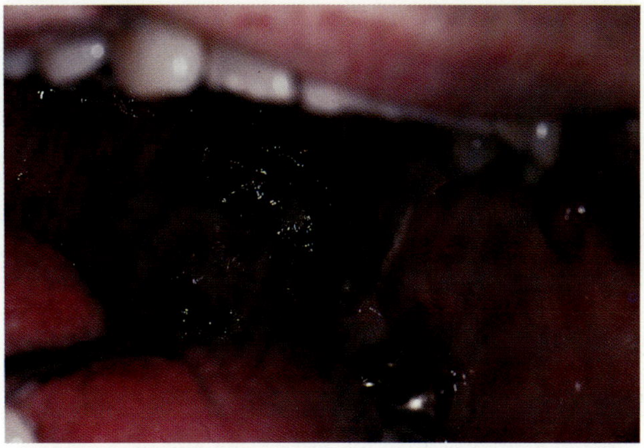

Figure 4–17. Fibrin coagulum day 1.

From the viewpoint of the microscopist, the laser wound (Fig. 4–16) has the following characteristics.[7,12,18,22] The superficial epithelium is homogeneously carbonized. Interspersed in the zone of thermal damage are "boiled away vesicles."[2] The deeper layers of epithelial cells show intercellular voids as a sign of thermal damage.[4] Denatured protein is found in the form of a coagulum near the wound surface.[23] However, there is minimal damage to adjacent tissue across an area of potentially reversible thermal injury of 150 to 300 μm. The amount of collagen found in the wound is diminished and epithelial regeneration is somewhat delayed and irregular.[20] However, during healing there is minimal inflammatory response, and compared with scalpel or cautery wounds, there are fewer myofibroblasts and very little wound contraction.[18,24,25] In vivo, reepithelialization occurs within 4 to 6 weeks, but may be as brief as 2 weeks in cases having ablation of less than 2 cm^2 of mucosa. During the entire healing process, tissues remain soft and pliable.

Not only are small blood vessels and lymphatics sealed by the laser, but nerve endings are "rounded off." This latter may account for some of the diminution in postoperative pain anecdotally reported, but this is not uniformly consistent. A fibrin coagulum forms in the first 24 hours (Fig. 4–17), which is slowly replaced without the occurrence of significant wound contraction.

SURGICAL TECHNIQUE

The oral mucosa is assessed and the requisite biopsies are obtained in the manner previously described. At the time of laser surgery, the vital staining is repeated. Local anesthesia is used unless the patient receives a general anesthetic. No pre- or perioperative antibiotics are given and no antiseptic preparation solution is used for the mouth. The face is protected with wet surgical drapes and the eyes are covered. If endotracheal intubation is utilized, the hypopharynx is packed with a wet gauze.

After identifying the extent of the pathology, the laser is set at an average power of 20 to 30 W for pulsed modes, and 15 to 20 W for CW mode. The spot size will vary between 2 and 3 mm in diameter. The clinical end point for ablation of the mucosa is to cause a "rapid bubbling of the epithelium which is opalescent in color and is accompanied by a crackling noise."[21] The lesion (Fig. 4–18) is outlined with a suitable margin of several millimeters and then parallel lines of application of the laser are placed within the marginal outline (Fig. 4–19). This is called rastering. After completion of this first layer of lasing, there should be almost no carbonization. If the wound appears blackened, there has been excessive heat conduction because of prolonged contact between the laser beam and the tissue as a result of excessively slow hand speed in moving the handpiece or microscope joystick-directed laser beam across the lesion. The more heat conducted, the greater the desiccation occurring at surgery.

A moist gauze is now used to wipe away the treated area of mucosa. This allows one to assess the depth of penetration of the laser. A pale pink base that does not bleed indicates removal of the epithelium at the level of the basement membrane (Fig. 4–20). If there are scattered droplets of blood, then the superficial aspect of the submucosal plane has been breached. If the depth of penetration is too superficial, a second raster is applied to reach the required depth, which results in removal of the entire thickness of the epithelium (Figs. 4–21 and 4–22). In areas of thick hyperplasia as for nicotine stomatitis or fibroepithelial hyperplasia of the palate (see Chapter 6), several layers of rastering may be required. The submucosal layer is identified both by the appearance of blood vessels and by the appearance of tissue of granular appearance and yellow color. At the conclusion of surgery the abnormal tissue has been removed and there should be no bleeding except where it was necessary to extend tissue removal into the submucosa, as may be required in this case of papillary hyperplasia of the palate where four rasters are needed for complete tissue removal. The fibrin coagulum that formed within the first 24 hours is still present at one week (Fig. 4–23). Complete mucosal reepithelialization and healing has occurred within 5 weeks (Fig. 4–24).

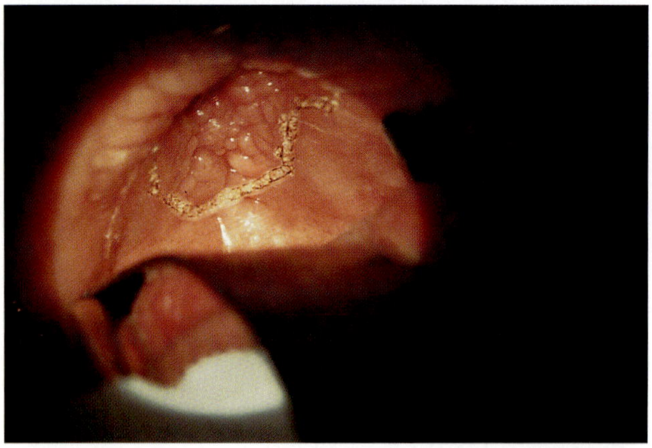

Figure 4–19. Outline of lesion with RSP, CO_2 laser.

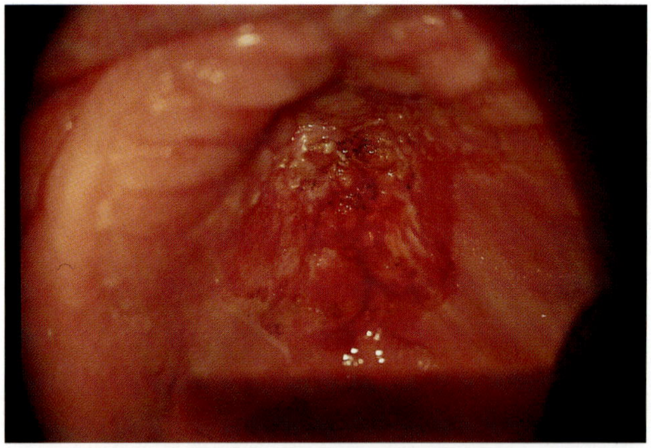

Figure 4–20. First layer of treated tissue wiped away with a moistened gauze sponge (16×).

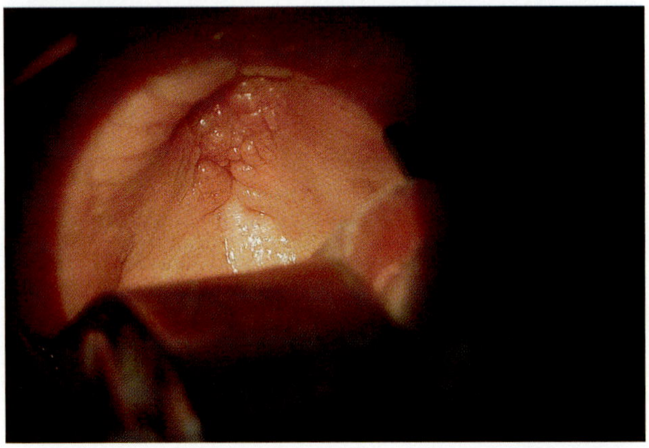

Figure 4–18. Lesion: papillary hyperplasia of the palate (10×).

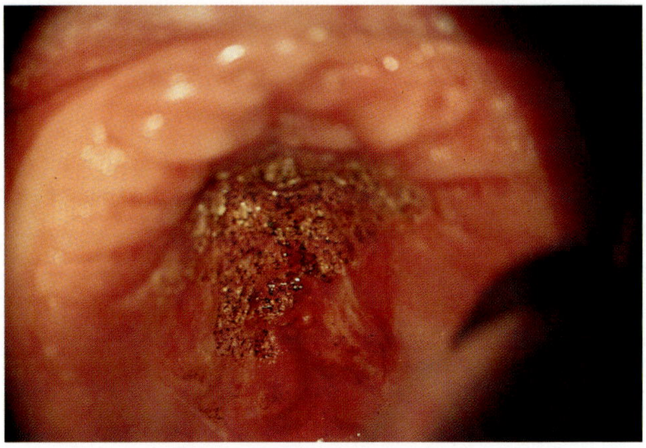

Figure 4–21. Second raster (16×).

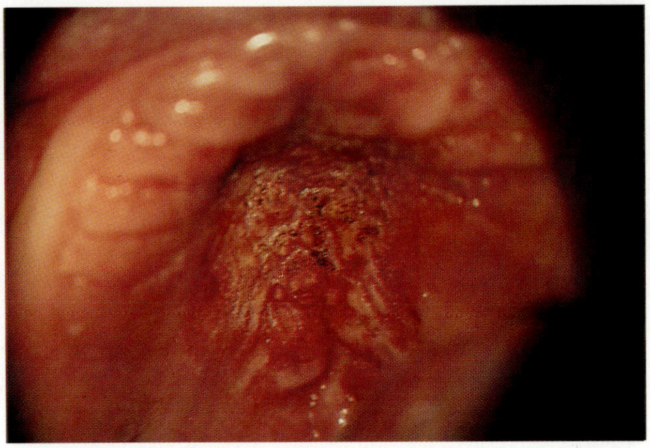

Figure 4–22. Residual lesion after wiping away tissue treated by second raster (16×).

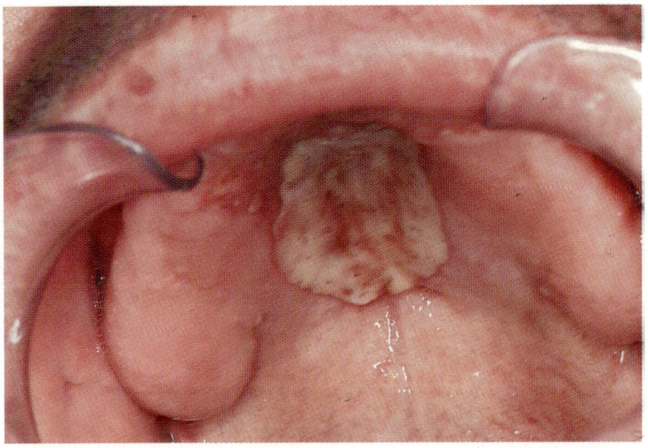

Figure 4–23. Fibrin coagulum still present after one week. Reepithelialization commencing from wound periphery.

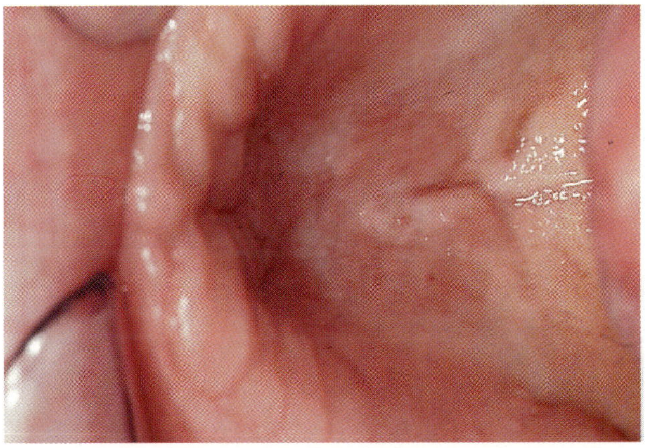

Figure 4–24. Reepithelialization complete after 5 weeks. Condition remained stable for the next 28 months when the patient was lost to recall examination.

HEALING

Epithelial resurfacing is rapid. A fibrinous coagulum forms within the first 24 hours, which is progressively replaced by epithelium originating from the wound edge. Ablation of less than 2.0 cm^2 of mucosa uniformly results in complete epithelial resurfacing in less than 3 weeks. Larger mucosal ablations (5.0 cm^2 or more) require between 4 and 5 weeks. However, in one patient, even an extensive insult of more than 60 cm^2 still required only 6 weeks for complete resurfacing. The major cause for delayed healing is from the creation of charring (carbonization) of the tissue. This occurs as a function of time of contact of the laser beam with the target tissue. Repeated application of the laser without removing the char from the previous exposure will dramatically increase heat transfer to the nontarget tissue. This will retard healing. Postoperative complications potentially include bleeding, infection and damage to teeth, lips, etc., or ignition of the endotracheal tube by laser "mishaps." In the treatment of 148 leukoplakias by ablation technique in the series from Sinai Hospital of Detroit, there were three cases of inadvertent single pulse laser hits to teeth (1) and lip (2). There were no serious complications.

RESULTS

Reports from the literature on the subject of recurrence after laser ablation of leukoplakia (dysplasia not specified), range from 4.5 to 22% at 3-year follow-up to 10 to 22% at 37- to 55-month follow-up.[2,5,15,18,26] Series with less than 2-year follow-up[26] may report spectacular results of lack of recurrence; however, this attenuates with time. Therefore, these patients require long-term surveillance, particularly if they continue to smoke and drink. There are no reports in the literature that laser treatment enhances malignant transformation of oral preneoplasia. One report reported recurrence in five of seven cases of leukoplakia,[27] a frequency that is not substantiated by reports of series with significant numbers of cases.[2,14,18,19,26,27]

LEUKOPLAKIA

The most important subset of oral preneoplasia (precancer) is *leukoplakia,* a clinical term describing a white lesion of the oral cavity that cannot be removed by wiping the mucosa with a gauze sponge, and to which no other specific diagnostic category may be assigned. Histologically leukoplakias may range from simple hyperkeratosis to intramucosal dysplasia or neoplasia. The ideal treatment is by free-beam CO_2 laser because ablation will completely remove the lesion. Furthermore, the mucosa will almost always reepithelialize in less than 4 to 6 weeks, with no scarring. There is no reduction of oral opening and the oral mucosa remains soft, moist, and pliable. This is particularly important because leukoplakia may affect many different locations within the oral cavity, may well recur, and may ultimately affect a large surface area of mucosa. Therefore, it is a great advantage to have the mucosa return to an undamaged state because retreatment may be necessary.

Although a recurrence rate of zero was reported from Semmelweis University in Budapest for a selected group of 126 patients with leukoplakias treated by ablative vaporization at 10 to 15 W [power density (PD) not specified] or by excision at 20 to 25 W (PD not specified), clinical follow-up had been quite brief, at only 16 to 28 months. This suggests that there is certainly no enhancement of malignant transformation by laser treatment during the early postoperative observation period. However, one must be mindful of the fact that most of the recurrences, which also may include progression to carcinoma, won't appear for about 30 months after identification of the index leukoplakia.[6]

My own series of 114 mucosal precancers occurring in 70 patients included 41 simple leukoplakias and 73 dysplasias that were treated by laser vaporization and followed for a minimum of 2 years to a maximum of 8 years. Of the dysplasias, 68% were located in the most dangerous sites for malignant transformation: floor of mouth, tongue, soft palate, anterior tonsillar pillar, and retromolar pad. This series is very heavily skewed toward high-risk leukoplakias, with 64% of all the index leukoplakias being dysplastic. Seventeen lesions in 70 patients escaped control after laser treatment, with eight relapsing as leukoplakias and nine transforming into cancer. Therefore, the overall failure rate (relapse, progression, or development of new lesions) during the 8-year period was 24.2% of which 12.9% (9/70) developed cancer and 11.3% relapsed as leukoplakias. Of the cancer occurrences, eight of the nine (88.9%) arose from areas of previous dysplasias. From the point of view of the individual lesions rather than patients, the failure rate was only 9.6% (11/114) during the first 6 years of observation, which compares favorably with laser success rates of 10 to 22% reported in the literature[5,18] after 37 to 55 months' surveillance.

Horch et al.[2] had a 22 to 28% recurrence rate for lesions treated by ablation with a handpiece. Roodenburg et al.[19] followed 70 patients with 103 leukoplakias, 33 of which were dysplastic and therefore probably at higher risk for recurrence or malignant transformation. Laser ablation was carried out using the microscopic technique at 10 to 15 W output (PD unspecified but probably approximately 375 w/cm^2). A recurrence rate of only 10% in 103 leukoplakias observed from 7 to 55 months after ablation was reported. There was no degeneration of any case into cancer and recurrence could not be correlated with degree of dysplasia.

Postoperatively, in all series listed above (over 700 patients) reepithelialization occurred within 3 weeks for all lesions smaller than 2 cm^2 and within 5 weeks for larger lesions. There was no scarring and no postoperative swelling, although soreness occasionally interfered with food intake. About one third of patients required analgesics for the first 24 hours after surgery, and only the rare patient required analgesics after day 5.[26] However, there was an unpredictable subset of patients that required no analgesics immediately after surgery, but that later required two or three days' use of analgesics, generally between days 3 and 5. Narcotics are rarely required, with nonsteroidal analgesics being the drug of choice. All patients were treated as outpatients, using local or general anesthesia or intravenous sedation, as dictated by site and extent of lesions, by patient emotional needs, and by the need to use the microscope.

Five case reports demonstrate the technique.

CASE 1: LIP LEUKOPLAKIA WITH DYSPLASIA

A 59-year-old white man with a leukoplakia containing areas of dysplasia of the lower lip was referred for removal of his lesion (Fig. 4–25). Vital staining with TN (Fig. 4–26) resulted in a mildly positive stain. The handpiece delivery system (Fig. 4–27) was chosen using a spot size of 2.5 mm (1.8-mm vaporization spot), 92 PPS superpulsed mode, PD = 617 W/cm^2, 216 mJ/pulse, P = 20 W, superpulsed by the 125-mm handpiece, TEM_{00} (transverse electromagnetic mode). Note the guide tip extension of the handpiece, which indicates that the laser is at its focal point at the tip of the handpiece. Moving the tip away from the target tissue results in reduction of the power density. The initial raster (Fig. 4–28) results in crackling and bubbling of the epithelium with slight brown discoloration of the treated mucosa. After wiping away the treated mucosa (Fig. 4–29) one may judge the thickness of tissue removal by observing the border of the untreated mucosa. The slightly yellow color of the base of the treated area indicates that tissue removal has included the basement membrane.

Any residual area requiring biopsy for assessment may be excised with the scalpel (Fig. 4–30) and bleeding from the base of the biopsy site may be controlled with the laser. A biopsy from an area of laser treatment at a magnification of 100× (Fig. 4–31) demonstrates that heat artifact is restricted to a thickness of approximately 0.21 mm. Note that the epithelium has been completely removed as was desired. At the conclusion of surgery, wiping away the treated mucosa (Fig. 4–32) demonstrates a clear demarcation between the normal epithelial border and the de-epithelialized treatment region. The dark brown area on the left of the illustration shows the discoloration secondary to the heat effect from application of the laser to control bleeding at the base of the area excised by the scalpel. At 13 days postoperative (Fig. 4–33) fibrin is present covering the wound surface and there are some signs of reepithelialization occurring. By 22 days (Fig. 4–34) healing is about 50% complete and by one month (Fig. 4–35) reepithelialization has been completed and maturation is occurring. At 5 months the lip looks normal (Fig. 4–36).

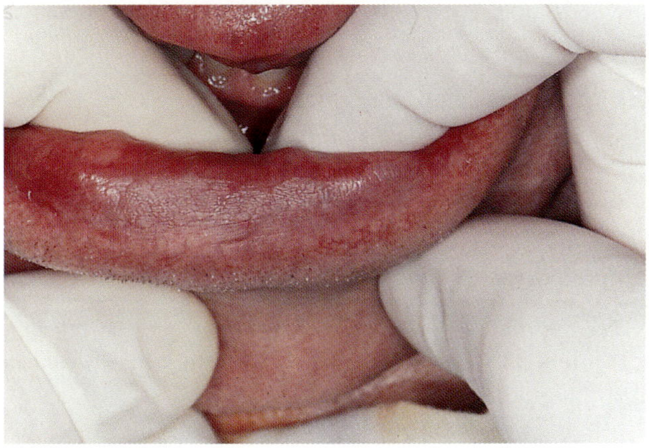

Figure 4–25. Dysplastic leukoplakia of lower lip.

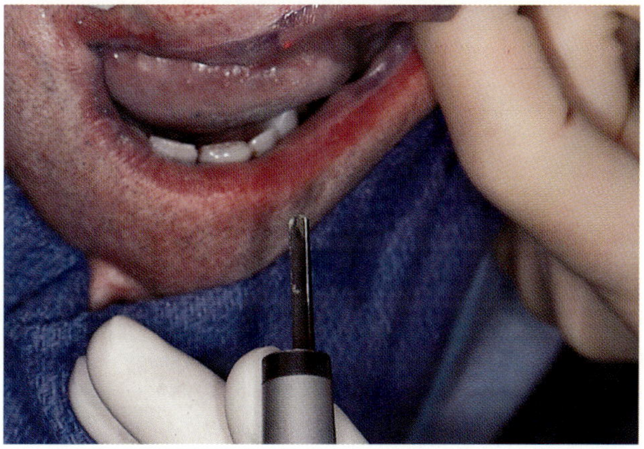

Figure 4–27. Laser handpiece in position to start treatment.

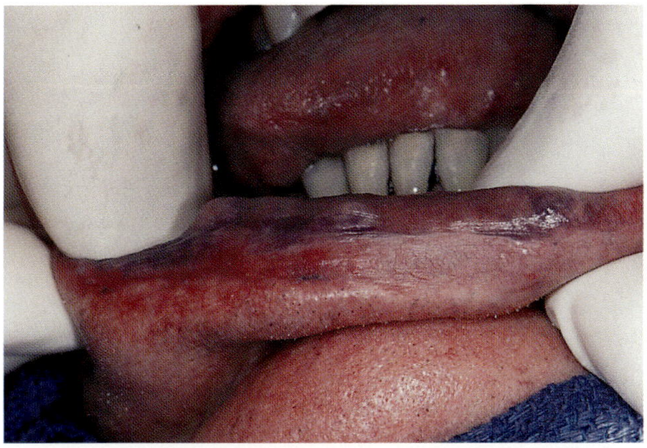

Figure 4–26. Vital staining with TN is mildly positive.

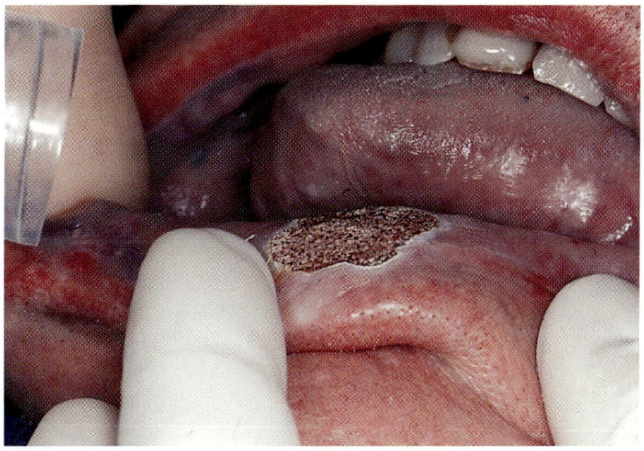

Figure 4–28. First raster at PD = 460 W/cm^2 (2.5 mm HeNe guide spot, 1.8-mm vaporization spot, 92 PPS superpulsed, average power of 20W, 216 mJ/pulse 1.1-ms pulse width with 125-mm handpiece).

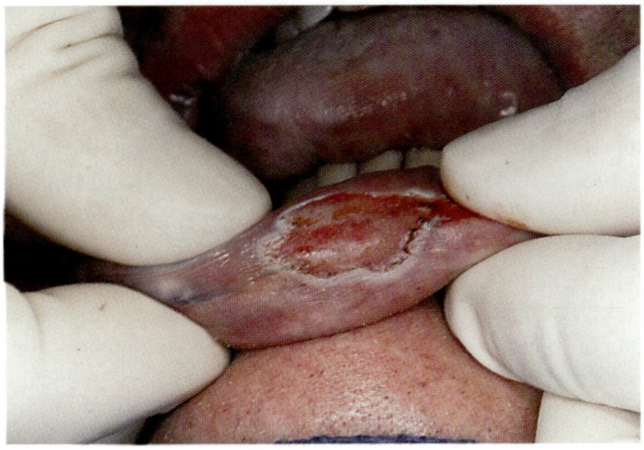

Figure 4–29. Tissue treated by first raster removed by wiping with wet gauze. Note sharp border of untreated mucosa. Full thickness of mucosa has been removed.

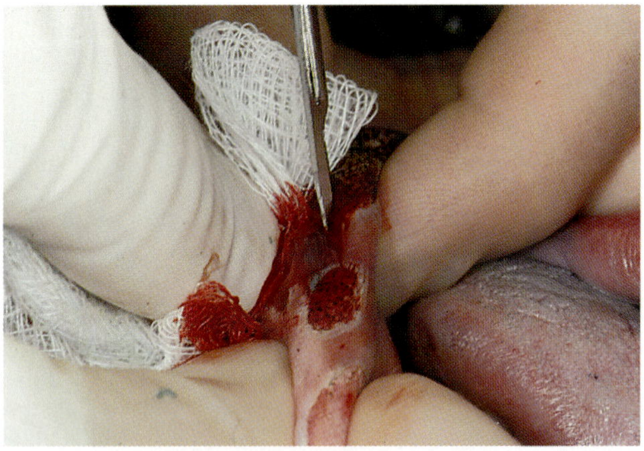

Figure 4–30. Selected, TN stained tissue sampled by excisional biopsy.

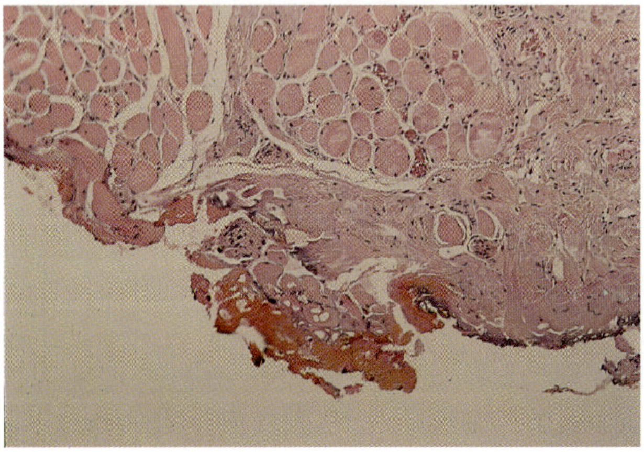

Figure 4–31. Heat effect at base of treated area at edge of biopsy sample: depth of thermal damage is 0.21 mm.

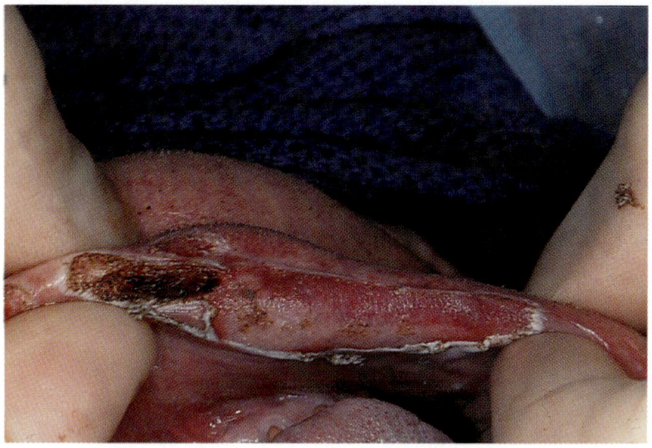

Figure 4–32. Completion of treatment. Dark color on right from coagulation of base of biopsy area with laser.

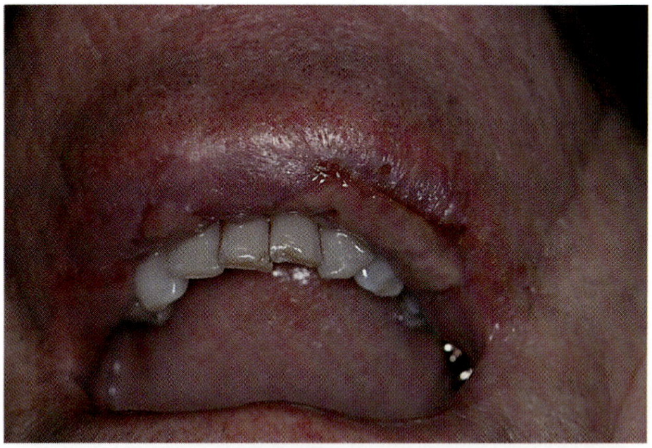

Figure 4–33. Healing at 13 days. Fibrin still covers wound.

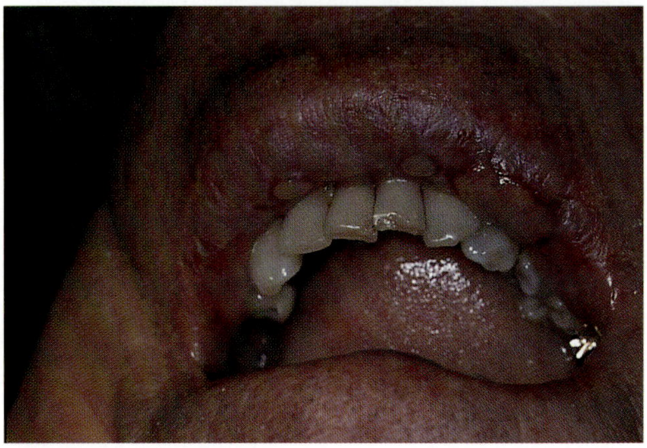

Figure 4–34. Healing at 22 days. Reepithelialization is prominent.

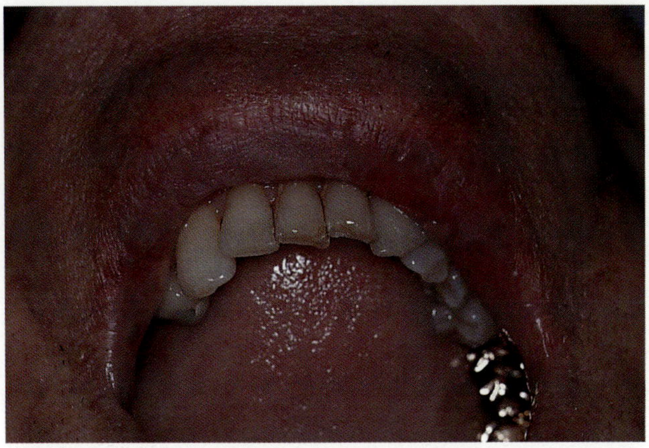

Figure 4–35. Thirty-three days. Reepithelialization has been completed and mucosa has started to mature.

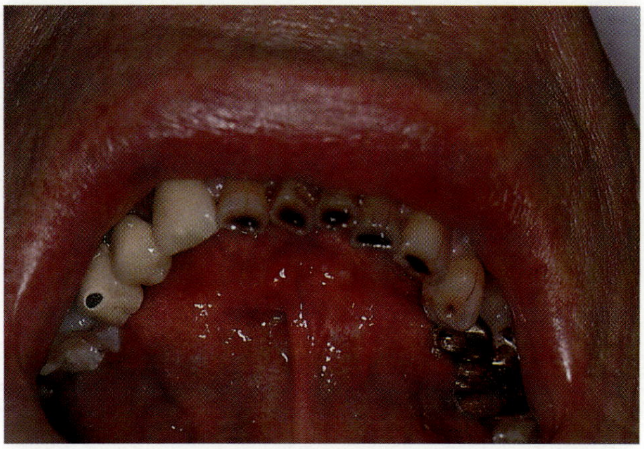

Figure 4–36. Five months. Maturation completed during second month. Mucosa has been stable for 12 months.

CASE 2: LEUKOPLAKIA, ANTERIOR FLOOR OF MOUTH AND LINGUAL GINGIVA

A 56-year-old man presented with a very subtle erythroleukoplakia of the anterior floor of the mouth centered on the lingual frenulum and extending onto the lingual gingiva (Fig. 4–37). Staining with TN was mildly positive. Treatment: The lesion was ablated with a CO_2 laser using the handpiece (125 mm focal length), average output power 15 W, RSP at 104 PPS, and PD approximately 375 w/cm^2. To ablate the lingual gingiva a front surface mirror was used to change the direction of the beam (Fig. 4–38). Spot size was between 2.5 and 3.0 mm, average output power 20 W at 58 PPS. The "slower" beam was used to permit easier coordination of energy delivery between the handpiece, mirror, and target tissue.

Ablation of the mucosa included the region directly adjacent to the orifices of the submandibular ducts. Note the absolute absence of charring of the native tissue at the site of ablation after removal of the layer of treated tissue (Fig. 4–39). Consequently uncomplicated complete epithelialization occurred within 30 days (Figs. 4–40 to 4–43). There was no transient obstruction of the submandibular salivary glands, no loss of attached gingiva, and no recurrence at 6 years' follow-up examination (Fig. 4–44).

Six years after treatment, an erythroplakia reappeared that was restricted to the lingual frenulum and the same laser vaporization procedure was repeated to remove the second erythroleukoplakia. Again, healing was uncomplicated, with complete epithelial resurfacing having occurred in approximately 30 days. At reoperation the tissue both of the floor of the mouth and of the lingual gingiva was noted to have the same characteristics of plasticity and response to the laser energy as had been the case for treatment of the index lesion, i.e., there was no long-term damage to the native tissue from the first operation 6 years before.

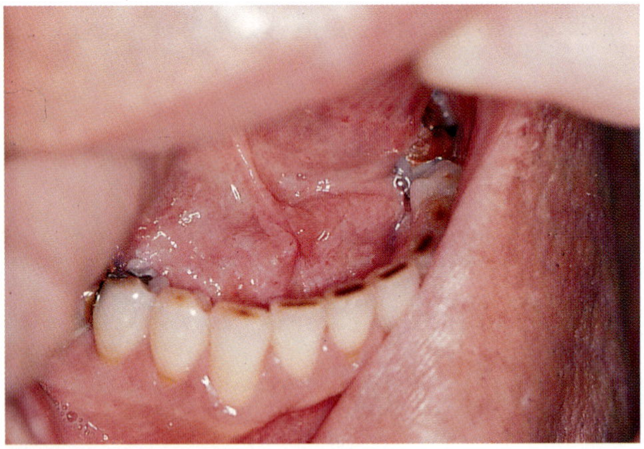

Figure 4–37. Subtle erythroleukoplakia of floor of the mouth originating at the base of the frenulum and extending over the submandibular duct orifices across the lingual sulcus and onto the lingual gingiva.

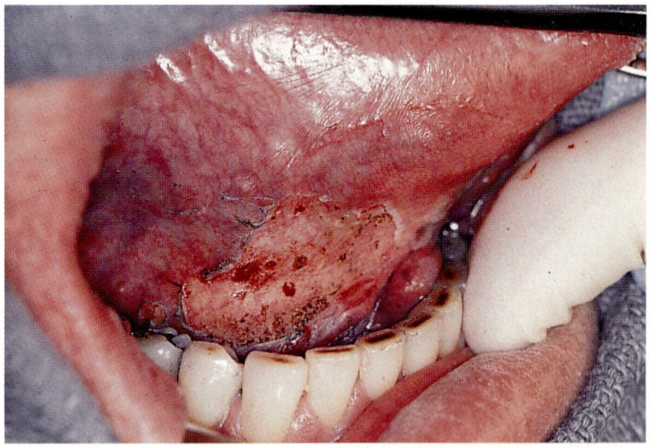

Figure 4–39. Lingual gingiva, sulcus, and area over ducts ablated.

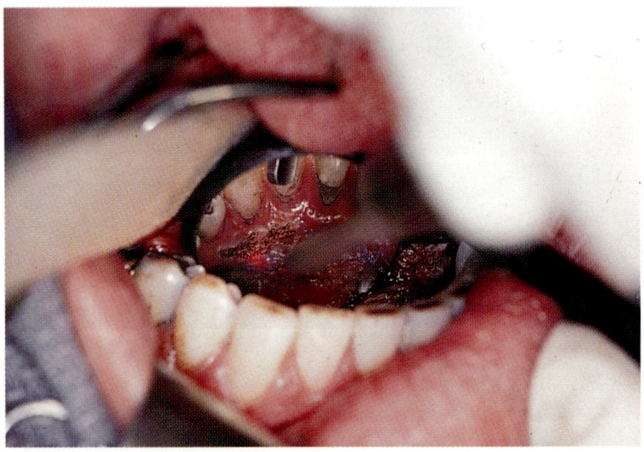

Figure 4–38. Use of front surface mirror to redirect the beam. Spot size is enlarged until PD is low enough not to damage the mirror.

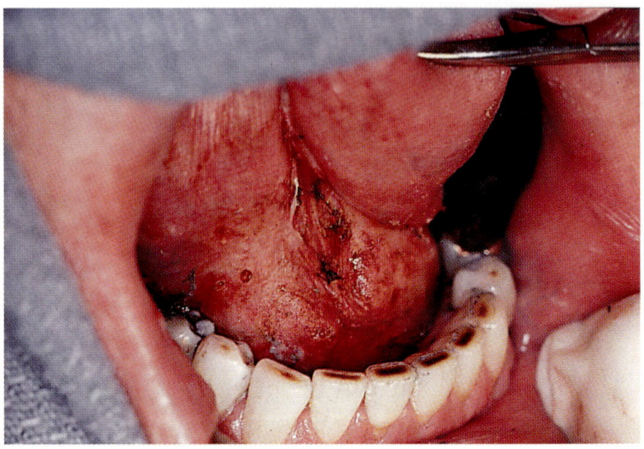

Figure 4–40. Note sharp demarcation between normal epithelium and ablated area. Few areas of pinpoint bleeding indicate deeper penetration of beam. Note absolute absence of charring of base of ablation region.

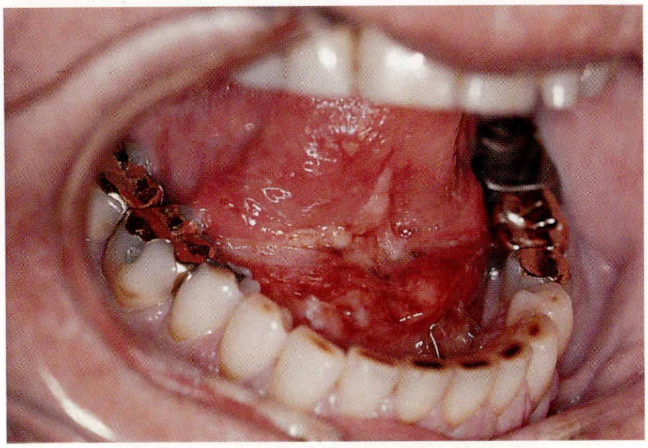

Figure 4–41. First postoperative day. Note deposition of fibrin within the wound.

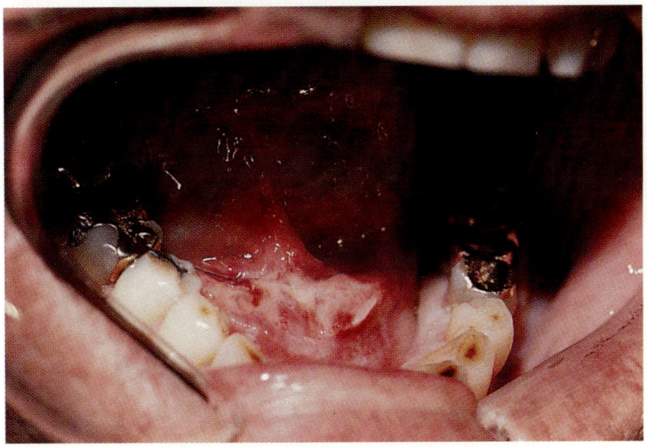

Figure 4–42. Postoperative: 10 days. Reepithelialization well established.

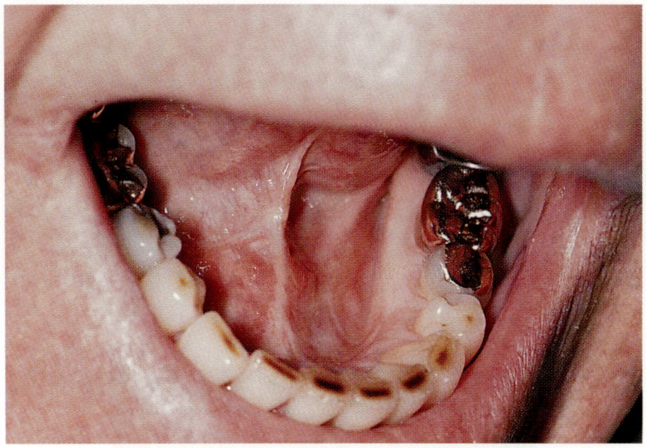

Figure 4–43. Postoperative: 30 days. Epithelialization complete.

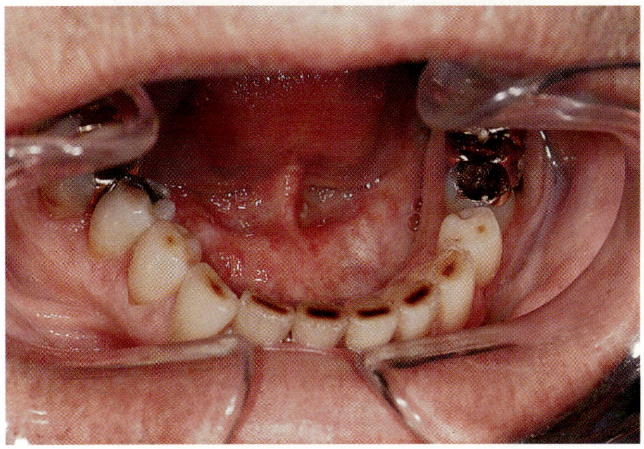

Figure 4–44. Postoperative 11 months. No loss of lingual attached gingiva.

CASE 3: BUCCAL MUCOSA

A 54-year-old white woman with a 35-pack-year cigarette smoking habit who did not drink alcohol presented with a leukoplakia of the buccal mucosa. The preoperative biopsy was interpreted as hyperkeratosis with mild atypia. The left buccal mucosa demonstrated a 2 × 3 cm area of leukoplakia that stained mildly positive with toluidine blue (TN). The microscope-guided superpulsed CO_2 laser was used with the power density adjusted to achieve the desired effect of creating opalescent crackling of the mucosa. This required an estimated average power density of approximately 585 W/cm^2 (15 W) average beam output power, HeNe aiming beam spot size approximately 2 mm, and a true spot size of 1.6 mm, 46 PPS with a pulse width of 4.2 ms. The worst area of the mucosa was excised for another histologic interpretation. The mucosa had completely resurfaced in 4 weeks (Figs. 4–45 to 4–48).

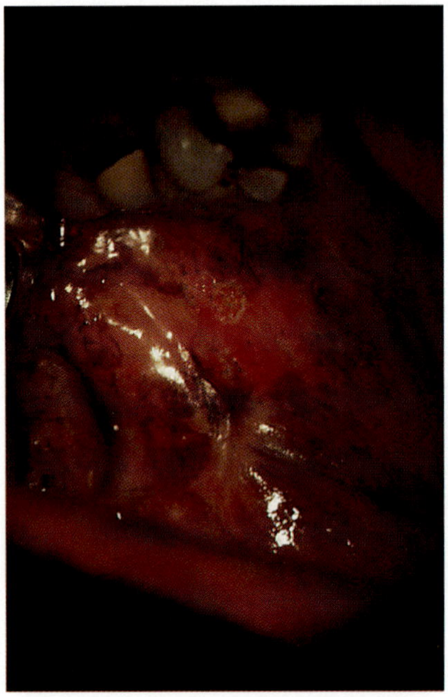

Figure 4–45. Buccal mucosa: area of mildly positive staining with TN indicates "worst" area of lesion (10×).

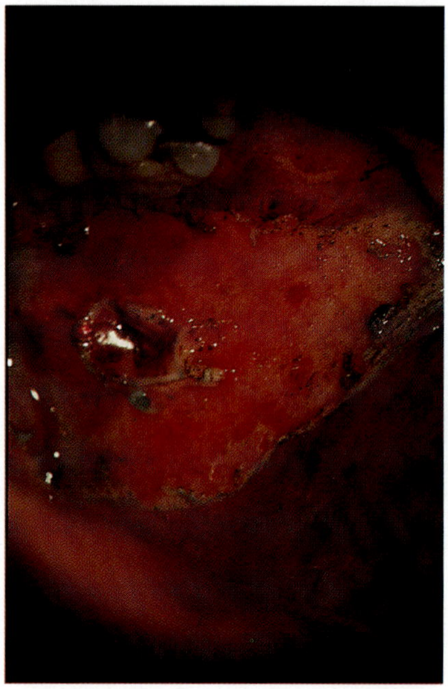

Figure 4–47. Tissue subject to first raster removed. Note lack of bleeding after ablation of epithelium only. Note sharp demarcation between normal epithelium and treated area (16×).

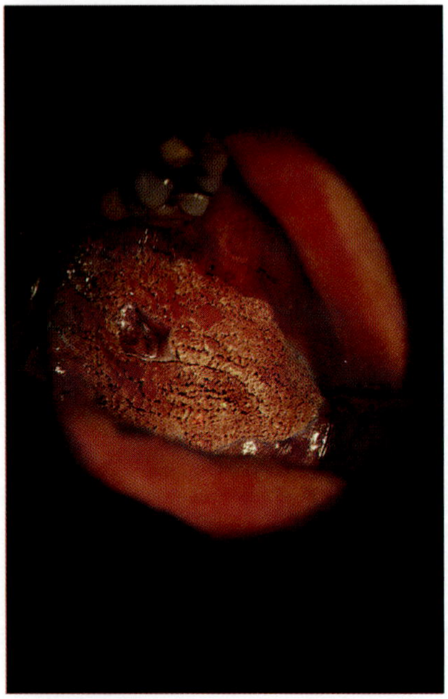

Figure 4–46. First raster completed. Mildly stained area saved for excisional biopsy (6×).

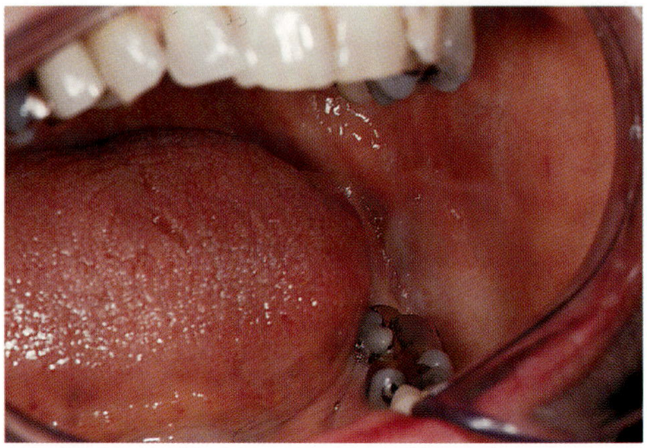

Figure 4–48. Mucosa completely healed at 4 weeks. Patient still is disease free at 4.5 years.

CASE 4: BUCCAL MUCOSA

A 58-year-old white man with erosive lichen planus and lichenoid dysplasia of both buccal mucosae. Protocol: Vital staining with TN resulted in a mildly positive result. Lesion removed in two rasters at an average power of 15 W, true RSP mode, HeNe spot of 2.5 mm (true vaporization spot size of 1.8 mm), giving an estimated PD of 463 W/cm^2 at 150 mJ/pulse at PRR = 118 Hz (Figs. 4–49 to 4–54).

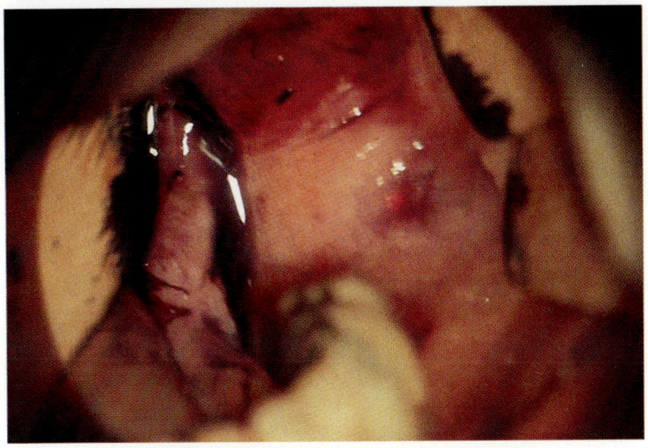

Figure 4–49. Mildly positive staining with TN. Red HeNe aiming beam centered on stained tissue (6×).

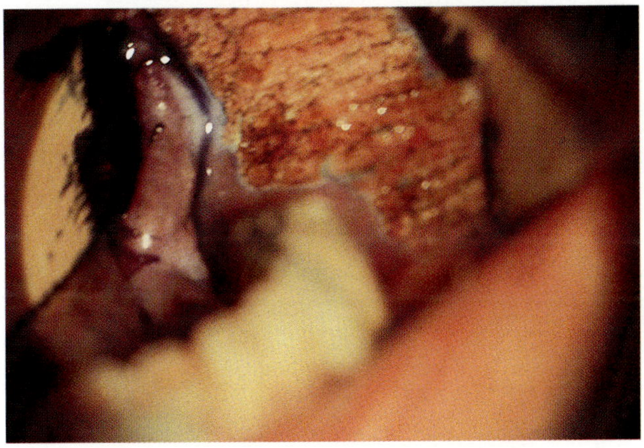

Figure 4–50. First raster completed. Note symmetry of "rows" of tissue ablated. There is no charring. Note distinct boundary between normal mucosa and treated area.

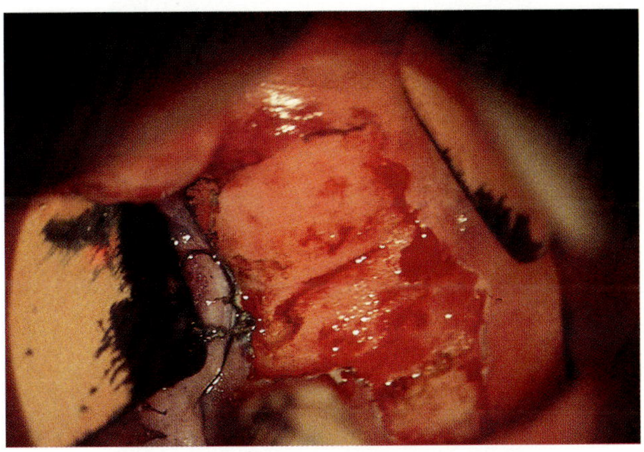

Figure 4–51. Rastered area wiped away with moist gauze sponge. A few areas of bleeding noted indicating extension of laser effect into submucosa.

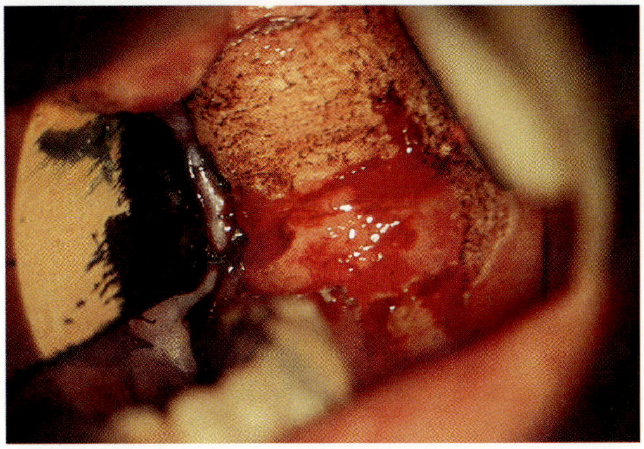

Figure 4–52. Second raster halfway completed. Note color change in upper one half of treatment field. The yellow color indicates second plane of ablation has been achieved at the level of the submucosa.

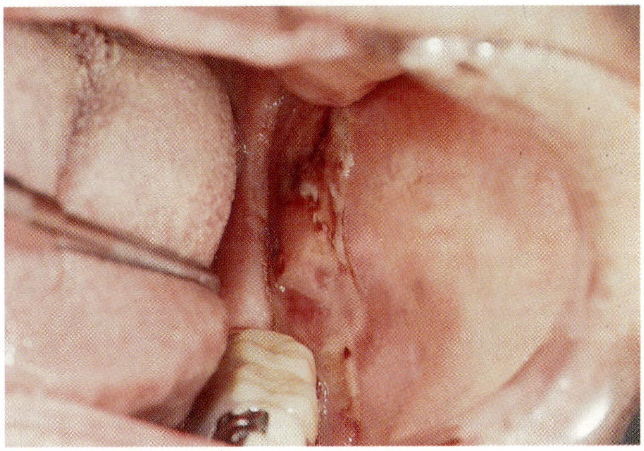

Figure 4–53. Epithelialization quite pronounced at 7 days. Epithelialization 80 to 90% complete at 13 days. Process complete within 28 days.

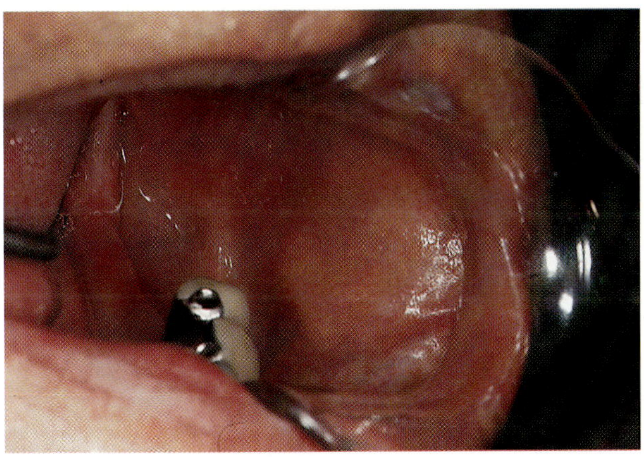

Figure 4–54. Two years. Mucosa is supple. Treated area appears normal.

CASE 5: LEUKOPLAKIA OF TONGUE

This 28-year-old white woman with no risk factors developed a TINOMO squamous cell carcinoma of the left posterolateral tongue border and a dense leukoplakia simplex covering much of the anterior dorsal tongue surface (Fig. 4–55). Three previous biopsies of the "worst"-appearing areas of her dorsal tongue demonstrated hyperkeratosis with mild atypia. Incisional biopsy of the tongue cancer was interpretated as well-differentiated squamous cell carcinoma.

Examination under anesthesia and vital staining also revealed a third white lesion of the left buccal mucosa. This stained only faintly with toluidine blue. No prophylactic antibiotics were administered.

The dorsal tongue lesion was vaporized with a true rapid superpulsed CO_2 laser and 46 PPS, average power of 20 W, spot size of 2.0 mm at a fluence of approximately 435 mJ/pulse width, a peak pulse power of 500 W, at a pulse width of approximately 4.2 ms, and an interpulse distance of 19 ms. Two rasters were applied with the target tissue being wiped free of debris between applications. There was almost no char and no bleeding (Figs. 4–56 to 4–58). The cancer was then removed with the same laser at 30 W average power using the handpiece in focus at 0.3 mm spot size for incision and defocused to control bleeding. The partial glossectomy wound was sutured closed. Estimated blood loss for the resection was 15 mL. Reepithelialization of the surface of the tongue was 100% complete at 27 days. Mild hyperkeratosis was present immediately after healing was completed.

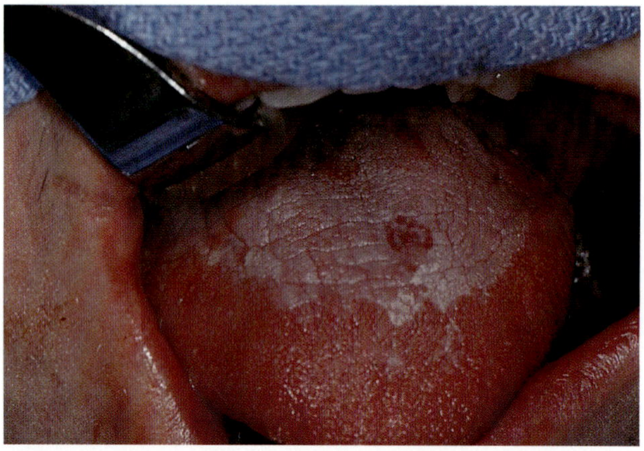

Figure 4–55. Leukoplakia affecting majority of surface area of dorsal tongue.

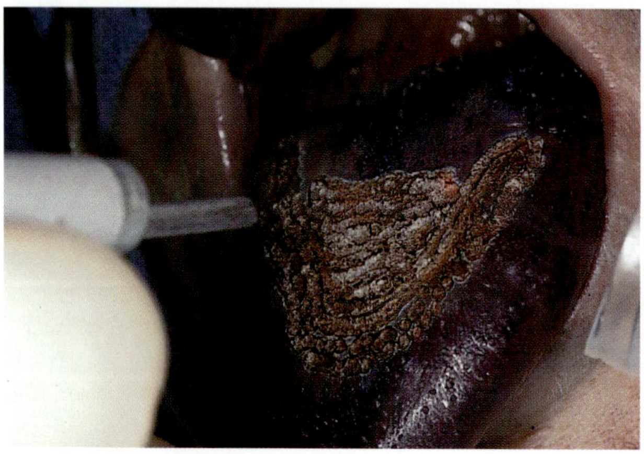

Figure 4–56. First, horizontal, raster used to remove surface epithelium. Note HeNe aiming spot of approximately 2.0-mm diameter. Rastering half completed.

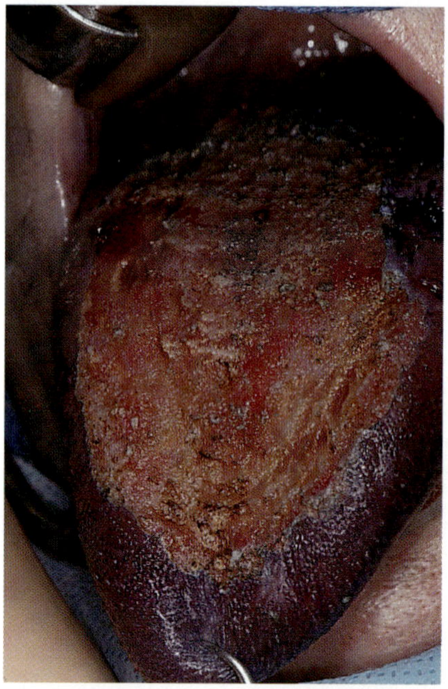

Figure 4–57. Debris removed by wiping with gauze sponge. Note yellow color in central portion where vaporization was deeper especially in center area which had stained positively with TN.

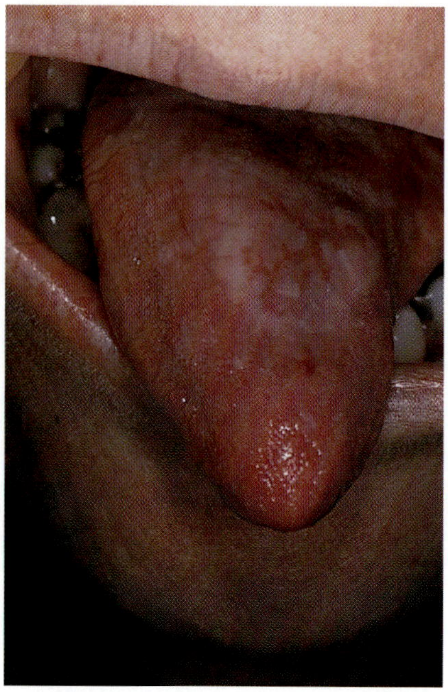

Figure 4–58. Surface reepithelialized at 3 weeks. Mature mucosa shown at 9 weeks.

REFERENCES

1. Kramer IR, El-Labban N, Lee KW. The clinical features and risk of malignant transformation in sublingual keratosis. *Br Dent J* 1978;144(6):171–180.
2. Horch H, Gerlach KL, Schaefer H. CO_2 laser surgery of oral premalignant lesions. *Int J Oral Maxillofac Surg* 1986;15: 19–24.
3. Mashberg A, Meyers H. Anatomical site and size of 22 early asymptomatic oral squamous cell carcinomas: a continuing prospective study of oral cancer. *Cancer* 1976;37:2149–2157.
4. Mincer HH, Coleman SA, Hopkins KP. Observations on the clinical characteristics of oral lesions showing histologic epithelial dysplasia. *Oral Surg* 1972;33:389–299.
5. Panders AK, Verschueren RCJ, Vermey A, et al. Laser surgery for superficial lesions for the oral mucosa. In: *Lasers in Biomedicine and Surgery.* Berlin: Springer; 1980.
6. Pindborg JJ. *Oral cancer and precancer.* Bristol, England: Wright; 1980.
7. Bouquot JE. Reviewing oral leukoplakia clinical concepts for the 1990's. *J Am Dent Assoc* 1991;122:80–82.
8. Pindborg JJ. Personal communication. September 1994.
9. Banoczy J. Follow-up studies in oral leukoplakia. *J Maxillofac Surg* 1977;5(1):69–75.
10. Bouquot JE. Common oral lesions found during a mass screening examination. *J Am Dent Assoc* 1986;112(1):50–57.
11. Mashberg A, Samit A. Early detection, diagnosis and management of oral and oropharyngeal cancer. *CA* 1989;39:67–88.
12. Bouquot J, Weiland L, Ballard D, et al. Leukoplakia of the mouth and pharynx in Rochester, MN, 1935–84: Incidence of clinical features and follow-up of 463 patients from a relatively unbiased patient pool. *J Oral Pathol* 1988;436.
13. Browne RM, Potts AJC. Dysplasia in salivary gland ducts in sublingual leukoplakia and erythroplakia. *Oral Surg Oral Med Oral Pathol* 1986;62:42–48.
14. Clayman L. Management of mucosal premalignant lesions. *Oral Maxillofac Clin North Am* 1994;6(3):431–443.
15. Mashberg A. Final evaluation of tolonium chloride rinse for screening of high-risk patients with asymptomatic squamous carcinoma. *J Am Dent Assoc* 1983;106:319–323.
16. Mashberg A. Tolonium (toluidine blue) rinse—a screening method for recognition of squamous carcinoma: continuing study of oral cancer IV. *JAMA* 1981;245:2408–2410.
17. Miller RL, Simms W, Gould AR. Toluidine blue staining for detection of oral premalignant lesion and carcinomas. *J Oral Pathol* 1988;17:73–78.
18. Frame JW, Das Gupta AR, Dalton GA, et al. Use of the carbon dioxide laser in the management of premalignant lesions of the oral mucosa. *J Laryngol Otol* 1984;98:1251–1260.
19. Roodenburg JL, Panders AK, Vermey A. Carbon dioxide laser surgery of oral leukoplakia. *Oral Surg Oral Med Oral Pathol* 1991;71:670–674.
20. Fisher SE, Frame JW, Browne RM, Tranter RMD. A comparative histological study of wound healing following CO_2 laser and conventional surgical excision of canine buccal mucosa. *Arch Oral Biol* 1983;28:287–291.
21. Clayman L. Management of mucosal premalignant lesions. *Oral Maxillofac Surg Clin North Am* 1994;6(3):431–445.
22. Clayman L, Fuller TA, Beckman H. Healing of continuous wave and rapid superpulsed carbon dioxide laser induced bone defects. *J Oral Surg* 1978;36:932–937.
23. Fisher SW, Frame JW. The effects of carbon dioxide surgical laser on oral tissues. *Br J Oral Maxillofac Surg* 1984;22: 414–425.
24. Mihashi S, Jako GJ, Incze J, et al. Laser surgery in otolaryngology: interactions of CO_2 laser and soft tissue. *Ann NY Acad Sci* 1976;267:263–294.
25. Loumanen M, Lehto VP, Meurman JH. Myofibroblasts in healing laser wounds of rat tongue mucosa. *Arch Oral Biol* 1988;33(1):17–23.
26. Gaspar L, Szabo G. Manifestation of the advantages and disadvantages of using the CO_2 laser in oral surgery. *J Clin Laser Med Surg* 1990; Feb: 39–43.
27. Braun RE, Liebow C. Clinical evaluation of tumor promotion by CO_2 laser. In: SPIE Vol 1424: *Lasers in Orthopedic, Dental and Veterinary Medicine.* 1991:138–144.

5 Papillomas and Human Papillomavirus

Richard Reid, Myron Strasser

Although controversial, evidence from immunoperoxidase and DNA hybridization studies have implicated human papillomavirus (HPV) as the etiologic agent for many diseases within the oral cavity. The possible relationship of HPV to the development of squamous cell cancer (SCC) of the head and neck merits an expanded discussion of HPV in this chapter. Well-established association of HPV with oral cavity disease includes condyloma acuminatum (HPV 45),[1,2] verruca vulgaris (HPV 6 and 16),[2–4] squamous papilloma (HPV 6, 11),[2,5] focal epithelial hyperplasia (HPV 13 and 32)[1,2,4] and squamous cell carcinoma (HPV 16 and 18).[1,2,6–12] Human papilloma virus has also been detected in diseases that do not show obvious viral stigmata, such as ameloblastoma (HPV 16, 18),[13–15] leukoplakia (HPV 16),[1,2,9,12,16] lichen planus (HPV 16),[1,2,12] white sponge nevus (HPV 16),[17] and odontogenic keratocyst (HPV 16).[18] In head and neck surgery as in other specialties, carbon dioxide (CO_2) laser surgery is gaining increasing acceptance in the treatment of such HPV-associated lesions as condyloma acuminatum, verruca vulgaris, squamous papilloma, and leukoplakia. The use of the CO_2 laser as an alternative instrument for excision is also useful in the resection of oral squamous cell cancer.[17,19,20]

BASIC VIROLOGY

Taxonomy

Papillomaviruses are small, double-stranded DNA viruses[12,21,22] that manifest qualitatively similar biologic characteristics. All papillomaviruses exhibit a similar pattern of genetic organization. DNA sequencing studies have shown that broadly equivalent areas of protein coding potential, known as open reading frames (ORFs), are preserved through the genome.[22] However, the actual nucleotide sequences within these ORFs are widely disparate; hence, individual papillomaviruses show enormous differences in species specificity, site predilection, and degree of oncogenicity. Human papillomaviruses compose the largest group, with more than 50 known types[3,6,23] (Fig. 5–1).

DNA Organization

The papillomavirus genome is a closed, circular, double-stranded DNA molecule, with a molecular length of 7,900 base pairs and a molecular weight of 5200 d. The viral DNA is combined with histones (derived from the cellular pool of the natural host) to form a small chromosome of which the viral DNA constitutes only 12% of the virion by weight.

When the nuclear proteins are stripped away, the viral DNA assumes a supercoiled shape (form I). Supercoiling is visible on electron microscopy and is also detectable by electrophoretic migration because of the relatively rapid mobility of these tight circular molecules. Cleavage of only one DNA strand by bacterial enzymes (restriction endonucleases) results in a relaxed circle, form II (Fig. 5–2), while cleavage of both strands at a single site produces a linear molecule form III,[20] which migrates more slowly in electrophoresis gels (Fig. 5–2C).

Viral Genetic Function

As previously mentioned, alignment of sequenced papillomavirus DNAs revealed a highly conserved pattern of protein-coding potential—the ORFs. In essence, each of these ORFs represents a viral gene. Virus-specified proteins apparently determine such characteristics as host range, tissue tropism, and the clinicopathologic consequences of infection.

The papillomavirus genome can be subdivided into three functional portions. The "early" or "E" region is the longest segment, representing about 45% of the viral genome. This region contains five ORFs that code for proteins; these either induce cell transformation or control viral DNA replication. The "late" or "L" region, which comprises about 40% of the viral genome, contains two ORFs that are essential to vegetative viral replication. The third region of the genome is the upstream regulatory region (URR). This is a noncoding segment, representing about 15% of the viral genome. It contains the origin of DNA replication, several promoters (sequences needed to initiate viral RNA synthesis), and several enhancers (sequences that increase the rate of RNA transcription). The URR is located between the end of the L1 ORF and the beginning of the E5 ORF. The URR is the genetic interval most likely to be divergent among viral types, and some of these differences have been correlated with changes in virulence and oncogenicity.[21,22]

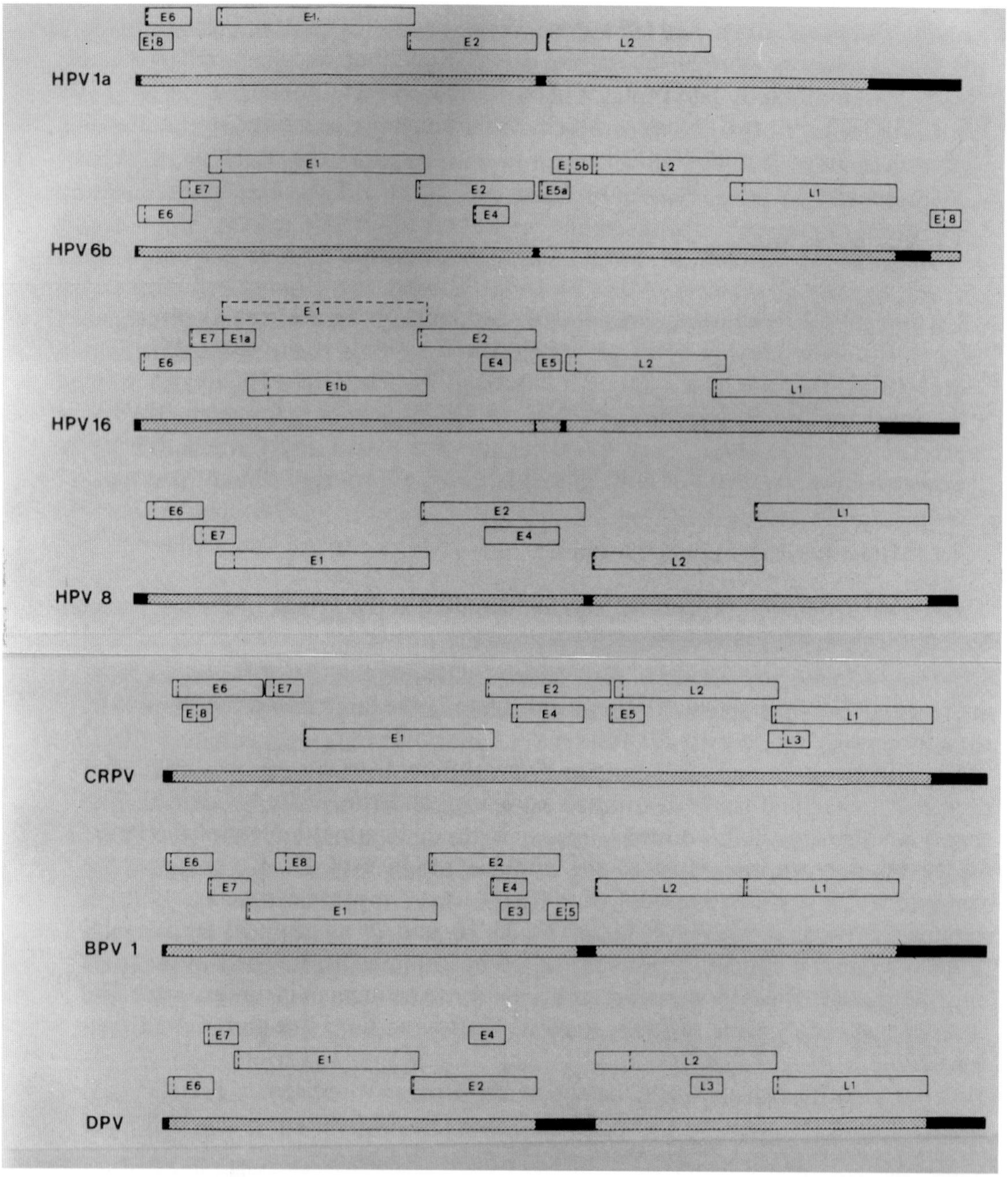

Figure 5–1. Genome organization of human papillomaviruses (HPV) 1a, 6b, 8, 16, bovine papillomavirus (BPV) 1, cottontail rabbit papillomavirus (CRPV), and deer papillomavirus (DPV). Open reading frames were displayed by means of the computer program FRAMES[34] and are indicated by open bars. Dotted lines within the frames represent the first methionine codon, which could serve as a start point of translation. In HPV 16 the E1 frame appeared to be split in the originally published sequence.[35] A continuous E1, which was found in four new isolates, is indicated by dotted lines. Stippled areas of the genome bar represent coding sequences and black regions stand for so-called non-coding regions. (From reference 35, with permission.)

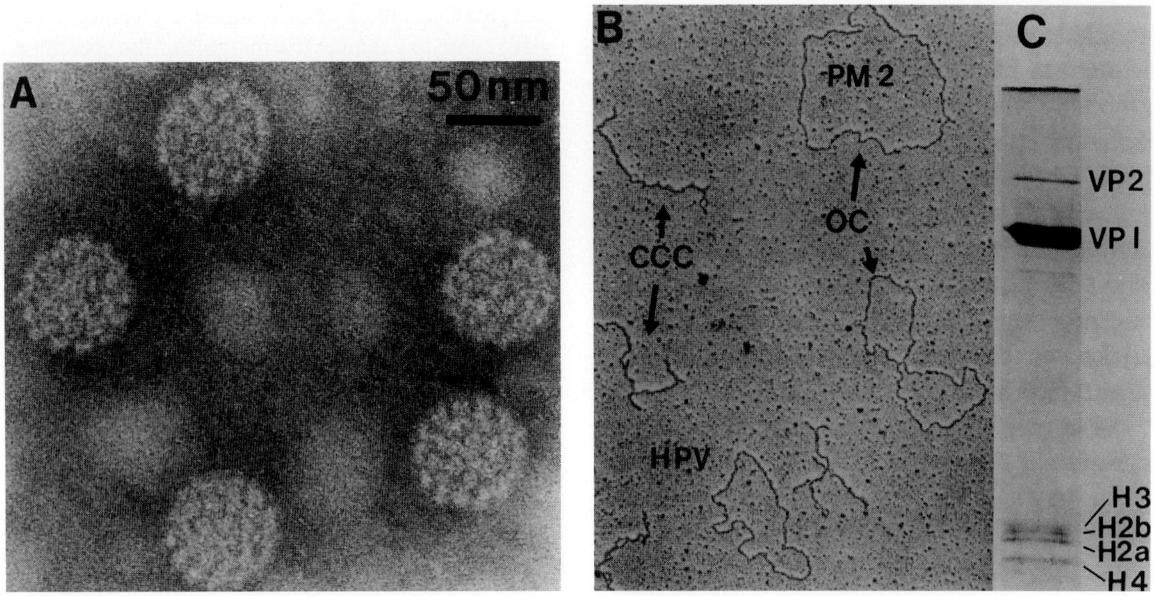

Figure 5–2. **(A)** Structure, **(B)** genomic DNA, and **(C)** protein pattern of papillomavirus particles. Capsids were stained with phosphotungstic acid. DNA was extracted by phenol treatment. DNA of phage PM2 was included as a size standard (97 kd). The molecules appear as supertwisted covalently closed circles (CCC) or open circles (OC). Proteins were separated by polyacrylamide gel electrophoresis after disruption of viral particles by sodium dodecyl sulfate (SDS). VP1 and VP2@ represent structural proteins of the capsid shell. Histones H3, H2b, H2a, and H4 are associated with the viral DNA and appear in preparations of DNA-containing capsids. (From reference 35, with permission.)

PATHOPHYSIOLOGY OF INFECTION

Inoculation

Inoculation occurs when material containing relatively large numbers of virus particles (e.g., exfoliated superficial cells or keratin fragments) lodge in sites of microtrauma within a susceptible epithelium. HPV virions penetrate to the basal layer of the damaged epidermis, where they then shed their outer protein capsid. The viral genome crosses the cell membrane and is then transported to the cell nucleus. There the infecting genome is translated and transcribed, thereby producing various virus-specific proteins. Transforming proteins induce conducive host cell functions, while regulatory proteins control viral gene expression.[22]

Incubation Phase

Initially the virus exists as a self-replicating extrachromosomal plasmid, termed an episome. Proteins specified by the early viral genes result in an initial burst of episomal replication, producing additional viral genomes that will gradually transfect neighboring cells. Because these episomal viral plasmids are programmed to replicate with each cell division, there is little dilution of viral copy numbers over the succeeding years.[22]

Active Expression Phase

Many exposed individuals will remain in long-term latent infection; however, in susceptible hosts, viral colonization may lead to active viral expression. Capture of the host cell results in pronounced alteration in cell growth in the basal layers, increased replication of the viral genome in the middle layers, and viral cytopathic effects in maturing cells. Such progression from episomal to productive viral replication depends upon the interplay of cell permissiveness, viral type, host susceptibility, and cofactor activity. Two basic types of cell–virus interaction are recognized: vegetative (productive) and transforming (nonproductive). Patients with high-grade dysplasia and those in whom oncogenic HPV subtypes are identified are at risk for higher recurrence rates after treatment.

CLINICAL AND LABORATORY EVALUATION

Comprehensive history-taking can help in establishing the diagnosis of HPV-related oral lesions. Consider, for example, a patient presenting with multiple painless, sessile, soft whitish papules on the lower labial mucosa and lateral tongue border (Fig. 5–3). Knowledge that such a patient has an Inuit ancestry would raise a high degree of suspicion for focal epithelial hyperplasia. When a definitive diagnosis cannot be established by history and clinical examination, a specimen must be obtained for microscopic and/or other laboratory evaluation. The decision to perform incisional versus excisional biopsy depends on such considerations as lesion size, location, and possible diagnosis of cancer.

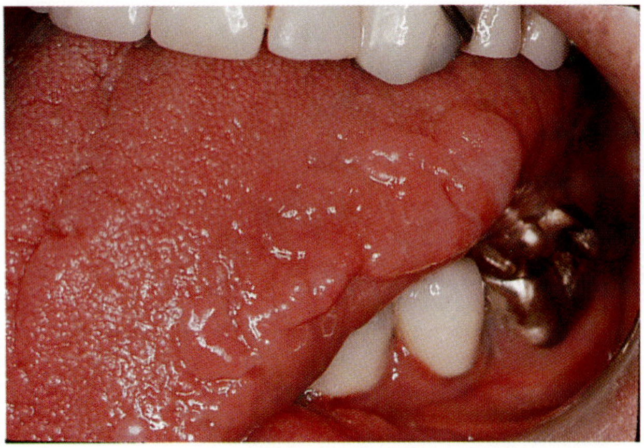

Figure 5–3. Focal epithelial hyperplasia of lateral tongue. (Photo courtesy of Scott Boyd, D.D.S., Ph. D.)

If the area under investigation is large or if one suspects malignancy, incisional biopsy is preferred. Conversely, small lesions that appear clinically benign may be excised. For both cases, tissue is sent to the pathology laboratory for routine processing. In the majority of cases, an oral pathologist will make a firm diagnosis with the light microscope, aided by clinical description and historical details. In difficult cases, if identification of the specific HPV is needed, ancillary testing is available. Viral analysis of formalin fixed tissue is done by either polymerase chain reaction or in situ DNA hybridization.[2,3,8,9,14,24–27] Greater sensitivity can be achieved by filter hybridization of fresh tissue (e.g., a cellulose swab or a frozen biopsy sample). Virus testing is still expensive and is not available for routine use.

CARBON DIOXIDE LASER

Excision and vaporization are the two techniques employed in soft tissue surgery. Excision is the preferable mode for removal of oral lesions, because this method permits histologic confirmation of the diagnosis and establishment of margins that are clear of cytopathic changes. The pathologist is able to examine the margins of the specimen because the laser destroys tissue in a precise manner, causing a central zone of tissue vaporization, and only 100 to 200 μm of tissue necrosis adjacent to the points of impact.[28,29] In contrast, during vaporization strategic tissue biopsies need to be obtained prior to vaporization. Laser vaporization (ablation) or painting away of the oral lesions are performed in a layer by layer method (rastering).[30] Carbonization produced by vaporization should be wiped away to improve visualization of the lased areas and to decrease crater temperature, thereby decreasing thermal conduction into the adjacent tissue.[7] Tissue irradiance of this carbonized material raises the temperature from 100°C (the boiling point of water) to more than 600°C (the temperature of a red-hot coal).[31] After the surgeon is confident that the lesion has been completely removed, a carbonized layer should remain to help maintain hemostasis of the small vessels that have been sealed by the laser[20] if the depth of removal extends into the submucosa. A fibrous coagulum replaces the carbonized layer after approximately 24 hours. Epithelialization of the laser wound occurs at approximately 1 week if its surface area is less than 1.0 cm^2. Larger wounds take 4 to 5 weeks to reepithelialize.[32] Many authors have noted that laser wounds heal slower than scalpel wounds, being delayed from 2 to 4 days.[19,32]

There will be slight but pathologically unimportant shrinkage at the base of the specimen being removed for biopsy.

Disadvantages of using the CO_2 laser include higher cost for the equipment, limited availability, slower healing of the laser wound, and the possibility of the HPV DNA being liberated in the plume of laser vapors.[33] It is mandatory to use a high-speed suction system to evacuate the vaporized material. The potential infectivity of virus particles found in the effluent plume is under intense investigation at present.

WARNING: If you smell the plume through the mask, there is a chance of inhaling particulate matter that may carry virus particles or whole virions. Although there is lack of consistent proof of the infectivity of these particles, prudence in regard to mask selection is strongly recommended.

CASE 1: PAPILLOMAS

(Courtesy Lewis Clayman, D.M.D., M.D.)

A 5-year-old African-American girl presents to her family doctor because of recurrent lip biting. Examination shows a 5-mm "wart" on the inner aspect of the mucosal surface of her left lower lip. With the lip in repose, this abuts a second similar lesion affecting the interproximal papilla between the left lateral incisor and canine teeth (Fig. 5–4). These are "kissing" lesions. A similar lesion is also noted adjacent to the upper right lateral incisor. A clinical diagnosis of oral papillomas is made. The parents are reported to be free of oral or genital papillomas by report from their family physician.

The patient is brought to the operating theater for photoablation by vaporization with the CO_2 laser. General anesthesia with oral endotracheal intubation was chosen because of the patient's age. The lip lesion was treated first with a true superpulsed beam with a peak power of 500 W delivering an average power of 10 W at 58 pulses per second with an average power density (PD) of 440 W/cm^2 at a spot size of 1.5 mm. The first raster removed the superficial mucosa. Part of the lower lip papilloma was excised with the laser in a focused mode (PD = 1250 W/cm^2) at a spot size of 0.3 mm. The remainder of the lesion was vaporized using two rasters to ablate just below the basement membrane. Figure 5–5 illustrates the depth achieved after wiping away the remainder of the treated mucosa. The lower incisor was protected with a metal matrix band (of the type used for placing interproximal amalgam restorations), and the interproximal gingiva was ablated at a power density of 500 W/cm^2 (Fig. 5–6). An additional 1 × 3 mm lesion of the left buccal mucosa was similarly ablated. Estimated blood loss was nil. Histopathologic and viral studies demonstrated oral papillomas positive for HPV 6 and 11. At 3-month follow-up assessment, the "kissing" lesions of the left lower lip and gingiva had recurred. The gingival lesion was now 7 mm in maximum dimension and a 5 × 2 mm plantar papilloma had recurred on the left lower lip. These were retreated using the same laser parameters as before. At 14 days, the mucosa had completely resurfaced with normal epithelium. One year later, there was no recurrence (Fig. 5–7). However, 2 years later, there was reactivation or reinoculation of the left lower lip lesion. The gingival lesion had not recurred.

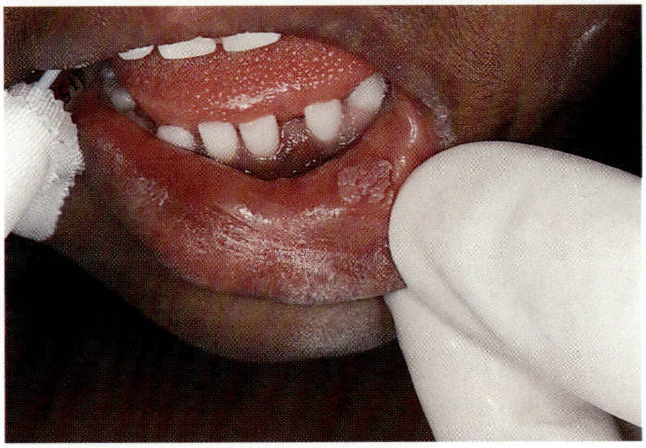

Figure 5–4. Five-year-old girl with contact papillomas of left mucosal surface of lower lip and left interproximal gingiva between left lower lateral incisor and canine.

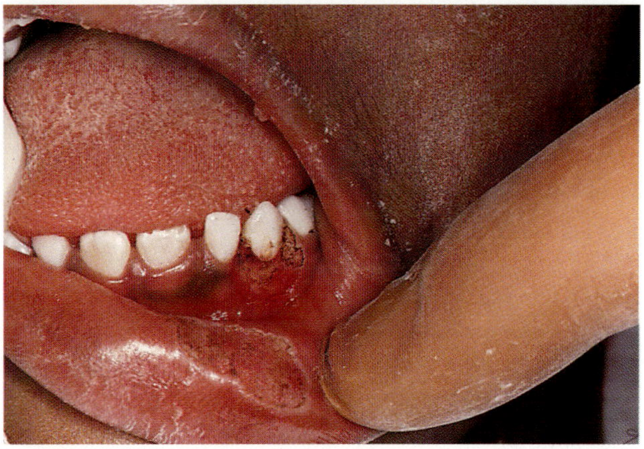

Figure 5–6. Gingival site after wiping away treated tissue.

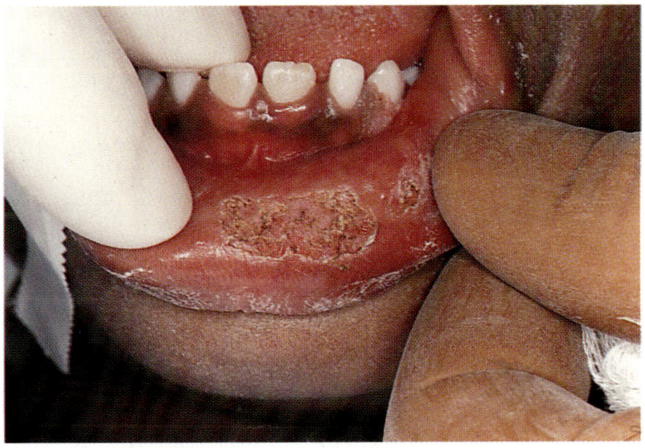

Figure 5–5. Lip site after wiping away char.

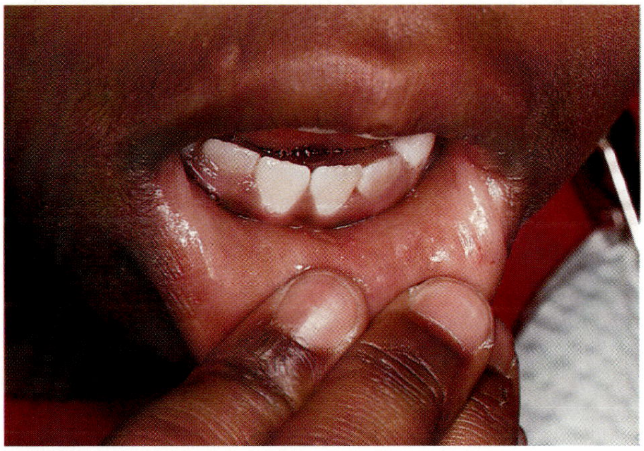

Figure 5–7. Lip: no recurrence at one year. Gingival site: no recurrence at one year, even after trauma of eruption of the succedaneous tooth.

CASE 2: EXTENSIVE ORAL PAPILLOMATOSIS ON A RENAL TRANSPLANT RECIPIENT

(Courtesy Lewis Clayman, D.M.D., M.D.)

This 56-year-old African-American man presented with a chief complaint of inability to wear dentures because of "growths" in his mouth (Fig. 5–8).

Twenty years earlier, maxillary split-thickness skin grafting and vestibuloplasty had been performed to aid in denture retention. Since then, progressive maxillary ridge resorption had resulted in the loss of all alveolar bone. The anterior nasal spine was now the most prominent feature of the residual ridge. Eighteen months before, his chronic renal failure had been successfully treated by a cadaver renal transplant. Following the institution of cyclosporine immunosuppression therapy, he developed extensive papillary hyperplasia of all of his oral mucosae, which precluded his ability to wear dentures. His list of illnesses active at the time of consultation included diabetes mellitus, hypertension, glaucoma, gout, and hypothyroidism. His transplanted kidney was functioning well. Current medications included: cyclosporine, prednisone, Imuran, lente insulin, Cardizem, Synthroid, Zantac, colchicine, potassium iodide, and ferrous sulfate. He was HIV negative. The histopathologic diagnosis of a representative biopsy of the papillomas of the maxillary alveolar ridge was verruciform hyperplasia. This sample was positive for HPV 6 and 11. The treatment recommendation for removal of the diseased oral mucosa by CO_2 laser in several stages was explained to the patient, and he agreed to therapy.

The first treatment was performed using general anesthesia and nasoendotracheal intubation. Aerodigestive endoscopy demonstrated mucosal changes extending into the pyriform recesses bilaterally, but not involving either the true or false vocal cords. Antibiotic prophylaxis with cephalothin was administered because of the renal transplant. No local anesthetics were used. The Sharplan 743 CO_2 laser with the microscope delivery system was used for the maxilla and tongue in a defocused superpulsed mode with a 3.0-mm spot size at 90 W average output power at 60 pulses per second. The PD was approximately 1280 W/cm^2. The treatment field included the entire maxillary and mandibular ridge, labiobuccal sulci, and palate for a total treatment area of approximately 60 cm^2 (Fig. 5–9). The entire dorsal tongue was similarly treated over an area of approximately 28 cm^2. The buccal mucosae, commissures, and upper and lower lips were treated at an average output power of 20 W superpulsed, using the handpiece delivery system with a spot size of approximately 1.6 mm at 120 pulses per second for an average power density of 780 W/cm^2. Estimated blood loss was 250 mL and operating time was 130 minutes.

Postoperatively, the patient took only two analgesic pills during the first 8 days after treatment. On day 8 there was epithelial resurfacing of about 20 to 30% of the mucosa. The most uncomfortable area of his mouth was the palate. By day 19 there were signs of regrowth of hyperplastic tis-

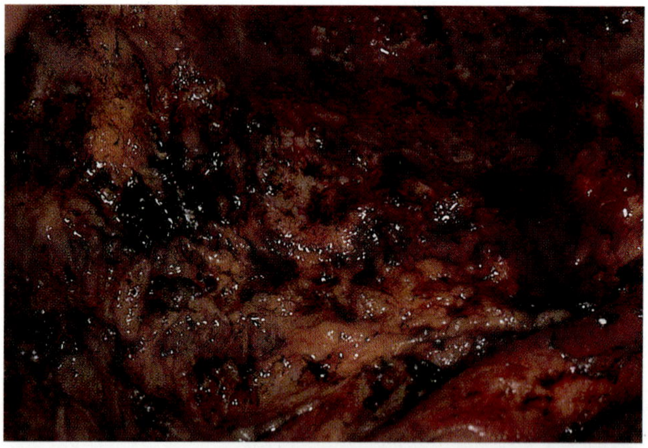

Figure 5–9. After first treatment using the microscope delivery system with a defocused beam in the superpulsed mode at an average power output of 90 W delivered at 60 pulses per second at 150 mJ/pulse with a spot size of 3.0 mm, the PD was 1280 W/cm^2. Estimated blood loss was 250 mL for treatment of more than 120 cm^2 of oral mucosae.

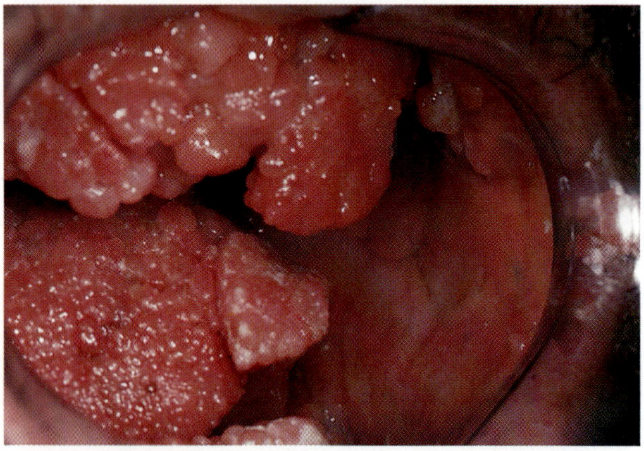

Figure 5–8. Extensive papillomatosis and verrucous hyperplasia of maxilla, buccal mucosa, alveolar ridges, and tongue. Palate and commissures also affected.

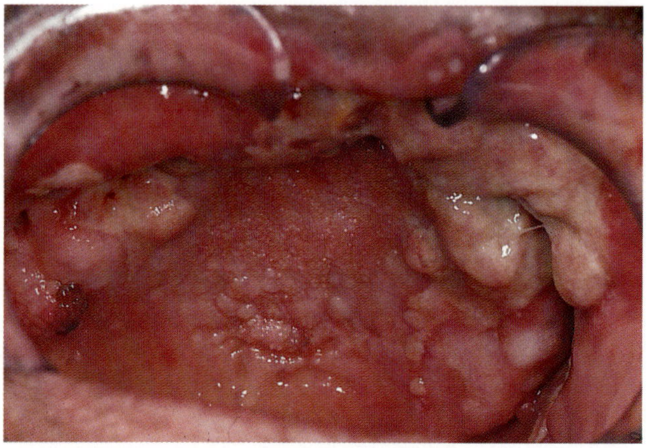

Figure 5–10. Maxillary alveolus and palate 19 days after treatment.

sue in the maxilla (Fig. 5–10). The mandible had reepithelialized to about 60% of normal, and he was completely pain-free. By day 25 epithelialization was 80% complete. By day 40 resurfacing was more than 90% complete, but there was approximately a 20% recurrence level of mucosal hyperplasia. At this stage the patient developed an attack of Herpes zoster in a left thoracic dermatome. By day 70 there was approximately 50% recurrence in the maxilla and there were minor areas of recurrence in the retromolar pad bilaterally, the oral commissures, and the floor of the mouth (Fig. 5–11). The areas of recurrence were treated as before. The total surface area of the treatment field was 53 cm^2, which represented approximately half of the surface area of the initial treatment (Fig. 5–12).

Examination and palpation under anesthesia did not demonstrate any scarring or loss of resiliency of the oral mucosa. Reepithelialization covered approximately 30% of the treatment area by day 14. The entire retreatment area was about 80% reepithelialized 31 days after treatment. There was slight scarring at the commissures but none intraorally. The patient remained disease free for 3 months, at which time minor recurrences were noted at the right mandibular alveolar ridge and left oral commissure. Using local anesthesia and intravenous sedation at a PD of 796 W/cm^2 (parameters: HeNe guide spot size = 2.0 mm; average output power = 25 w, PRR = 156 PPS with defocused 125-mm handpiece), these two areas were retreated. After 2 months, small recurrences were observed at the left commissure (2 × 7 mm) and the midline of the hard palate (3 × 4 mm). These areas were completely reepithelialized in 24 days after a third retreatment cycle. One year later the patient remained disease free in the palate but had a minor recurrence in the lateral tongue and left oral commissure (Fig. 5–13).

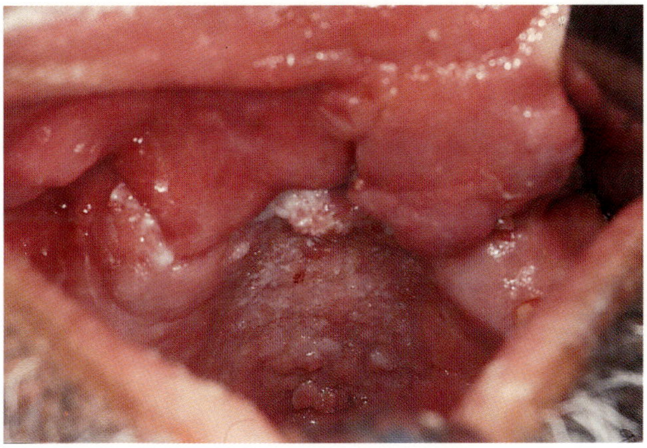

Figure 5–11. Recurrent disease 70 days after initial treatment.

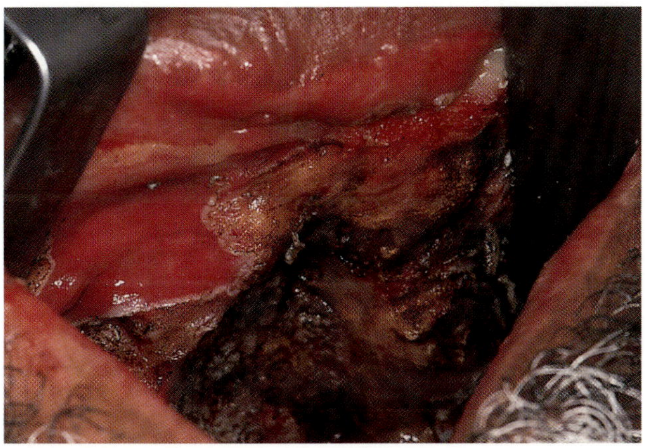

Figure 5–12. Retreatment again using the microscope delivery system, superpulsed at a PD of 780 W/cm^2.

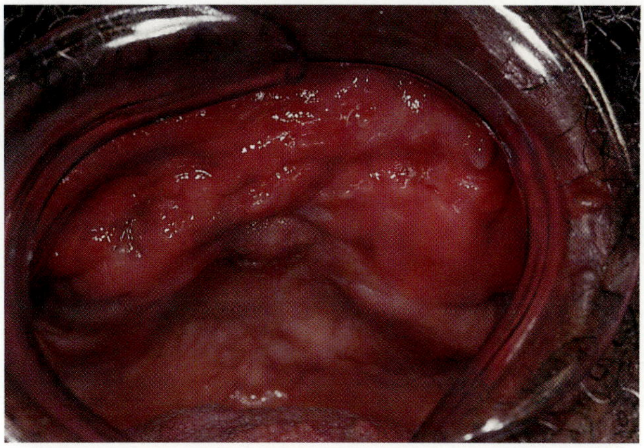

Figure 5–13. One year after treatment and 5 months after maxillary ridge augmentation with corticocancellous block iliac crestal bone.

REFERENCES

1. Pogrel M, Yen C, Hansen L. A comparison of carbon dioxide laser, liquid nitrogren cryosurgery, and scalpel wound in healing. *Oral Surg Oral Med Oral Pathol* 1990;69:269–273.
2. Shroyer K, Gree R. Detection of human papillomavirus DNA by in situ DNA hybridization and polymerase chain reaction in premalignant and malignant oral lesions. *Oral Surg Oral Med Oral Pathol* 1991;71:708–713.
3. Pecaro B, Garehim W. The CO_2 laser in oral and maxillofacial surgery. *J Oral Maxillofac Surg* 1983;41:725–728.
4. Duncavage J, Ossoff R. Use of the CO_2 laser for malignant disease of the oral cavity. *Lasers Surg Med* 1986;6:442–444.
5. Eversole L. Viral infections of the head and neck among HIV-seropositive patients. *Oral Surg Oral Med Oral Pathol* 1992;73:155–163.
6. Greer R, Eversole L, Crosby L. Detection of human papillomavirus-genomic DNA in oral epithelial dysplasias, oral smokeless tobacco associated leukoplakias, and epithelial malignancies. *J Oral Maxillofac Surg* 1990;48:1201–1205.
7. Reid R. Physical and surgical principles of laser surgery in the lower genital tract. *Obstet Gynecol Clin North Am* 1991;18:429–474.
8. Sachs S, Borden G. The utilization of the carbon dioxide laser in the treatment of recurrent papillomatosis: report of the case. *J Oral Surg* 1981;39:299–300.
9. Scully C, Cox M, Prime S, Maitland N. Papillomaviruses: the current status in relation to oral disease. *Oral Surg Oral Med Oral Pathol* 1988;65:526–532.

10. Watts S, Brewer E, Fry T. Human papillomavirus DNA types in squamous cell carcinomas of the head and neck. *Oral Surg Oral Med Oral Pathol* 1991;71:701–707.
11. Woods K, Shillitoe E, Spitz M, Schantz S, Adler-Storthz K. Analysis of human papillomavirus DNA in oral squamous cell carcinomas. *J Oral Pathol Med* 1993;22:101–108.
12. Broker T. Structure and genetic expression of papillomaviruses. *Obstet Gynecol Clin North Am* 1987;14:329–405.
13. Garden J, O'Banion K, Shelnitz L, Pinski K, Bakus A, Reichmann M, Sundbery J. Papillomavirus in the vapor of carbon dioxide laser-treated verrucae. *JAMA* 1988;259:1199–1202.
14. Reid R. Physical and surgical priniciples governing carbon dioxide laser surgery on the skin. *Dermatol Clin* 1991;297–316.
15. VanHeerden W, VanRenoburg E, Raubenheimer E, Venter E. Detection of human papillomavirus DNA in an ameloblastoma using the in situ hybridization technique. *J Oral Pathol Med* 1993;22:109–112.
16. Eversole L, Laipis P. Oral squamous papillomas: detection of HPV DNA by in situ hybridization. *Oral Surg Oral Med Oral Pathol* 1988;65:545–550.
17. Cox M, Eveson J, Porter S, Maitland N, Scully C. Human papillomavirus type 16 DNA in oral white sponge nevus. *Oral Surg Oral Med Oral Pathol* 1992;73:476–478.
18. Cox M, Eveson J, Scully C. Human papillomavirus type 16 DNA in an odontogenic keratocyst. *J Oral Pathol Med* 1991;20:143–145.
19. Ficarra G, Miliani A, Adler-Storthz K, Woods-Francis K, Del Mistro A, DeRossi A, Riccardi R, Ravina A, DeMaio E. Recurrent oral condylomata acuminata and hairy leukoplakia: an early sign of myelodysplastic syndrome in an HIV-seronegative patient. *J Oral Pathol Med* 1991;20:398–402.
20. Marguard J, Racey G. Combined medical and surgical management of intraoral condyloma acuminata. *J Oral Surg* 1981;39:459–461.
21. Bradley PF. Thermal surgery in the management of maxillofacial malignancy. *Oral Maxillofac Surg Clin North Am* 1993;5:331–346.
22. Premoli-de-Percoco G, Galindo I, Ramirez JL, Perrone M, Rivera H. Detection of human papillomavirus related to oral verruca vulgaris among Venezuelans. *J Oral Pathol Med* 1993;22:113–116.
23. Chang F, Syrjanen S, Kellokoski J, Syrjanen K. Human papillomavirus infections and their associations with oral disease. *J Oral Pathol Med* 1991;20:305–317.
24. Kahn M. Demonstration of human papillomavirus DNA in a peripheral ameloblastoma by in situ hybridization. *Hum Pathol* 1992;23:188–191.
25. Reid R, Keye WR, ed. *Laser Surgery in Gynecology and Obstetrics.* Chicago: Year Book, 1989:46–99.
26. Young S, Min K. In situ DNA hybridization analysis of oral papillomas, leukoplakias and carcinomas for human papillomavirus. *Oral Surg Oral Med Oral Pathol* 1991;71: 726–729.
27. Zeuss M, Miller C, White D. In situ hybridization analysis of human papillomavirus DNA in oral mucosal lesions. *Oral Surg Oral Med Oral Pathol* 1991;71:714–720.
28. Pick R, Colvard M. Current status of lasers in soft tissue dental surgery. *J Periodontol* 1993;64:589–602.
29. Pick R, Pecaro B. Use of the CO_2 laser in soft tissue dental surgery. *Lasers Surg Med* 1987;7:207–213.
30. Kellokoski JK, Syrjanen SM, Chang F, Yliskoski M, Syrjanen KJ. Southern blot hybridization and PCR in detection of oral human papillomavirus (HPV) infections in women with genital HPV infections. *J Oral Pathol Med* 1992;21:459–464.
31. Pogrel M, McCracken K, Daniels T. Histologic evaluation of the width of soft tissue necrosis adjacent to carbon dioxide laser incisions. *Oral Surg Oral Med Oral Pathol* 1990;70:564–568.
32. Kellokoski JK, Syrjanen SM, Syrjanen KJ, Yliskoski M. Oral mucosal changes in women with genital HPV infection. *J Oral Pathol Med* 1990;19:142–148.
33. Frame J. Removal of oral soft tissue pathology with the CO_2 laser. *J Oral Maxillofac Surg* 1985;43:850–855.
34. Devereau Q, Ustrell V, Pickart C, Rechsteiner M. A 26 S protease subunit that binds ubiquitin conjugates. *J Biol Chem* 1994; 269 (10): 7059–7061.
35. Papillomaviruses: particles, gerome organisation and proteins. In Syrjanenk, Gissman L, Koss LG (eds.) *Papillomaviruses and Human Disease.* Heidelberg, Germany: Springer-Verlag, 1987, pp 1–18.

6 Soft Tissue Excision Techniques

Lewis Clayman, Paul C. Kuo

GENERAL PRINCIPLES OF CLINICAL LASER APPLICATION

Surgical lasers are instruments with their own specific indications for applications. Consideration must be given to the nature of the lesion to be treated, its anatomic location and functional implications after laser treatment, as well as the benefits, risks, and alternate modes of treatment available.

Careful observation of the target tissue is well advised during laser application, particularly with the free-beam CO_2 laser where there is no tactile feedback and the depth of penetration is shallow. The beam should be directed perpendicular to the target tissue unless dissection of tissue underlying the lesion is desired. When using the continuous or rapid pulse modes, the surgeon should work expeditiously and with even strokes. Both the power density and the fluence may change with small variations in operative technique and may affect clinical outcome in sensitive areas, such as facial skin. Be aware of tissue that is in the path of the laser beam beyond the target tissue. Protection of the underlying tissue should be provided in anticipation of any laser beam that may "escape" inadvertently after cutting through the target. Recall that the width of the laser cut corresponds to the beam diameter, the depth depends in part on the power set, and the degree of coagulation necrosis on the duration of laser exposure.

The no-touch technique with a free-beam laser theoretically offers the added advantage of limiting transplantation of malignant[1] or infected cells because in the process of thermovaporization and thermocoagulation, the heat produced sterilizes the surgical field. In addition, blood vessels and lymphatics adjacent to a target tumor are also sealed. Some controversy may exist on the subject of tumor promotion by CO_2 laser since there is a report of seven cases of oral leukoplakia being treated by CO_2 laser of which five recurred.[2] However, this is not supported by more substantial series with longer follow-up[3,4] where the rate of recurrence or progression of leukoplakia is reported as to be as high as 28%. The CO_2 laser was also not found to promote tumor growth in a mouse-melanoma model,[1] nor was it found to promote metastases in a mouse adenocarcinoma model.[5]

USE OF CO_2 LASER IN INCISIONAL PROCEDURES

To use the CO_2 laser as a precise cutting instrument, the spot size at its focal point should be small, approximately 0.2 to 0.3 mm. A focus guide probe, along with a coaxial helium-neon (HeNe) guide beam are helpful in acquiring evenness in the cut when a laser handpiece is used. A pulsed CO_2 laser with a fluence of greater than 4 J/cm^2 delivered with a pulse width shorter than the thermal relaxation time of approximately 950 μs, allows precise tissue ablation with minimal lateral thermal damage.[6,7] This can best be achieved with a minimum energy of approximately 150 mJ/pulse. Where the target tissue can tolerate a wider zone of coagulation necrosis, such as incisions made in oral mucosa, a continuous wave (CW) laser may be used. At higher power densities the surgeon will have to work rapidly to minimize unwanted thermal damage. Charring will inevitably occur in inverse relationship to incisional speed. This char must be wiped away with wet sponges or cotton swabs as intentional or inadvertent second exposures on the desiccated charred tissue cause severe heat transfer. This results in creation of a burn in the target tissue. Traction and countertraction of tissue with sponges, forceps, or sutures will facilitate precise surgery just as it does for conventional technique. The target tissue should be examined to see if the desired depth is reached. As with a scalpel, several passes may be necessary to achieve this. Although this is a "no-touch" technique, the loss of tactile sensation with which surgeons are so familiar with traditional surgical instruments is easily overcome by visual feedback and a bit of practice.

Frenectomy (Maxillary, Mandibular, Lingual)

Maxillary frenectomy can be accomplished using incision and/or ablation. Either CW mode at 3 to 5 W with a 0.2-mm spot size for incision or a pulsed mode at 20 W, 50 to 60 pps, and 2.0-mm spot for ablation size can be used. Topical anesthetic is usually adequate but infiltration technique may be preferred. With the upper lip everted and the frenum stretched taut (Fig. 6–1), a short (3–5 mm), vertical incision is made through the mucosa of the midportion of the frenum. Horizontal releasing incisions are then developed

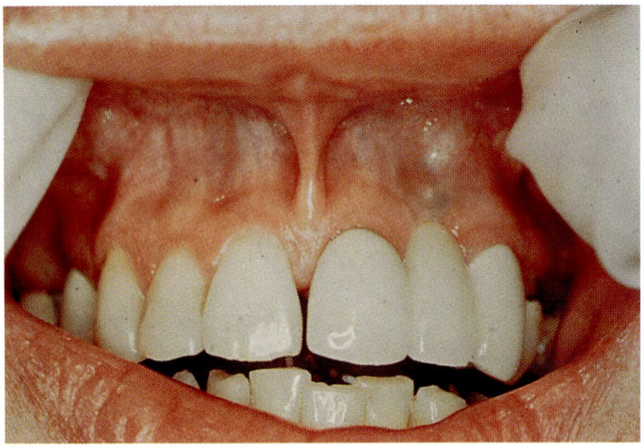

Figure 6–1. Low attachment of maxillary frenum.

through the mucosa on both sides of the frenum, which may extend to the periosteum. A diamond-shaped mucosal wound is developed as the lip-mucosal attachment is released. The fibrous band between the central incisors, if present, is then vaporized. The field should be dry (Fig. 6–2). Any small bleeding vessels encountered can be vaporized or welded closed by withdrawing the handpiece to increase the spot size and decrease the irradiance. Any char that develops should be wiped away with a wet gauze to prevent heat accumulation that may cause excessive lateral thermal damage on reapplication of the laser beam. Warm saline with hydrogen peroxide rinses are prescribed. No dressing is necessary. The wound develops a fibrinous coagulum in 24 hours and reepithelialization occurs in $\frac{1}{2}$ to 3 weeks (Fig. 6–3). Alternatively, a contact Nd:YAG laser using a fine scalpel tip at 8 to 12W CW may be used, following the same surgical technique.

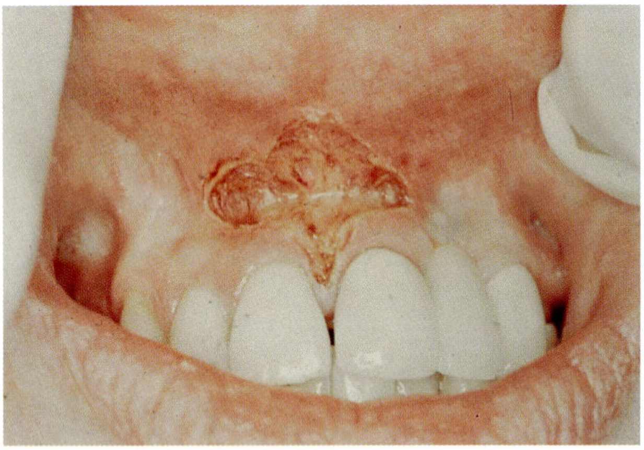

Figure 6–2. After 3- to 5-mm vertical incision and superior and inferior horizontal incisions a diamond-shaped dissection is created. Notice absence of char after use of rapid superpulsed CO_2 laser.

Vestibuloplasty

Other incisional procedures include vestibuloplasty and sulcus extension. Submucous vestibuloplasty is more commonly performed for the atrophic mandible, where denture adherence and stability is problematic. With the lower lip retracted and the mucosa stretched, the junction of the attached gingiva and the alveolar mucosa is noted. Using a focused, small beam spot of 0.2 mm at 6 W CW, an incision is made along the junction from the midline of the mandible posteriorly to the first molar areas bilaterally. Attempts should be made to identify the position of the mental foramen from where the mental nerves emerge. Supraperiosteal dissection can be carried out with the laser to the desired depth. Care should be taken to avoid the mental nerves. Because of the shallow depth of penetration of the laser, the soft tissue overlying these nerves can be dissected precisely, thereby avoiding damage to the mental nerves in their extraosseous course. The use of a split-thickness skin graft to surface the wound and inhibit vestibular loss from upward migration of the mimetic muscles during healing is

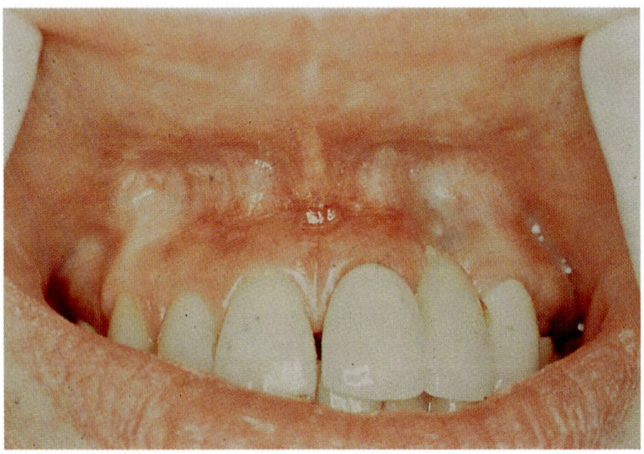

Figure 6–3. Treatment area healed at 24 days.

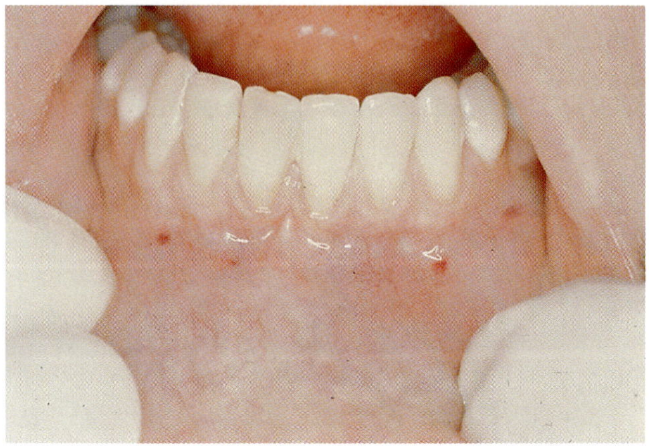

Figure 6–4. High frenal attachment in mandible.

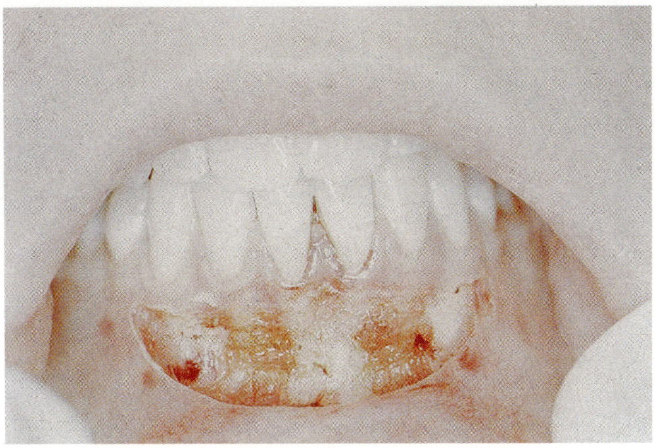

Figure 6–5. Linear dissection using 0.2-mm spot at 6 W CW function. Expanding dissection to compensate for expected regression after submucosal vestibuloplasty technique.

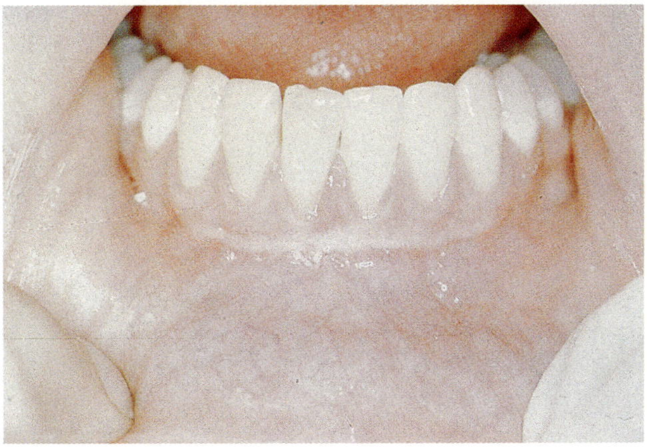

Figure 6–6. Healed treatment area at 5 weeks. High frenal attachment has been lowered, but as expected without mucosal free grafting, some loss of vestibular depth has occurred.

advisable. The flanges of the existing denture are extended and relined to use as a surgical stent for 7 to 10 days. Routine oral hygiene is adequate thereafter (Figs. 6–4 to 6–6).

USE OF THE CO_2 LASER IN EXCISIONAL PROCEDURES

The CO_2 laser offers a number of advantages when used as an excisional instrument, particularly for small to moderate-sized mucosal, submucosal and cutaneous lesions. The procedure is usually simple and straightforward. The excisional depth can be easily controlled. A good specimen can be obtained with little damage to the margins, although one must include an additional 1 to 2 mm of marginal tissue more than would otherwise be adequate with conventional scalpel excision, to allow for tissue lost by vaporization or damaged by coagulation necrosis. The surgical wound usually does not need to be sutured. An outline is rapidly made using repeated single pulses (175 mJ/pulse, 0.2-mm spot at 5 W) to circumscribe the desired target tissue. Following this outline, a laser incision is then made to the desired depth using the same method and laser setting as described previously. One edge of the cut margin can then be elevated with forceps and the lesion undermined and harvested at the correct depth of dissection with the laser. With the laser beam defocused, the surgical wound is briskly "painted" over in one pass (raster) to seal off lymphatic vessels and nerve endings and left open to heal by second intention. A fibrinous wound surface results and cellular infiltration begins after 3 days. Larger wounds can be packed with an antiseptic ointment (Balsam of Peru, Bips paste, neomycin, bacitracin, etc.) applied to ribbon gauze for 2 to 7 days.

FIBROMA

Fibromas commonly appear on the buccal mucosae, inner surface of the lip or lateral surfaces of the tongue. Presumably their origin is from trauma, particularly lip or cheek biting, although they may result as the final involutional form of a pyogenic granuloma (Figs. 6–7 to 6–9).

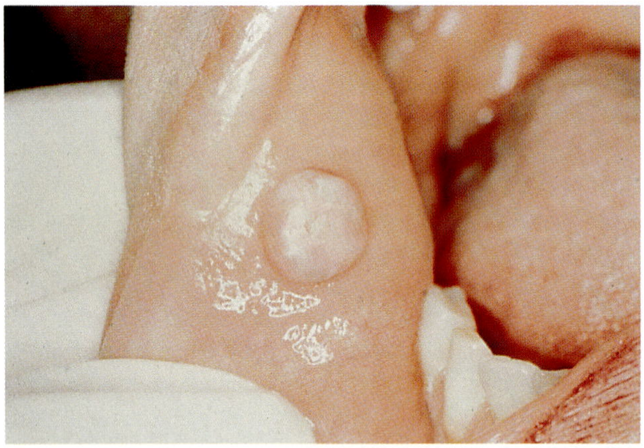

Figure 6–7. Large fibroma of cheek, quite close to commissure, probably initiated by repeat cheek biting.

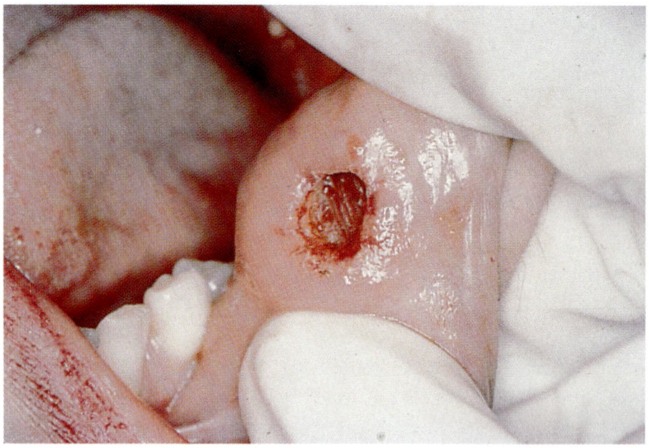

Figure 6–8. Defect left to heal by secondary intention after removing lesion with RSP CO_2 laser at 58 pps, 150 mJ/pulse, 0.2-mm spot size delivered with a handpiece at 6 W average output power (PD = 15,000 W/cm^2).

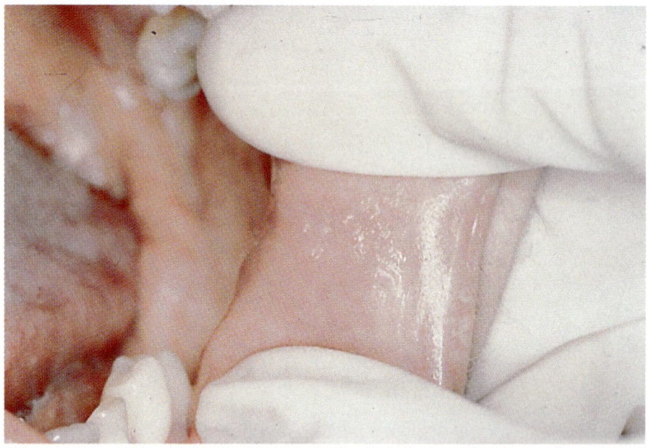

Figure 6–9. Cheek well healed by the 1 month recall visit.

FIBROEPITHELIAL POLYP

Removal of a fibroepithelial polyp of the tongue in a neonate is illustrated in Figures 6–10 to 6–13. The polyp arising from the dorsal midline of the anterior tongue was both interfering with suckling and causing consternation for the parents and the pediatrician. At approximately 7 weeks of age the patient was brought to the operating room where, using general anesthesia delivered by an oral endotracheal tube and without supplemental local anesthesia, the polyp was bloodlessly removed in one minute of operating time. Laser parameters were handheld CO_2 rapid superpulsed laser at 50 pps, evaporative spot size of 0.3 mm, average power output of 10 W [power density (PD) approximately 20,000 W/cm^2].

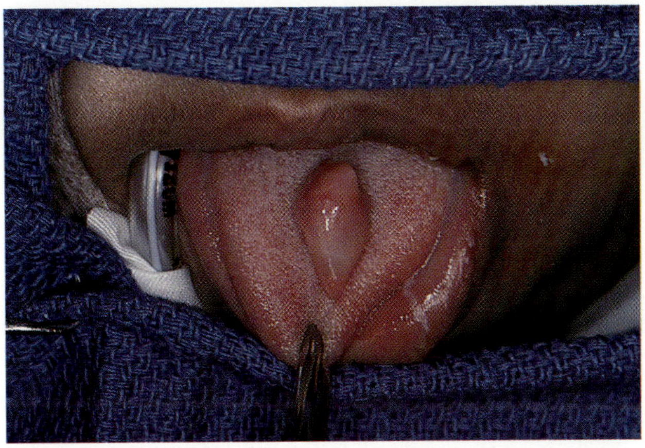

Figure 6–10. Fibroepithelial polyp of dorsal midline of tongue.

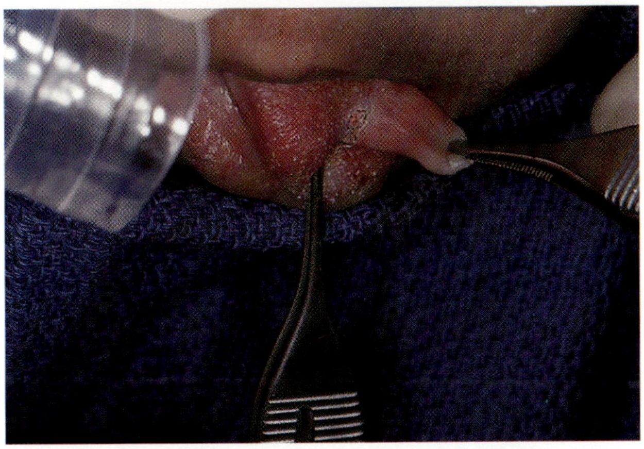

Figure 6–11. Lesion placed under traction as incision commences across base of lesion. Note HeNe guiding beam in center of incision.

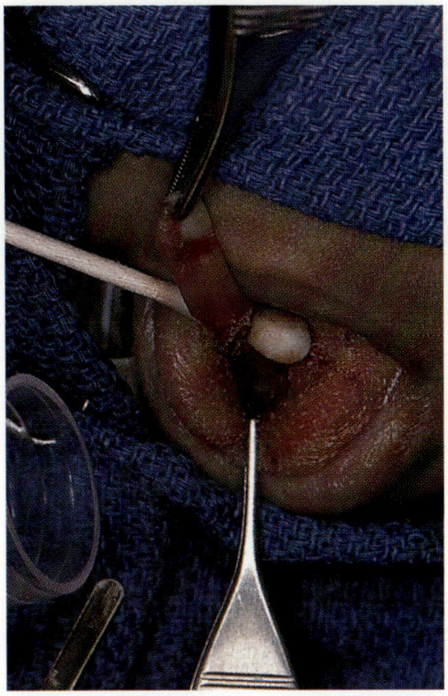

Figure 6–12. Transection almost complete, cotton swab placed behind target area to prevent unwanted laser contact with adjacent tissue as transection is completed. No bleeding occurred during surgery.

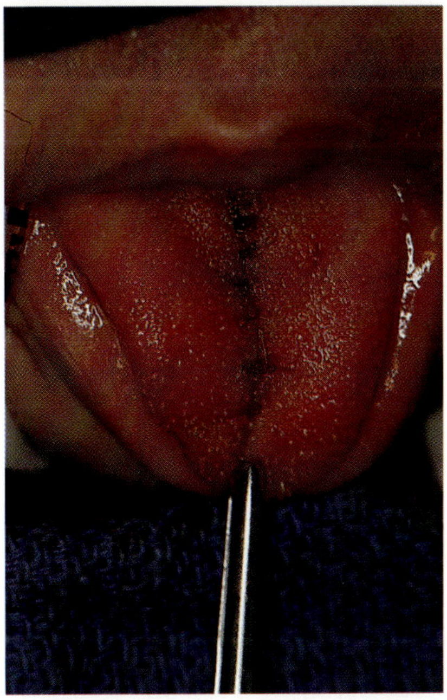

Figure 6–13. Primary closure of surgical site with resorbable suture.

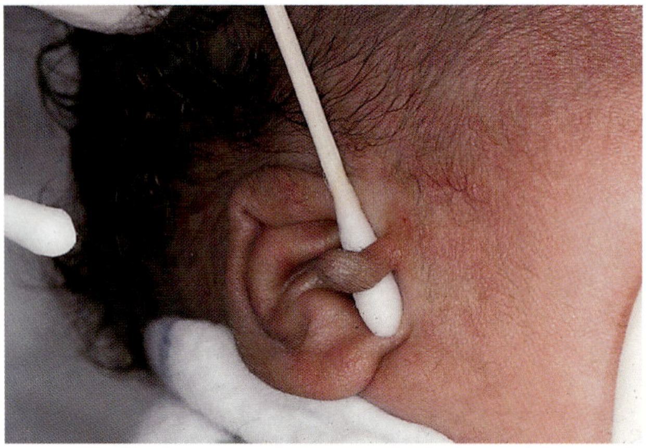

Figure 6–14. Ear tag lifted away from underlying normal skin by a cotton tipped applicator, which also protected the underlying normal skin.

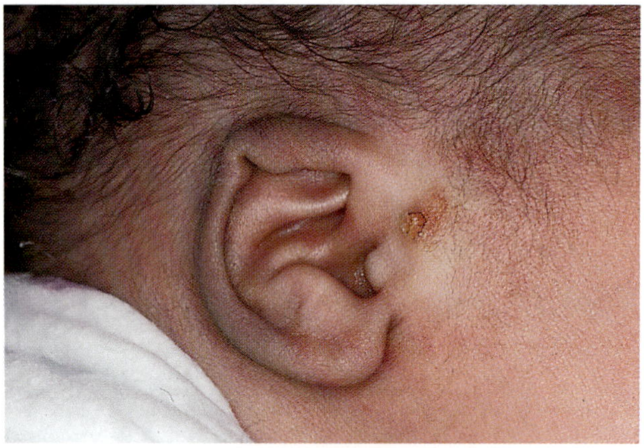

Figure 6–15. Surgical site at conclusion of laser surgery. Area was resurfaced in approximately 10 days.

EAR TAG

Skin tags occasionally occur in newborns as well as adults. In this illustrative case a consultation was received from the newborn nursery to remove an ear tag. Otologic and auditory examinations were normal.

The baby was brought to the laser lab where he was first fed. Then, after falling asleep the base of the lesion was infiltrated with 0.25 mL of 2% lidocaine. The lesion was then removed with the superpulsed CO_2 laser at 6 W average output power, 0.3-mm spot size using a handpiece at 118 pps. The operation required less than a minute and there was no blood loss (Figs. 6–14 to 6–15).

A similar case in an adult man from India is illustrated in Figures 6–16 to 6–18.

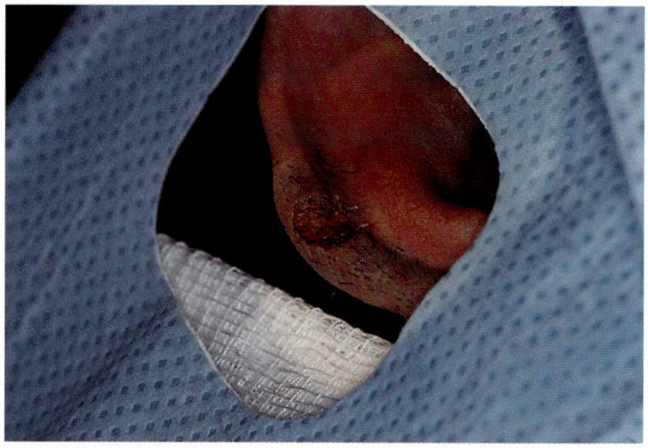

Figure 6–17. Base of treatment of area after excision of skin tag. Dissection performed after injection of local anesthetic at 6 W, 0.3-mm spot size, 118 pps in RSP mode. Note complete absence of char. Skin was completely healed by 17 days.

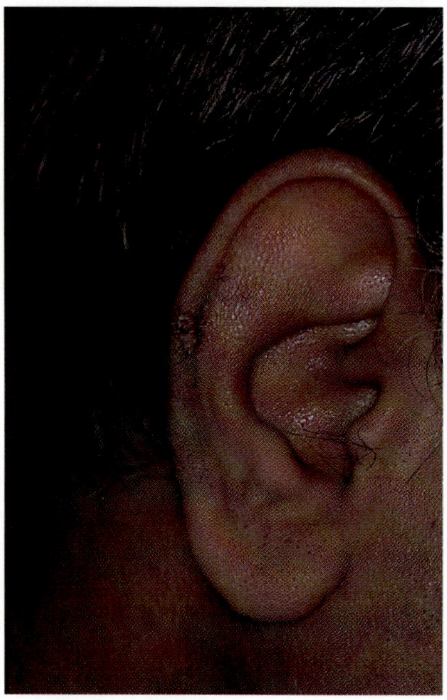

Figure 6–16. Skin tag along periphery of the helix of the right ear.

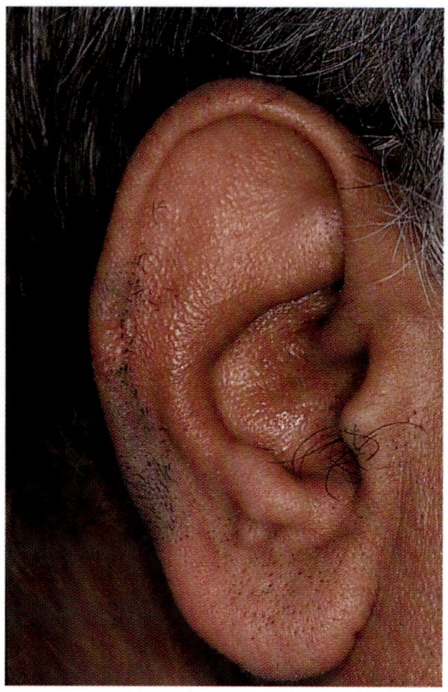

Figure 6–18. Long-term appearance 4 years later.

EXPOSURE OF IMPACTED TEETH

Although exposure of impacted teeth (soft tissue impaction) is easily accomplished in the dental operatory using local anesthesia and a loop cautery, there is less swelling, less postoperative pain, and less chance of thermal injury to the exposed tooth if the free beam CO_2 or the contact heodymium:yttrium-aluminum-garnet (Nd:YAG) laser is used (Figs. 6–19 and 6–20).

The CO_2 laser may be used at PD of approximately 10,000 W/cm^2 at 50 PPS, 10 W average output power and 0.3 mm spot size to incise around the impacted crown of the tooth. As dissection proceeds, the mucosal flap is elevated with tissue forceps until the underlying crown is identified. At this point, the handpiece is moved away from the tissue to diminish PD, thereby permitting dissection of the mucosa away from the crown without marring the enamel surface from inadvertent laser strikes at high PD.

Alternatively, as illustrated in Figures 6–19 and 6–20, the Nd:YAG laser in contact mode using a short scalpel tip at 5 to 10 W average output power is used to excise the gingival cuff. Rapid identification of the crown permits the operator to avoid inadvertently damaging it by excessive heating from the scalpel tip. There is no bleeding.

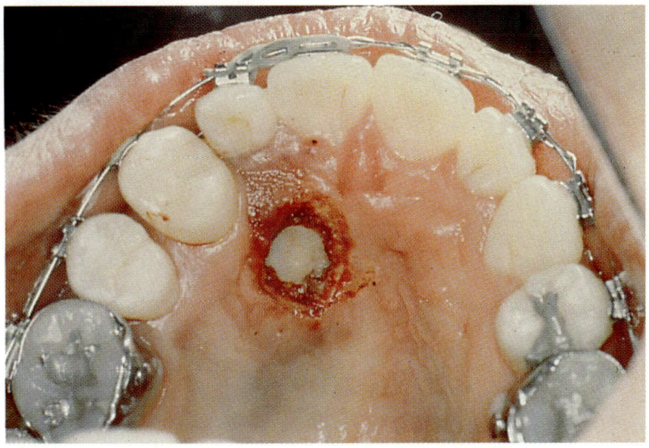

Figure 6–19. Crown of impacted tooth exposed. Note absence of bleeding.

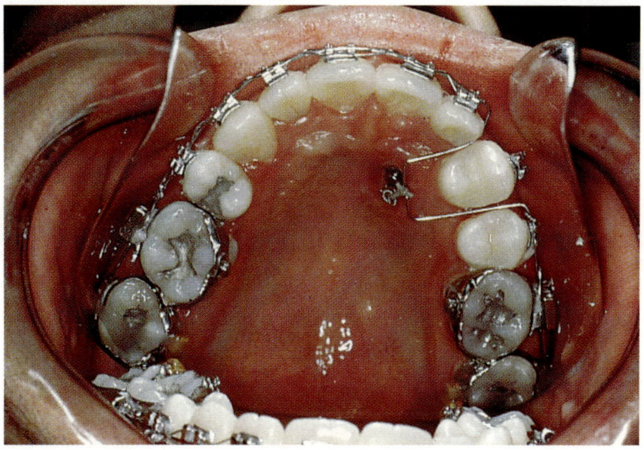

Figure 6–20. Mucosa well healed at 3 weeks. Bonded bracket ready to be used to start tooth movement.

FREE GINGIVAL GRAFTING

Lack of attached gingiva was treated by first dissecting away the alveolar mucosa with the CO_2 laser at 5 W average power, pulsed mode, 50 pps, 0.2-mm spot size. A completely bloodless and char-free base was obtained (Fig. 6–21). A free palatal graft was obtained with scalpel dissection and thinned with scissors to the correct thickness. This was secured to the recipient site with sutures (Fig. 6–22). The donor site was "sealed" to stop bleeding with one raster in the defocused mode. The graft was readily accepted and the mature graft is demonstrated at 6 weeks recall examination (Fig. 6–23).

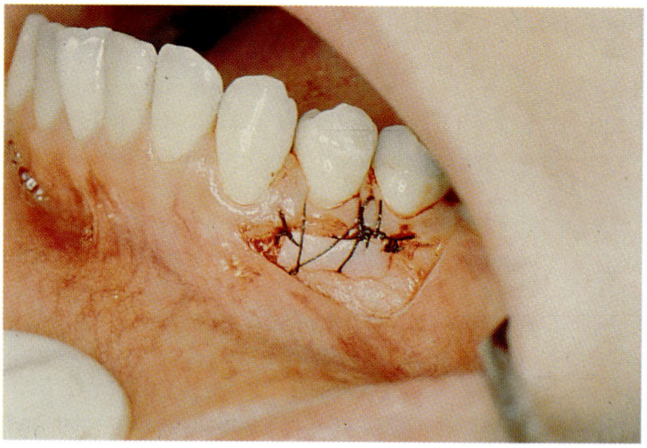

Figure 6–22. Free palatal graft secured in position.

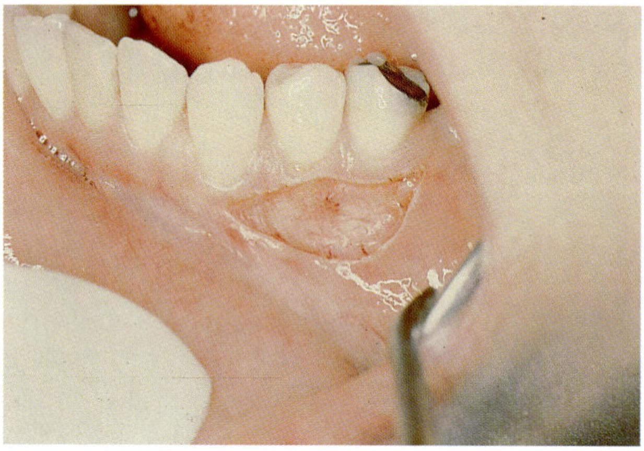

Figure 6–21. Recipient site prepared with RSP CO_2 laser with P = SW, PRR = 50 Hz, spot size = 0.2 mm.

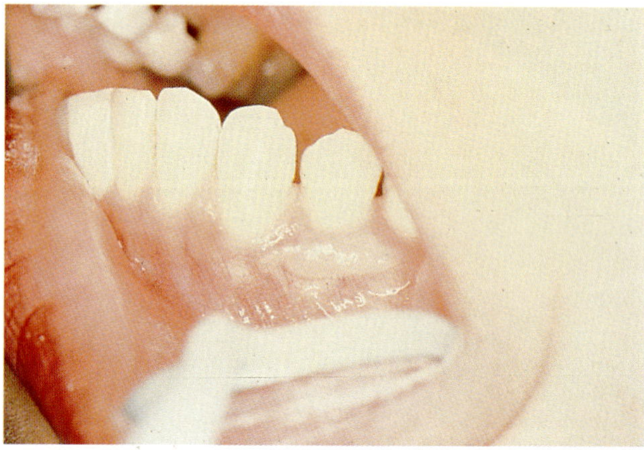

Figure 6–23. Mature graft. Complete "take" at 6 weeks.

HEMANGIOMAS AND VASCULAR MALFORMATIONS

Hemangiomas in the oral cavity are most effectively treated with the argon laser (see Chapter 3) by direct application after compressing the lesion with a glass slide or for larger lesions by intralesional introduction of the fiber. Large, higher-flow lesions are occasionally treated with the Nd:YAG laser. However, small, localized, low-flow lesions may be excised with the CO_2 laser. In the illustrated case (Figs. 6–24 to 6–27) a small vascular malformation of the labial sulcus was excised with the CO_2 laser.

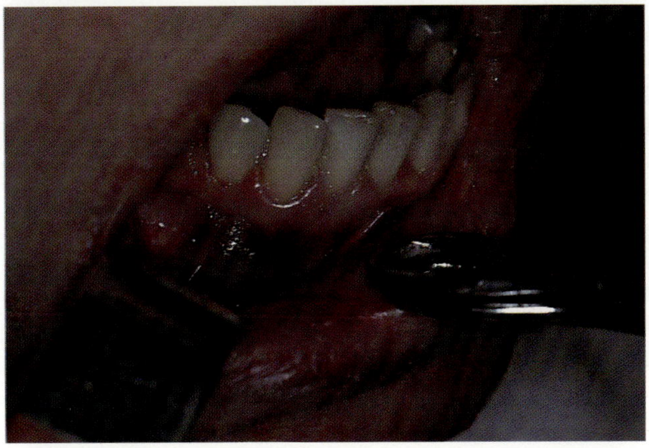

Figure 6–24. Small vascular malformation of labial sulcus.

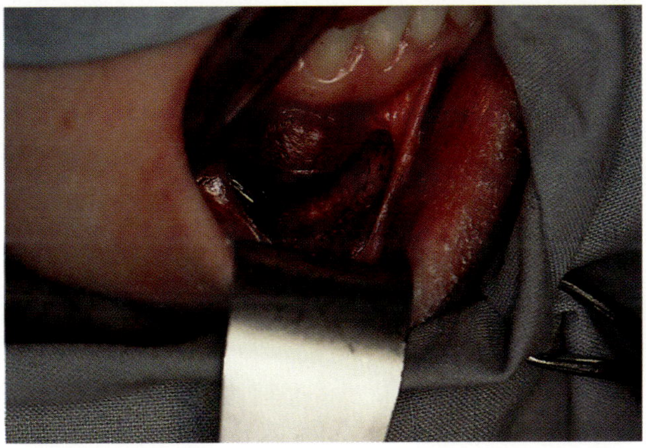

Figure 6–25. Dissection of the inferior mucosal flap. An absolutely dry field was achieved with RSP CO_2 laser, handheld at 118 pps, 150 mJ/pulse, at 10 W average output power, 0.3-mm spot size which was defocused when necessary to control small bleeding points.

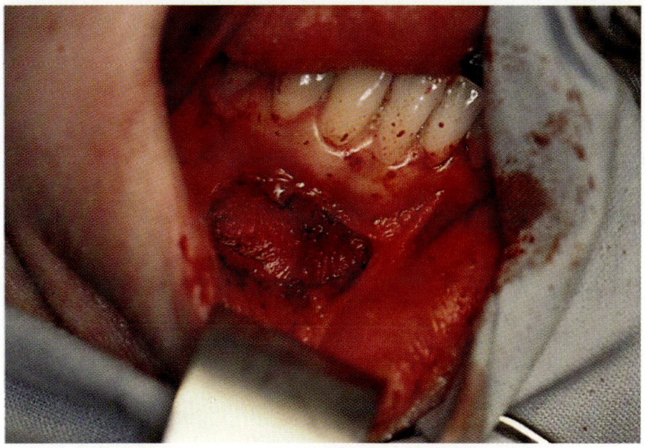

Figure 6–26. Dissection of the lesion itself.

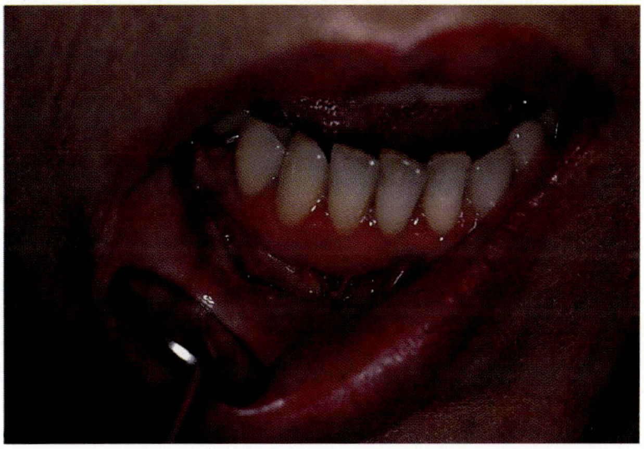

Figure 6–27. Two weeks postoperative, the wound was nearly healed with some contraction of the surgical site, which had been left open to heal by secondary intention. The surgical site was completely healed in an additional 2 weeks. Ten years later there was no recurrence.

USE OF THE CO_2 LASER AS A VAPORIZATION INSTRUMENT

Vaporization with the CO_2 laser is used when ablation of localized, superficial strips of tissue is desired. It works in a similar manner to incisional and excisional techniques except that a larger beam size is preferred. The PD used, which is best adjusted by varying the distance of the incident beam to target tissue, depends on the preference and experience of the surgeon. Slow vaporization with lower PD causes greater coagulation necrosis, increases pain and delays healing. On the other hand, vaporization can be achieved at a higher PD with little charring and minimal thermal effect on the adjacent tissue but also less photocoagulation for good hemostasis. In general, the power can be set from 15 to 30 W average power at 50 to 150 pps at 50 to 650 mJ/pulse. Usually approximately 100 to 150 mJ/pulse is used. A defocused spot size of 1 to 5 mm at the target is used. The target tissue is vaporized with a defocused beam in a "painting" (rastering) fashion. With deeper lesions it is better to ablate the entire surface of the lesion to the same shallow depth in layers, repeating the process until the desired depth is reached. Each treated layer is wiped away with a gauze sponge before applying the next raster. This prevents excessive overlapping of laser crater margins, which results in increased thermal damage, as can be the case when narrower areas are first vaporized to the desired depth. This is because of the Gaussian distribution of the laser energy curve (see Chapter 1) such that a laser crater may be clean in the center but charred at its periphery, especially when multiple passes are performed. This procedure is performed most accurately when the laser is used in conjunction with the microscope and efforts are taken to maintain a perpendicular relationship between the laser and the target tissue. However, careful use of the handpiece will usually produce satisfactory results. (For detailed examples of clinical use, see Chapter 4.)

GINGIVAL HYPERTROPHY

A 34-year-old African-American male recipient of a cadaver renal transplant receiving azathioprine, prednisone, diltiazem, doxazosin, captopril, clonidine, and cyclosporine was treated for hypertrophic gingivae. Key elements of laser technique for gingivoplasty include the use of a superpulsed CO_2 laser with the handpiece at a PD of 500 to 625 W/cm^2 by varying the spot size between 2.0 and 2.5 mm at 58 pps 600 mJ/pulse at an average power output of 25 W. A matrix band is secured around the cervical margin of the tooth below the free margin of the gingiva to protect the enamel and cementum from injury by the laser beam. Gingiva removed by each raster is wiped away to remove the carbonization prior to applying additional rasters with the laser (Figs. 6–28 to 6–32).

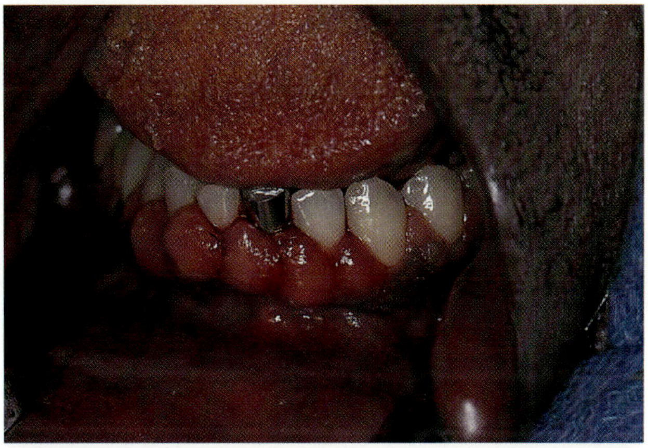

Figure 6–28. Gingival hypertrophy. Loss of normal interproximal gingival contour. Bulbous papillae and hypertrophy of marginal and attached gingiva.

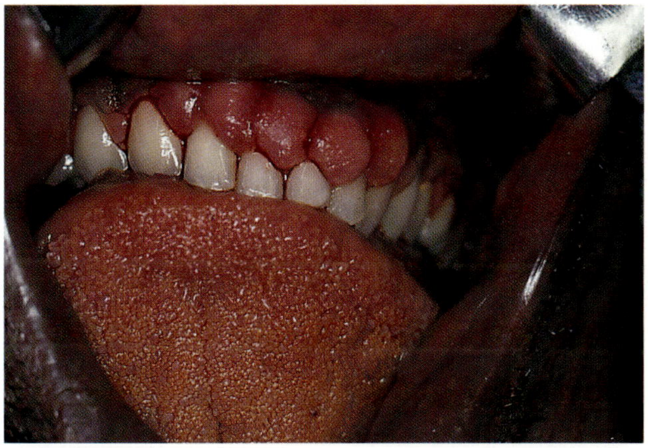

Figure 6–29. Tofflemire-type metal matrix band applied snugly around tooth at or below cervicoenamel junction.

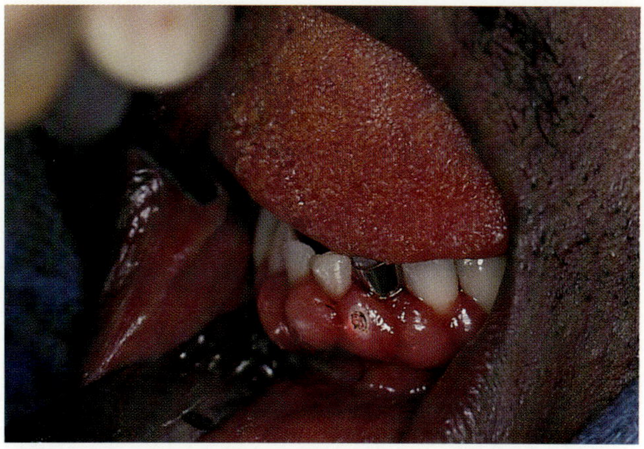

Figure 6–30. Series of test spots to assess for suitable PD to produce opalescent bubbling of first layer of tissue to be removed. Note red HeNe aiming beam adjusted to approximately 2.0-mm spot size.

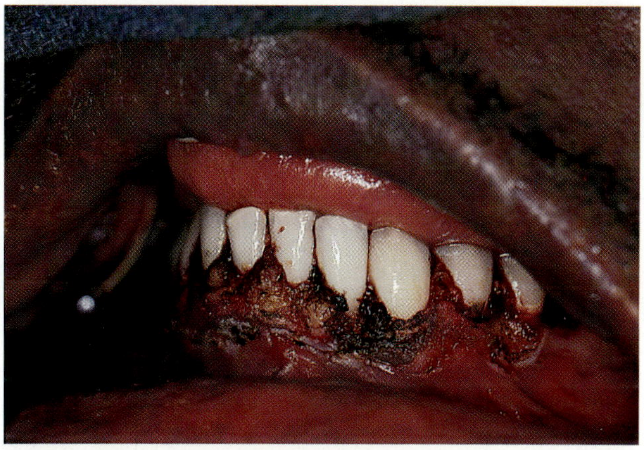

Figure 6–31. Gingivectomy complete; charred area consequent to defocused beam application to control bleeding.

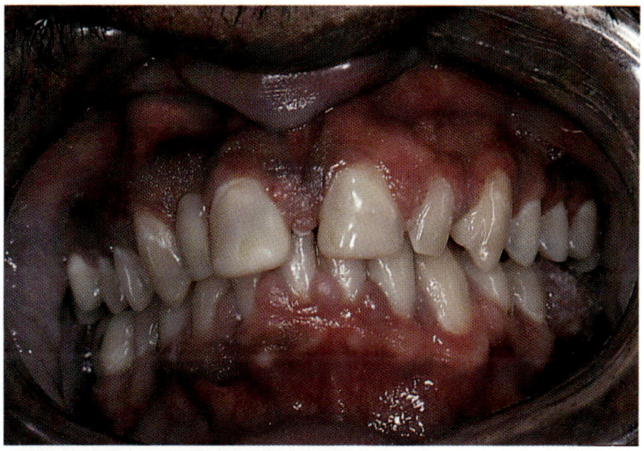

Figure 6–32. Six months follow-up. Patient has not received recommended dental prophylaxis every 3 months. Still on cyclosporine. Some recurrent hyperplasia present between the lower central incisors.

SEVERE GINGIVAL HYPERTROPHY

A 35-year-old woman with epilepsy has been taking diphenyl hydantoin in a stable dose for many years to control her seizure disorder. Gingival hypertrophy was extensive and was much more fibrotic than was the hypertrophy induced by cyclosporine illustrated in the previous case. A superpulsed CO_2 laser at 30 W average output power, with a 2- to 3-mm spot size was used. Blood loss was less than 5 mL and four quadrant gingivectomy, without the use of local anesthetic, required 60 minutes under general anesthesia (Figs. 6–33 to 6–36).

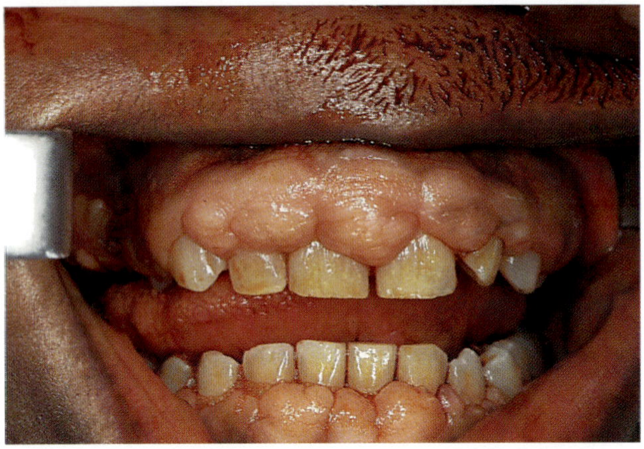

Figure 6–33. Severe gingival hypertrophy induced by phenytoin (diphenyl hydantoin).

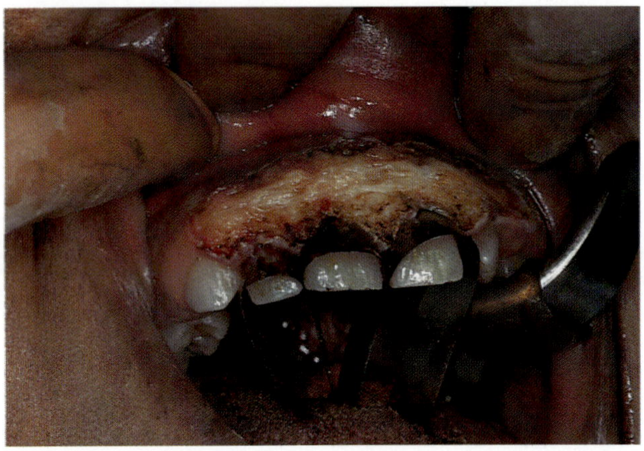

Figure 6–34. Removal of excess gingivae. Bone exposure was studiously avoided. Note placement of self-retained matrix bands.

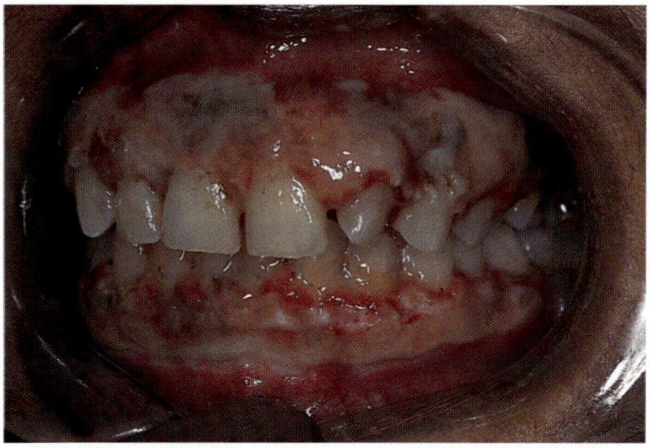

Figure 6–35. Healing gingivae at 1 week. At 2 weeks the wound was 50% epithelialized.

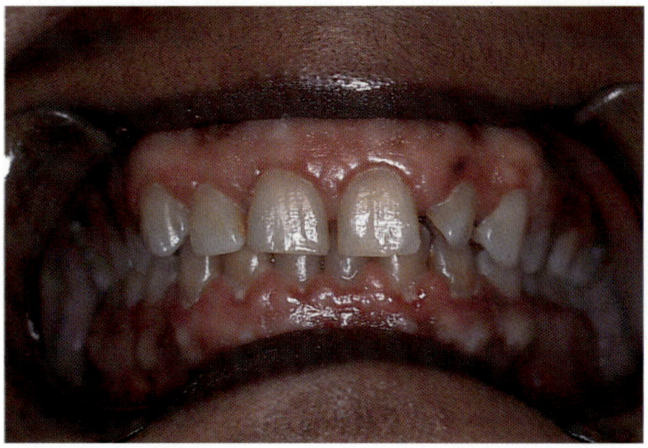

Figure 6–36. Two years postoperative.

FIBROEPITHELIAL HYPERPLASIA OF PALATE

A 65-year-old white woman with a history of rheumatoid arthritis, emphysema, and colon resection for adenocarcinoma presented with a complaint of a sore mouth under her upper denture. She smoked two packs of cigarettes per day, and took 2.5 g of aspirin per day, having completed a full course of gold therapy for her rheumatoid arthritis 8 months ago. She had a family history of an undefined "bleeding disease." Her coagulation profile was normal.

She has a 1.5-cm raised, reddish, irregular midline palatal lesion that, when biopsied, is reported to be representative of fibroepithelial hyperplasia of the palate. Ablation by vaporization with the CO_2 laser is chosen as the treatment of choice. Consequent to her medical history, this patient is admitted to the hospital on the morning of surgery and discharged the following day. She is treated under general anesthesia with nasoendotracheal intubation, no prophylactic antibiotics are used, and the surgical site is not prepared with antiseptic solutions. Local anesthetic with vasoconstrictor is administered for postoperative pain relief. At surgery, the CO_2 laser is used in the CW mode specifically to induce a greater than customary amount of lateral heat conduction to minimize bleeding. The parameters for the laser treatment are spot size 2.0 mm, power output 20 and 30 W, CW function, at average PDs, respectively, of 500 W/cm^2 and 750 W/cm^2. Surgical treatment requires two rasters at 750 W/cm^2 to remove all of the abnormal tissue followed by a third exposure at 500 W/cm^2 to coagulate the base of the lesion. Observation for 10 minutes by the clock at the conclusion of surgery shows no bleeding. Total surgical time including the period of observation is 27 minutes, and the estimated blood loss, measured prospectively, was 18 mL. The area ablated measured just over 15 cm^2.

Postoperatively, a single diflunisal tablet was taken for pain control on the evening of surgery. However, on days 1, 2, and 3 the patient required four analgesics (Synalgos) per day and a single dose of acetaminophen (500 mg), with 300 mg of codeine on the evening of day 3. She required similar analgesics for the next 4 days, and none thereafter.

By day 21, the operative site was 90% resurfaced with epithelium despite the heavy charring created at the base of the lesion by the coagulation of the base with the 30 W beam. Epithelialization was complete on day 26. There was no recurrence when she was discharged from follow-up observation 28 months after surgery (Figs. 6–37 to 6–46).

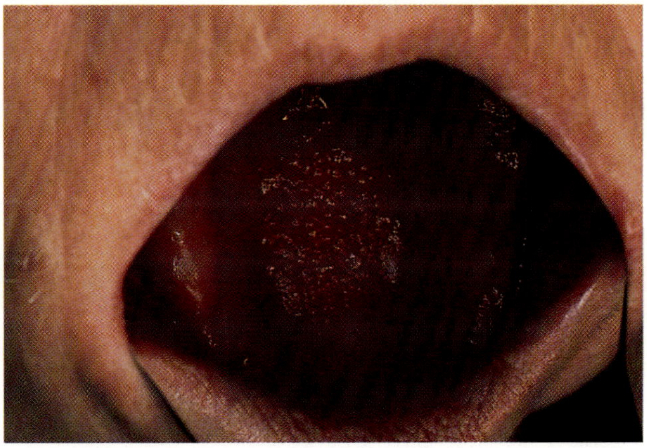

Figure 6–37. Fibroepithelial hyperplasia of palate.

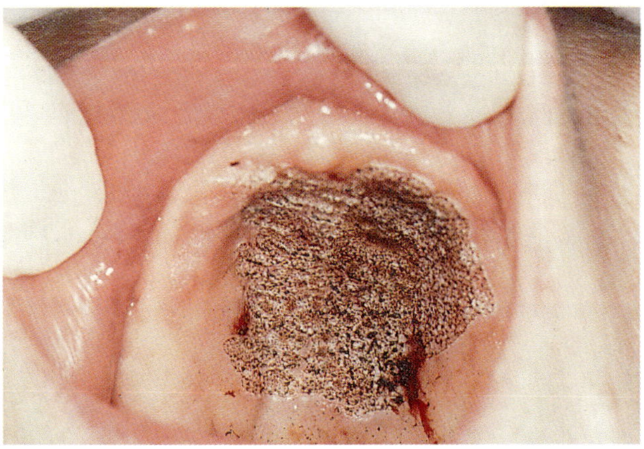

Figure 6–38. Completion of first raster, CO_2 laser in CW mode at 20 to 30 W.

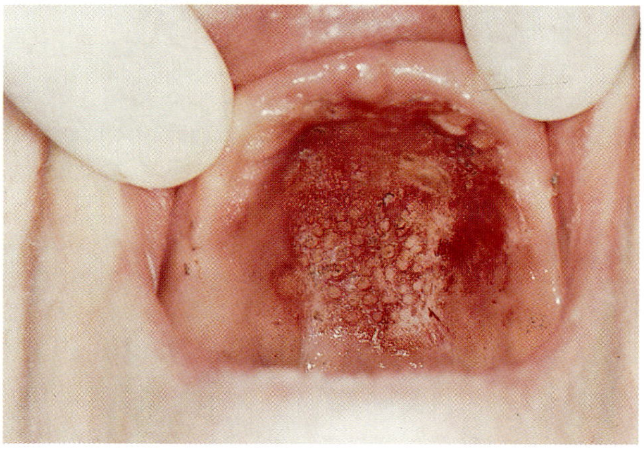

Figure 6–39. First raster after wiping away the char.

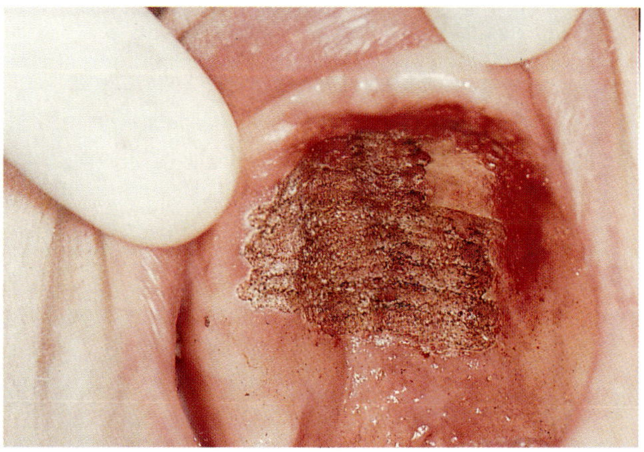

Figure 6–40. Last raster (third application of laser).

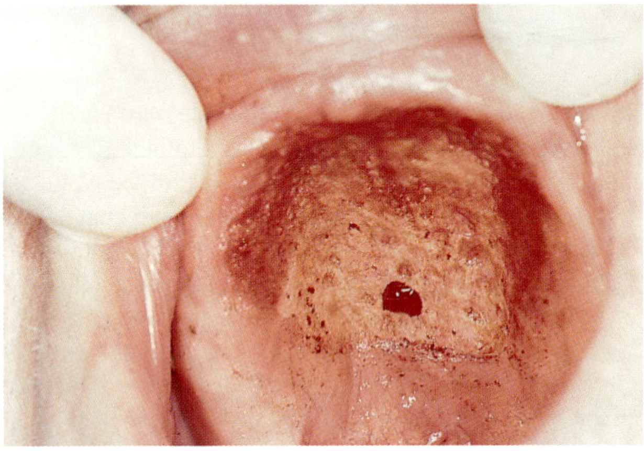

Figure 6–41. Last raster after wiping away the char. Note general yellow color as submucosa deep to minor salivary glands has been excised.

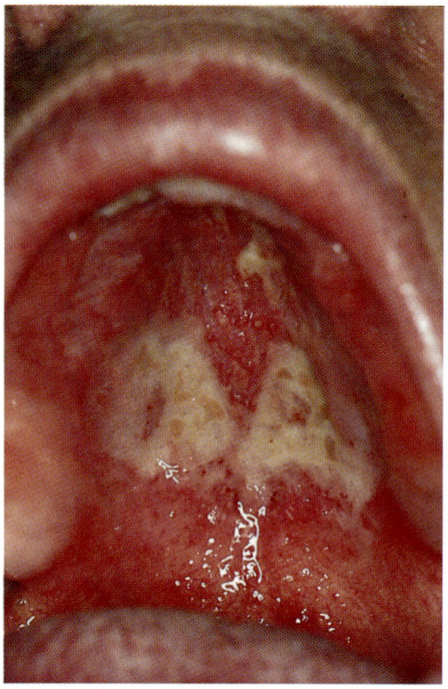

Figure 6–43. Day 6.

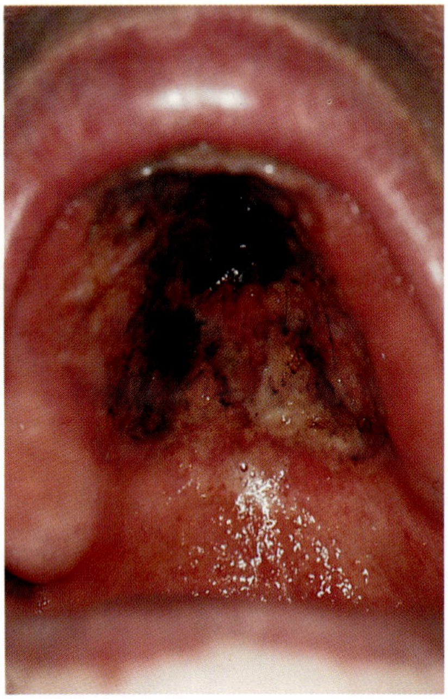

Figure 6–42. First postoperative day. Characteristic appearance of fibrin covering the wound.

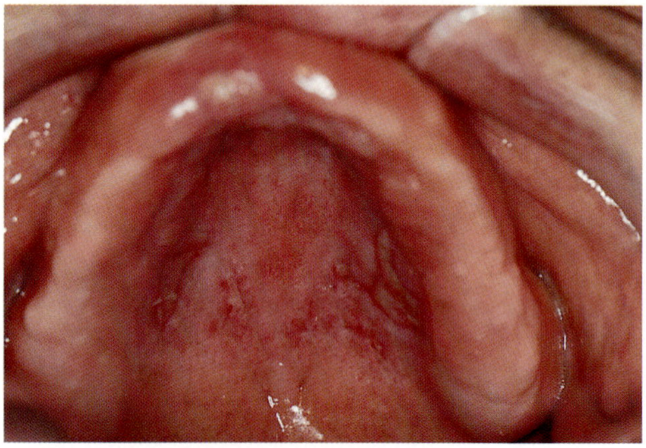

Figure 6–44. Day 19.

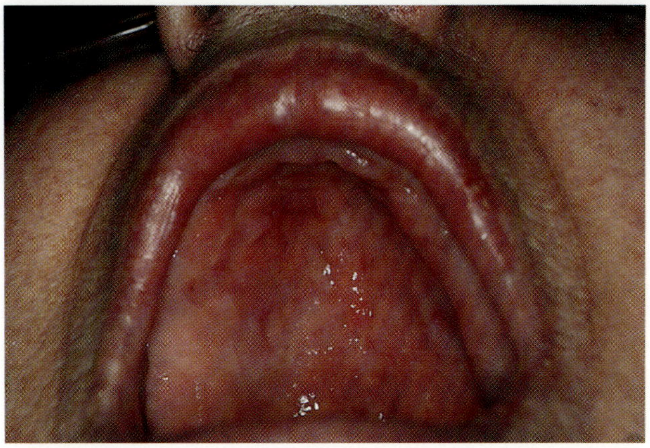

Figure 6–45. Day 26. Treatment area has become completely reepithelialized.

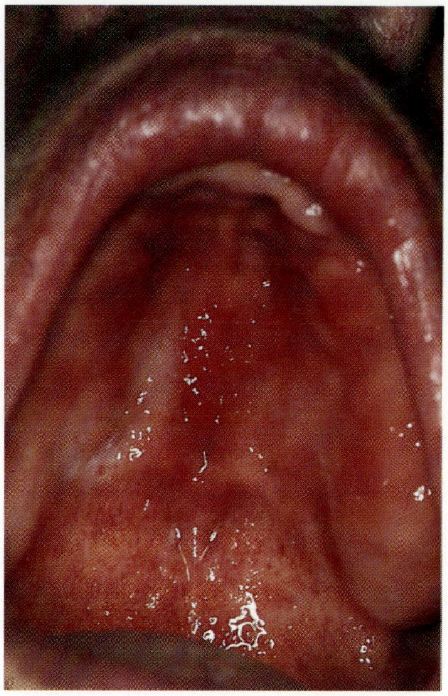

Figure 6–46. Long-term results; 15 months postoperatively mucosa has been stable.

FACIAL NEVI

A 38-year-old white woman sought consultation for removal of a nodular facial nevus present for the past 10 years. Vaporization technique with rapid superpulsed (RSP) CO_2 laser was chosen to reduce scarring. Laser parameters: RSP CO_2 laser (110 mJ/pulse) at 108 pps using the microscopic and microslad system. The laser spot size was 2.0 mm at an output power of 15 W and a PD of approximately 450 W/cm^2. The target site was anesthetized by infiltration of 1% lidocaine local anesthetic. No skin preparation was performed (Fig. 6–47). Two rasters were administered under 10× magnification and the surface of the target tissue was debrided with a wet gauze sponge after the first and second raster (Fig. 6–48). One year later there was only a faint depression at the treatment site and there was no change in skin color (Fig. 6–49).

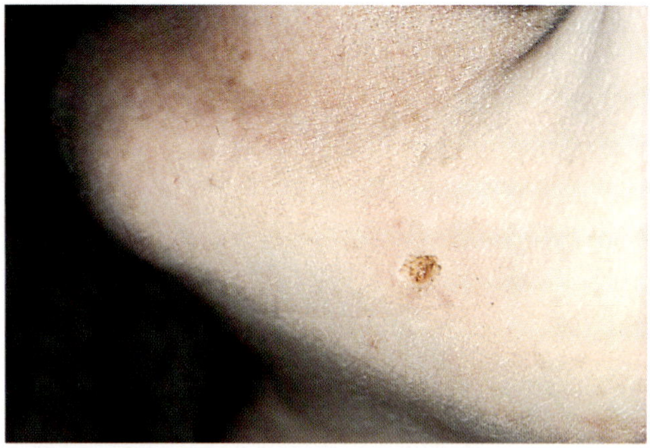

Figure 6–48. Treatment of nevus. After two rasters at PD = 450 W/cm^2, RSP CO_2 with microscope at 10× magnification.

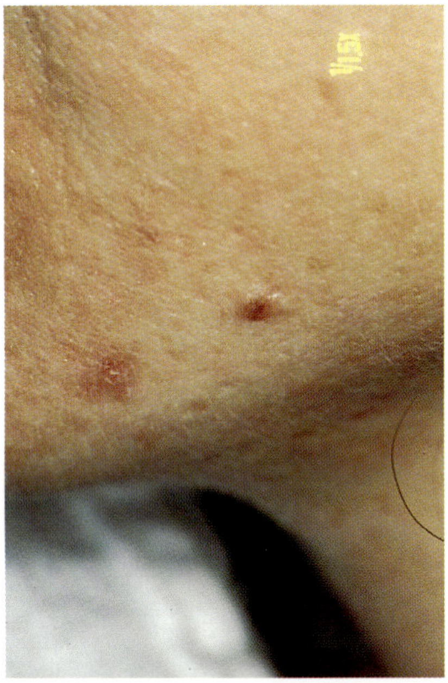

Figure 6–47. Facial nevus.

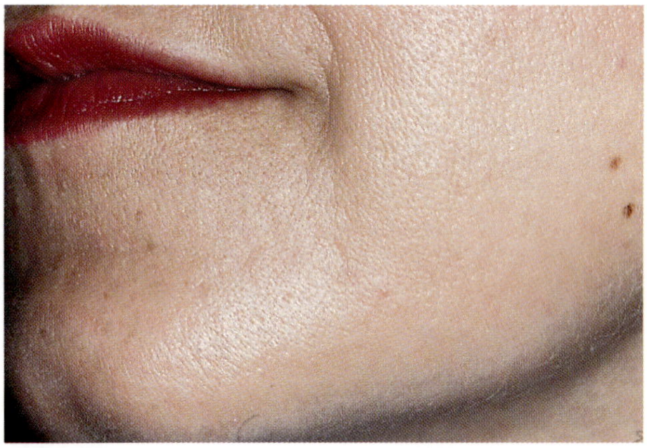

Figure 6–49. Result at one year. Very minor depression. Perfect skin color at treatment site.

SKIN RESURFACING IN AESTHETIC SURGERY

Skin wrinkles, or rhytides from excessive sun exposure, particularly those occurring on and around the lips and eyes, may be reduced by treatment with the CO_2 laser using an automated scanner such as the SilkTouch flash-scanner (Sharplan Lasers). This microprocessor controlled device creates char-free ablation by moving a high-irradiance beam at a rapid rate, thereby preventing the dwelling time at any one point scanned to be greater than the thermal relaxation time of the skin. The scanner can be attached to any CO_2 laser that provides a CW, collimated beam, and is capable of removing very shallow skin craters whose penetration level is restricted to the epidermis and upper dermis. The subjacent papillary and reticular dermis receives no thermal damage. The wrinkle is treated by ablating the area adjacent to the deepest point of the wrinkle fold with the laser set at 7 W average output power in the pulsed mode at 0.2-s cycles. This permits assessment of the laser effect after completion of a single cycle (one complete revolution of the flash scanner within its target circle). As always, the target tissue is removed with a saline moistened gauze sponge (Figs. 6–50 to 6–57). Pending the area to be treated, a second and third pass may be necessary to penetrate into or through the papillary dermis. Alternatively, a Computer Pattern Generator (Coherent Lasers) can be used with an ultrapulse CO_2 laser at 175 to 300 mJ/pulse and an average power of between 60 and 100 W. Benign cutaneous growths and atrophic scars and pits can be treated similarly (see chapter 4, White Lesions of the Lip.) Postoperative results are consistently good.

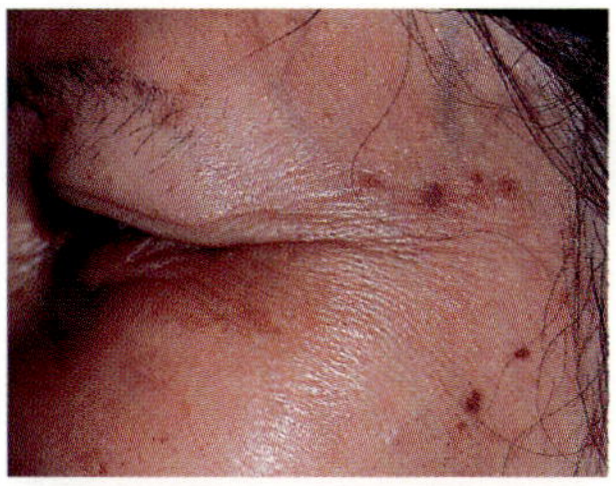

Figure 6–50. 62-year-old female with fine wrinkles in lower lid, lateral and infraorbital areas.

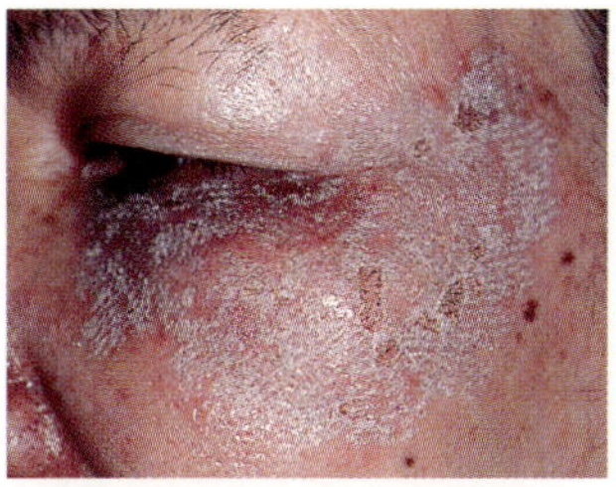

Figure 6–51. CO2 lasers resurfacing with Coherent Ultrapulse 5000C CPG scanner at 225 mJ, 60W, with one pass at moderate density over lower lid and 2-3 passes over lateral and infraorbital/malar areas.

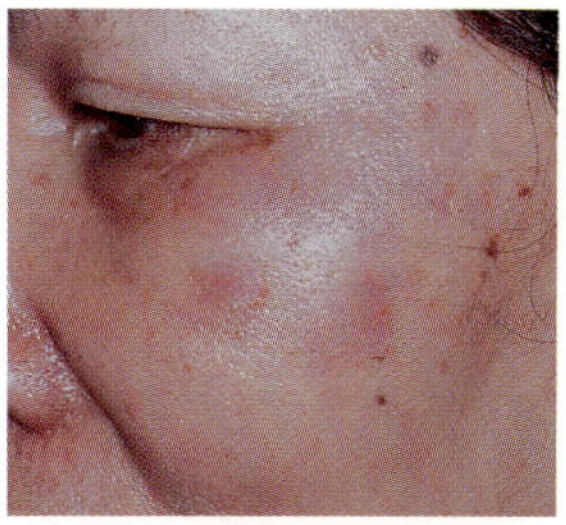

Figure 6-52. 3 weeks post surgery Note resolving edema and erythema.

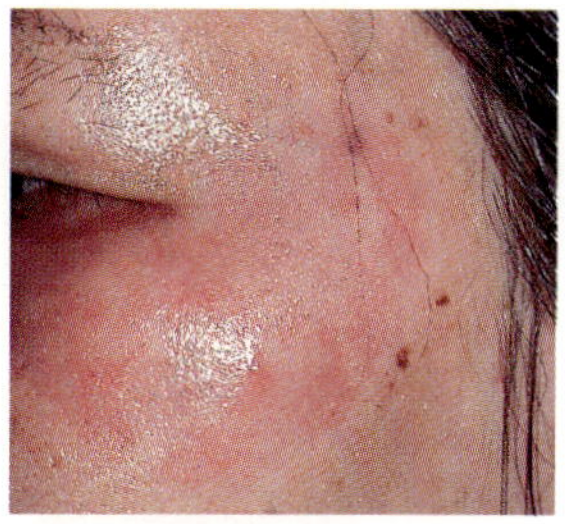

Figure 6-53. 6 months post surgery.

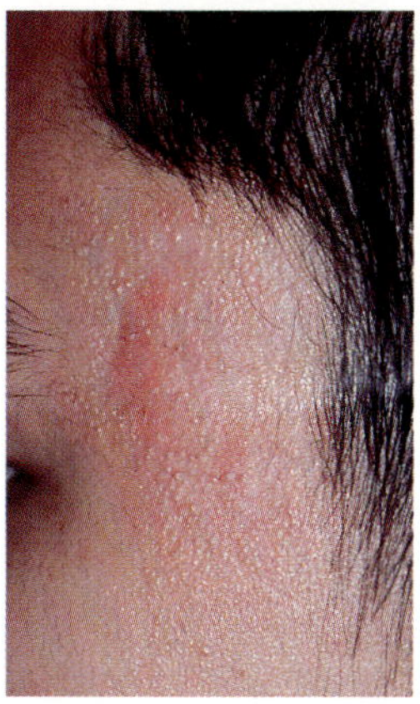

Figure 6–54. 18-year-old male with small area of burn scar, mildly raised, sustained 2 years prior, over right temporal area.

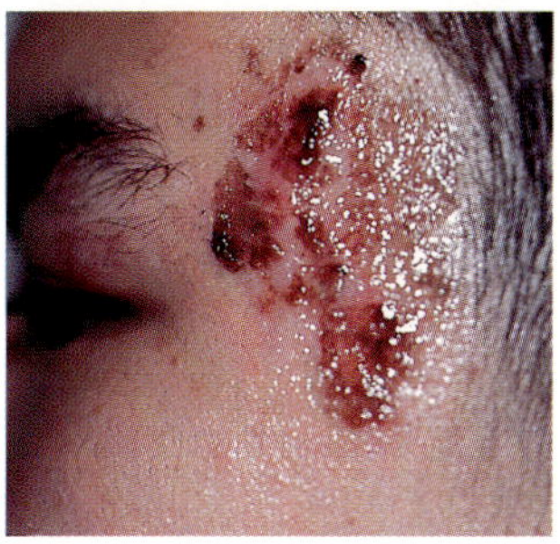

Figure 6–55. CO_2 laser resurfacing with the Coherent Ultrapulse 5000C CPG scanner at 300 mJ, 100W with 2 passes at moderate density.

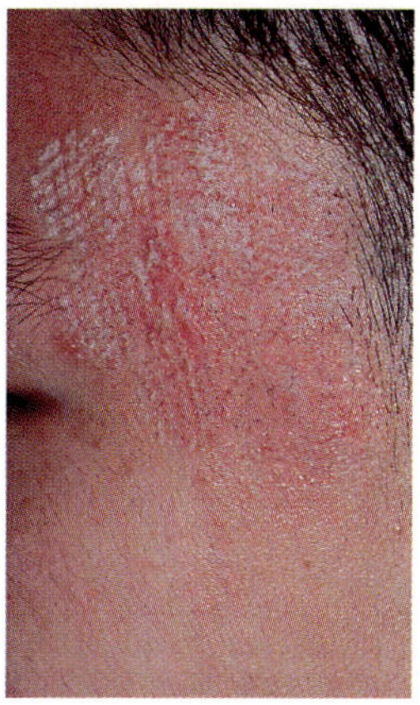

Figure 6–56. 1 week post surgery.

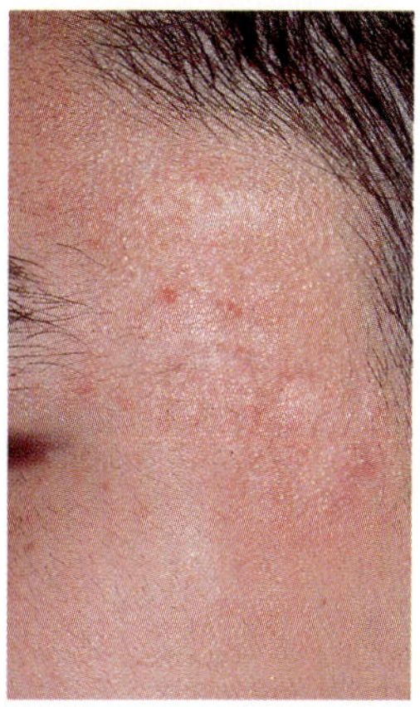

Figure 6–57. 2 months post surgery. Note smoothened area with the slight hypo-pigmentation, which is expected to improve in time.

COMBINATION USES

A combination of excision and vaporization techniques can be used in the treatment of certain diseases. In fact, the versatility of the CO_2 laser in its ability to incise, coagulate, and ablate by simply moving the laser handpiece into and out of focus is a major advantage of the instrument in its medical applications. As long as laser-tissue interaction principles are understood and adhered to, the desired tissue effect can be obtained.

Rhinophyma

Treatment of rhinophyma is an example. (Fig. 6–58) Previous treatment methods with dermabrasion was often incomplete, whereas electrocautery would leave significant scars. Recontouring with a scalpel is complicated and also difficult because of excessive hemorrhage. The CO_2 laser allows good precision and a dry field for easier sculpting. Thermal damage using the CW beam should be avoided. Excision with a small spot size at 5 W of power can be used in combination with vaporization in the defocused mode with multiple passes for recontouring. The presence of intact sebaceous glands should be noted on the deep margin to minimize scarring. Reepithelialization takes place in 3 to 5 weeks (Fig. 6–59).

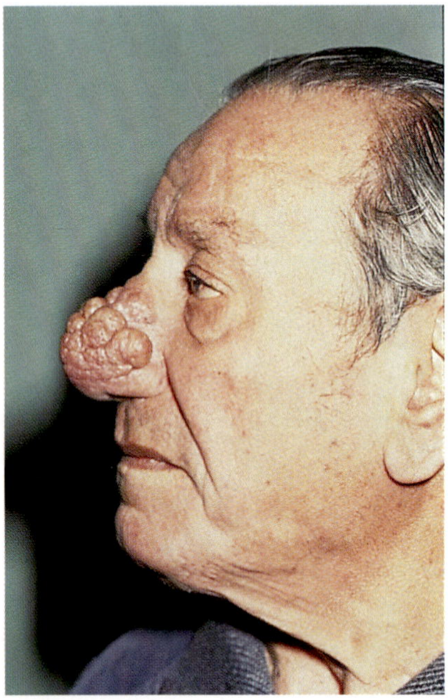

Figure 6–58. Rhinophyma. (Courtesy of Dr. Andrew Van Hassel.)

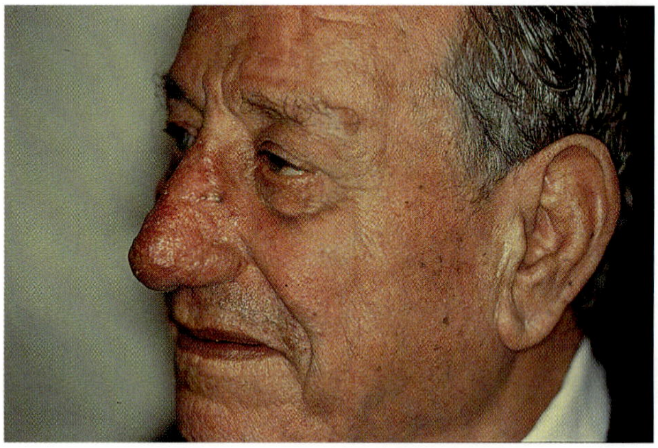

Figure 6–59. Postoperative result at 5 weeks.

EPULIS FISSURATUM

Epulis fissuratum, which consists of hyperplastic mucogingival folds from fibroepithelial proliferation secondary to ill-fitting dentures, prevents proper denture seating on a stable base. It responds well to laser excision with minimal postoperative discomfort and swelling. In this case, a defocused beam at 5 to 10 W CW is used to aid hemostasis and promote a dry field. Alternatively, a pulsed waveform at 20 W, PRR = 50–200 pps at 2.0 to 3.0-mm spot size may be used. The existing denture is relined with soft denture liner. The wound re-epithelializes in about 3 weeks with little loss or no loss of sulcus depth (Figs. 6–60 to 6–63).

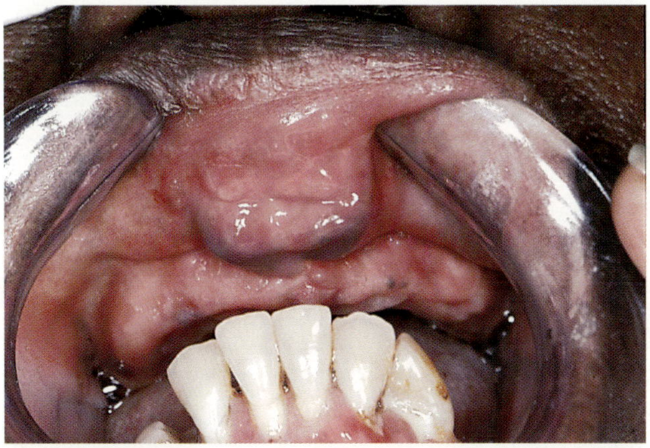

Figure 6–60. Epulis fissuratum secondary to a poorly fitting maxillary denture.

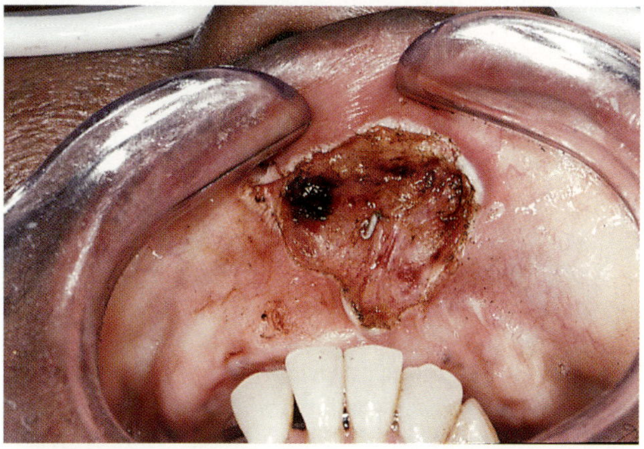

Figure 6–62. After treatment and wiping away treated area.

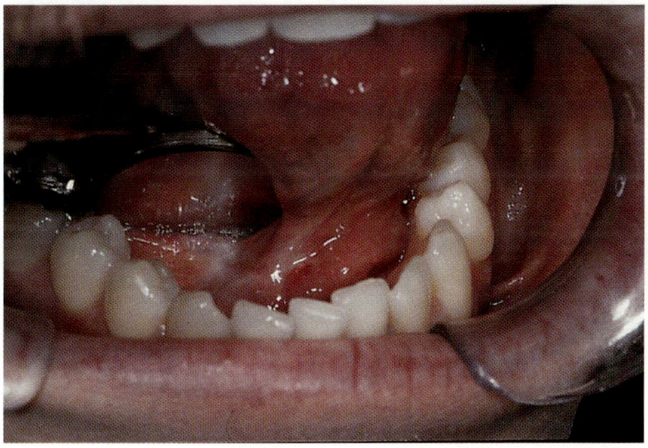

Figure 6–61. CO_2 handpiece. Focus mode used to excise much of the redundant tissue.

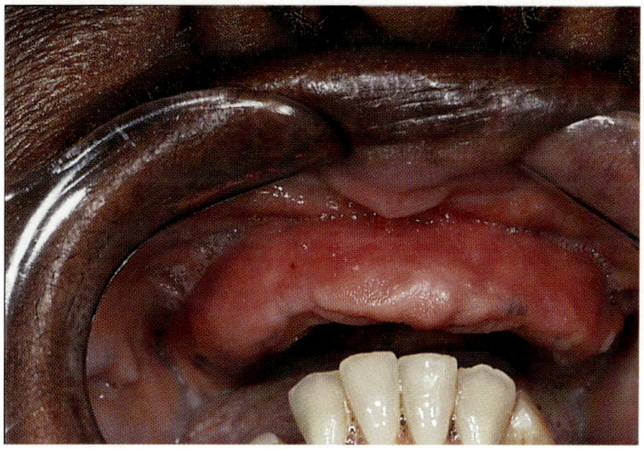

Figure 6–63. Three weeks. Sulcus deepened approximately 5 mm after frenectomy. Stability was maintained at a 6 month recall visit.

MUCOCELE

Mucoceles can be excised after mucoepidermoid carcinoma has been ruled out. At 6 to 8 W CW, the lesion is first unroofed. The gland is then propped up and excised in toto to prevent recurrence. Large ranulae are marsupialized by having the "roof" excised. The wound margin is then sealed with a defocused beam. Reepithelialization is complete in 2 or 3 weeks depending on the size of the wounds (Figs. 6–64 to 6–67).

Benign Pigmented Lesions

The CO_2 laser used in combination with scalpel surgery facilitates wound management and healing. Skin moles can be excised sharply with a scalpel flush to the skin. A pulsed laser at 3 W of power output with 200 mJ/pulse of energy using a 1- to 2.5-mm spot size can then be used to "paint" over the surgical wound to a slightly grayish color. The center of the wound may become slightly concave due to contraction of collagen fibers. The periphery or rim of the wound is then recontoured with the larger spot size and adequate energy/pulse to level raised areas. If residual pigment is present in the deep dermis, it can be left alone until such pigment rises to the surface of the dermis during healing. The area can then be resurfaced again.

Aphthous Stomatitis

A similar technique with the CO_2 laser can be used to primarily desensitize oral wounds. Mucosal donor sites in the palate can be glazed over to provide a thin layer of fibrinous coagulation. CW and defocused mode using a char and wipe technique is adequate here, as occasional minimal scarring can be well tolerated. Similarly, painful, ulcerative lesions can be removed and treated palliatively. Aphthous and traumatic ulcers are first painted over with topical anesthetic. A lower power, defocused CO_2 beam is then passed over the entire lesion including the red halo rim. The lesion heals in 2 to 3 weeks without pain. Likewise, lichen planus that causes burning and itching sensations can be treated with passes of CO_2 laser beam at lower power settings in

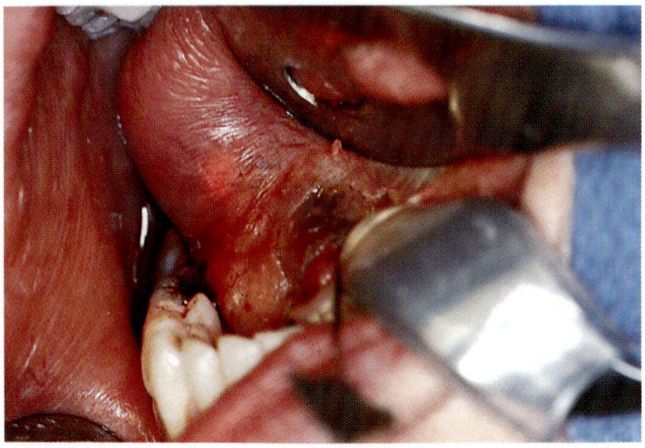

Figure 6–64. Recurrent mucocele of floor of mouth.

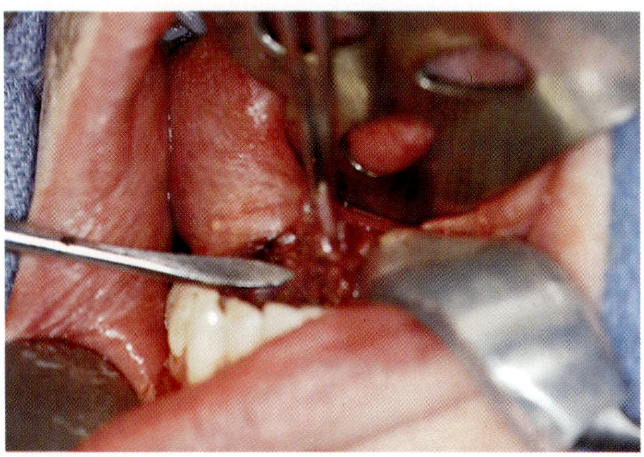

Figure 6–65. Hene guide beam beyond periphery of "roof" of mucocele, the central portion of the lesion is lifted with a forceps.

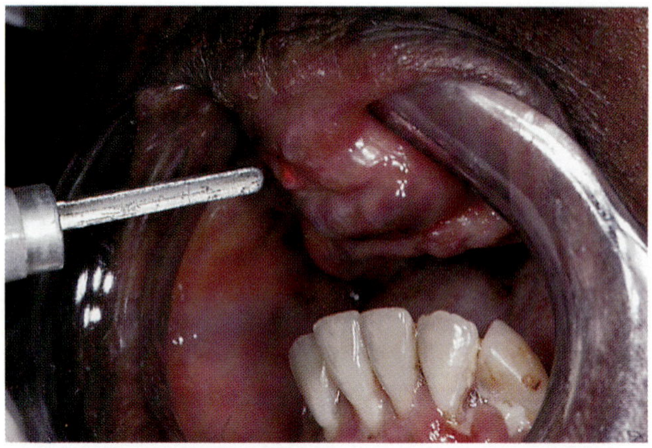

Figure 6–66. Part of sublingual gland ablated.

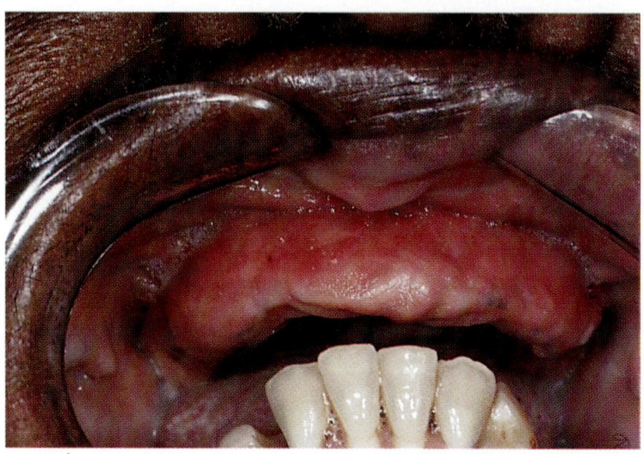

Figure 6–67. Three months. Slight scar at surgical site. No submandibular gland obstruction.

the defocused mode until the mucosal tissue begins to blister and turn white. This tissue can be peeled away with a hemostat and the underlying tissue assessed. Any remaining disease can be treated with a second pass. Improvement of symptoms varies from patient to patient. In general, some improvements can be expected with smaller lesions. The ultimate fate of the lesion, however, will be determined by the natural history of lichen planus.

WOUND CARE

The objective of postoperative wound care is to protect the wound, provide patient comfort, and promote healing. Wound care ideally should be simple such that the patient can perform the tasks at home. Smaller oral and pharyngeal wounds are left open, covered only with coagulum, which is the intermediate zone of coagulation necrosis. Carbonized eschar (char) should be wiped and removed. The coagulation necrosis widens in the first few postoperative days and sloughs, accounting for the delay in initial wound healing and possibly some increase in patient discomfort at that time. Larger oral wounds may be covered initially with gauze packing impregnated with a topical agent like Balsam of Peru, Whitehead's varnish, Bips paste, or an antibiotic ointment. Warm saline rinses four to six times daily and general oral hygiene care should be instituted. Skin wounds should be cleansed gently twice daily with a mild soap solution and topical antibiotic ointment applied. Extra protection with a dressing such as Duoderm is advisable until new epithelium is formed in 4 to 6 weeks. Sun exposure should be avoided for 6 to 12 months.

COMPLICATIONS

Laser-related complications in the orofacial area are minimal if proper precautions are taken. Many of the laser procedures are minor and can be performed under local or topical anesthesia. With the latter, care should be taken to monitor the pain tolerance of the patient and prevent patient movement. Supplemental O_2 should be avoided unless delivered through an endotracheal tube. Unintentional burns should be diligently avoided.

Charring is expected with laser burn. Charring promotes hemostasis but also can act as a heat sink and mask the depth of laser effect on tissues. The degree of thermal damage tolerance of the target tissue should be understood.

Long-term complications are related to regeneration of wound tissue. This includes granulation tissue, hypertrophic scar, wound contracture, and hypo- and hyperpigmentation. Management of these complications is similar to those resulting from scalpel or electrocautery surgery. Prevention of their formation by choosing the proper wavelength and parameters is paramount. Postoperative edema is usually minimal. However, both edema and pain will increase if poor technique results in excessive heating of the tissues during surgery.

The advantage of CO_2 laser usage is evident, particularly in treatment of widespread, superficial diseases, bloody procedures, and vascular tissues. It is useful as a surgical instrument in patients with bleeding disorders, patients who are on anticoagulants, patients in whom the use of epinephrine vasoconstriction is contraindicated, and in those patients who are on monitoring or pacemaker devices. It can also be helpful in infected surgical sites as it theoretically sterilizes during application.

REFERENCES

1. Oosterhuis JW. *Tumor Surgery with the CO_2 Laser. Studies with the Cloudman S91 Mouse Melanoma.* Groningen, Netherlands: Rijksuniversiteit; 1977:111.
2. Braun RE, Leibow C. Clinical evaluation of tumor promotion by CO_2 laser. In: SPIE vol 1424: *Lasers in Orthopedic, Dental, and Veterinary Medicine.* 1991:138–144.
3. Roodenburg JL, Panders AK, Vermey A. Carbon dioxide laser surgery of oral leukoplakia. *Oral Surg Oral Med Oral Pathol* 1991;71:670–674.
4. Clayman L. Management of mucosal premalignant lesions. *Oral Maxillofac Clin North Am* 1994;6(3):431–443.
5. Ammirati M, Rao LN, Morthy Ms, Buchmann T, Goldschmidt RA, Scanlon EF. Partial nephrectomy in mice with milliwatt carbon dioxide laser and its influence on experimental metastasis. *J Surg Oncol* 1989;41:153–159.
6. Absten GT. Physics of light and lasers. *Obstet Gynecol Clin North Am* 1991;18(3):407–427.
7. Rox Anderson R, Parrish JA. Selective photothermolysis: precise microsurgery by selective absorption of pulsed radiation. *Science* 1983;220:524–527.

7 Transoral Resection of Oral Cancer

Lewis Clayman

The most serious, life-threatening disease originating from the oral cavity is squamous cell carcinoma. Despite the potential for early detection, most oral cancers are still discovered in their late stages (stages III and IV). In the United States this results in approximately 8000 deaths per year.[1] The rate of new case formation is approximately 30,000 per year. Morbidity and late detection remain high largely because of the low rate of clinical examination by health care workers. The Centers for Disease Control (Atlanta, GA) estimates that in 1993 less than 14.3% of adults had ever had any type of simple screening examination for oral cancer. Of those people ever having been examined for oral cancer 54.4% had received this examination as part of a dental examination and 35% as part of a routine physical examination.[2]

Transoral resection of stages I and II oral cancer is a well-accepted treatment method in oncologic surgery. The specific surgical technique is less important than is the sound application of oncologic principles to achieve adequate resection of the tumor. The gold standard for outcome is the result achieved by scalpel resection. Any other technique such as electrosurgery, cryosurgery, or laser surgery must produce comparable or improved cure rates. Cure rates achievable with the surgical laser match those attributed to scalpel or electrosurgery, and also provide the significant advantages of better hemostasis, less postoperative edema, shorter hospital stay, diminished infection rates, and elimination of the need for split-thickness skin grafting. In addition, in theory, because of the laser's ability to seal small blood vessels and lymphatics, there is a reduced likelihood of inducing tumor microemboli during surgical extirpation of the tumor, which in turn reduces the chances of "seeding" the surgical site or the vascular or the lymphatic system.

SURVIVAL

The most recent survival statistics applicable to oral cancer are those published in 1994 by the National Cancer Institute of the United States National Institutes of Health for the period 1973 to 1991.[1] For the most recent interval in this series (1983 to 1990) the 5-year relative survival rate for oral cavity and pharynx is 52.3%. As expected, the survival is worse for regional disease (primary and neck involvement) at 41.5% and it is better for local disease (tumor, node, metastasis tumor staging—stage I: $T_1N_0M_0$, stage II: $T_2N_0M_0$) at 78.9%. Therefore, for transoral resection with the surgical laser to become acceptable, 5-year survival for local disease (stage I or II) must equal or exceed 78.9%.

Reports in the literature[3–6] regarding survival after transoral resection of localized oral cavity cancer using the CO_2 laser quote relative survival rates of 81 to 89% for previously untreated lesions. Collectively, 178 patients were studied, of whom 22 were monitored for 2 years and 156 were monitored for 5 years. As reported later in this chapter, in my own experience at Sinai Hospital of Detroit, 106 patients have been treated by transoral resection with the free-beam CO_2 laser. Of this group, 43 patients with 51 stage I or II oral cancers have been under surveillance for more than 5 years. The determinate 5-year survival rate is 92.3%.[7] Serendipitously, it is noted that for T_2 glottic cancer, a nonoral head and neck site, endoscopic excision with the free-beam CO_2 laser resulted in a 5-year local control rate of 94% with a 5-year survival rate of 78% with deaths attributable to either a second primary cancer or intercurrent disease.[8]

One of the questions to consider that could theoretically have a negative effect on local recurrence is the possibility that cancer cells that are not clinically apparent during surgery could become buried and maintain their viability after losing continuity with the epithelial surface from which they arose. This question was considered and investigated during studies of CO_2 laser ablation of the transformation zone in cases of cervical intraepithelial neoplasia. During colposcopic and histopathologic assessment it was noted that recurrent lesions did maintain contact with the surface epithelium. They did not lie dormant as buried crypts of abnormal epithelium that would then have the potential to grow into neoplasms later.[9]

Compared with patients having stages I and II oral cavity tumors that were treated by conventional surgery using transoral resection technique, the laser-treated cases did not show increased local recurrence or regional metastases. In concordance with the National Cancer Institute data individual studies from the literature reporting cure rates for conventional surgery of previously untreated localized tongue and floor of mouth cancer ranged from 86% to as high as 94% for 2 years for T_1 lesions and 69 to 86% for T_2 lesions.[1,5,10–12] At 5 years, the survival rate for T_1 floor of mouth cancer fell to 67 to 96% depending on whether the patients had originally been treated by radiotherapy or surgery, respectively.[11–13] For T_1 and T_2 oral tongue cancer treated by resection the 5-year survival was 77% and 65%, respectively, with no significant difference reported for transoral resection alone vs. transoral resection with elective neck dissection.[14] These survival statistics support the use of the surgical laser for transoral resection of localized (stages I and II) oral cancer without increasing the risk of local recurrence or regional spread.

When used as an alternative or as an adjunct to conventional surgery for larger T_3 and T_4 lesions, there were no adverse effects on either wound healing or tumor control.[3,15,16]

The most important negative aspect to consider in evaluating laser surgery is whether the laser beam itself might have any tumor-promoting effects that might enhance recurrence or spread to loco-regional or distant sites. Because the beam is applied only to clinically normal tissue at the resection margin and not on the tumor itself, any enhancement of spread would be expected to be a consequence of direct handling of the neoplastic tissue by retraction instruments. This being the case, one would not expect to find a diminished control rate with laser use and, in fact, the literature does *not* support such a negative outcome in surgical laser treatment of human oral malignancies.[3,17–19] A prospective clinical trial to evaluate such an effect for T_1 lesions where the laser cure rate exceeds 90% would require 342 cases in each arm of a study (conventional and laser) to detect a 5% survival difference at a $p < .05$ (at 80% power) (personal communication: Y Daoud, biostatistician, Sinai Hospital, Detroit). Such a study has never been done.

The issue regarding tumor promotion by direct application of laser light to the tumor itself is more controversial. Review of the literature of the biostimulatory effects of low-level laser light on fibroblasts and epithelial cells in tissue culture generally shows stimulatory effects at energy densities below 3.0 to 4.0 mJ/cm^2 and inhibitory effects above 4.0 mJ/cm2 (see Chapter 15). Animal solid tumor models have demonstrated conflicting results with hamster cheek pouch carcinoma responding by increasing tumor spread[20] and mouse melanomas not being affected by laser light.[21] Carcinomas in a rat liver model were not subject to increased metastases when exposed to milliwatt CO_2 lasers.[22] Mouse mammary carcinomas treated by contact neodymium: yttrium-aluminum-garnet (Nd:YAG) laser scalpel had lower local recurrence rates compared with conventional resection with a steel scalpel.[23] There are no animal data on squamous cell carcinoma response to irradiation with 10.6-μm laser light (CO_2).

FREE-BEAM CO_2

The transoral resection of oral cancer was first reported by Strong et al.[24,25] in 1979. They established the safety of microscope-guided CO_2 laser surgery coupled with the use of vital staining with toluidine blue and the use of frozen sections to control margins. This concept received further support by the early 1980s, particularly from Panjer et al.[3] and Carruth.[4] Two techniques were employed: hand-held probe and joystick micromanipulator coupled to an operating microscope. For both techniques irradiance must exceed 5,000 to 10,000 W/cm^2. Hemostasis requires a longer duty cycle than does ablation as discussed in the preceding chapter because a moderate amount of lateral thermal conduction is required to seal the microvasculature. This can be achieved by using a chopped continuous wave (CW) mode rather than rapid superpulsed (RSP). The chopped mode provides a reasonable compromise between a "cool" beam and the heat transfer to tissue required for hemostasis. This usually means acceptance of a zone of heat damage at the depth of the crater as well as along its side walls of about 0.5 to 1.0 mm.

Using a superpulsed CO_2 laser with a fluence of approximately 3 J/cm^2 at 2 Hz an estimated zone of tissue damage of nonablated tissue of 40 to 50 μm width is obtainable in a guinea pig skin model.[26] In vivo, at more realistic ablation rates of 50 to 150 pulses per second it is consistently noted that the zone of damage is less than 200 μm (see Fig. 7–8). This extent of heat damage of tissue adjacent to the beam in cancer resection is quite acceptable. In addition, its extent is much more controllable than is heat damage associated with electrosurgery. Both the handheld probe and the joystick micromanipulator result in safe excisional surgery; however, the microscope enhances control by magnifying the surgical field and thereby adding precision to the method of tissue removal.

DRY FIELD

Maintenance of a dry field depends on laser-tissue interactions as well as other tissue factors. The former is a time-dependent function of energy absorption and thermal conduction, and therefore hemostasis is enhanced by CW or chopped CW free-beam lasers compared with RSP lasers. Similarly, Nd:YAG delivered by conventional sapphire tip or by the silica contact probe of the Surgical Laser Technologies (SLT)[27–29] laser improves hemostasis significantly while still avoiding excessive heat damage (see Fig. 7–44). Enhancing hemostasis in tissue is abetted by the use of local anesthetic solution containing dilute (1:200,000) epinephrine or Pitressin (1.0 units/mL). It is well advised to wait 5 to 7 minutes for maximum vasoconstriction to occur prior to operating. These latter adjuncts add the benefit of intraoperative and postoperative analgesia in addition to the vasoconstriction that facilitates accurate surgery by maintaining a dry field.

Operating conditions are further improved by using the laser. The application of the laser energy to the tissue does not cause any movement of the tissue, particularly muscle, as is the case with electrocautery whose application induces strong muscle contractions. This is most apparent during surgery on the tongue. The result is that the target tissue lies passively during energy application, which enhances the precision of resection.

CO_2 AND CONTACT Nd:YAG

For transoral cancer resection, the two lasers of greatest value are the free-beam CO_2 and the various contact Nd:YAG lasers. Their utility becomes progressively more important as more aged patients come to surgery for resection of their oral cancers. Most of these patients have significant intercurrent diseases, particularly cardiovascular, pulmonary, and cerebrovascular, which make it preferable to perform their surgery using local and/or regional anesthesia techniques accompanied by intravenous sedation. Because operating in the oral cavity under these conditions places the airway at risk for obstruction from bleeding during surgery, maintaining a dry field becomes essential to the maintenance of a patent airway. Both the CO_2 and the YAG lasers permit the safe conduct of surgery under these circumstances. In comparison with the role of free-beam CO_2 the contact Nd:YAG laser when used at 15 to 25 W output power with an 800-μm conical tip was found to reduce bleeding and *not* to impair wound healing. When used for the resection of advanced-stage oral cancer that had been previously treated by radiation it was even found to reduce infectious complications, fistula formation, and distant flap complications.[29]

A prospective study of the use of free-beam CO_2 in the Department of Dentistry/Oral and Maxillofacial Surgery at Sinai Hospital was initiated in 1988 to evaluate its efficacy for the transoral resection of stages I and II oral cancer. The first parameter to be examined was blood loss resulting from partial glossectomy and floor of mouth resection. There were 12 tongue lesions treated with the free-beam CO_2 laser (study group) and 10 treated with scalpel or electrosurgery (conventional group). The average blood loss for the conventional group was 122 mL and that for the laser-treated group was 60 mL. Both groups received local infiltration anesthesia with lidocaine 0.5% and epinephrine 1:200,000. For floor of mouth cancer, the 10 patients treated conventionally all had local anesthetic with vasoconstrictor, and their average blood loss was 190 mL. The laser-treated group consisted of five patients who did not receive vasoconstrictor whose blood loss was 90 mL and three who did receive vasoconstrictor whose average blood loss was 38 mL for the same operation. The trend was toward reduced blood loss for the laser-treated patients. The floor of mouth resections for both groups did not include removal of bone. All operations for tongue and floor of mouth were performed on patients having general anesthesia with the airway maintained by nasoendotracheal intubation.

AVOIDING GENERAL ANESTHESIA

Surgical Protocol

The anatomic site was injected with lidocaine or bupivacaine containing epinephrine 1:200,000. For floor of mouth cases, Pitressin (1.0 unit/mL) was also added to the local anesthetic. The cancer itself was not manipulated but the area around the tumor that would later constitute the margin was infiltrated with the anesthetic solution. The drapes were then applied and a hypopharyngeal gauze pack was inserted. For operations performed using sedation instead of general anesthesia, a gauze pack was placed as a throat screen rather than as a hypopharyngeal pack. No "prep" solutions were used and no preoperative or intraoperative antibiotics were given unless they were required for prophylaxis because of cardiac valvular disease or the presence of metallic orthopedic implants. Neither systemic nor locally applied steroids were given. Traction using sutures or instruments to aid visibility during surgery was applied as necessary. (See case reports for details.)

Since 1988, there have been 13 patients with T_1 or T_2 oral carcinomas, seven of which were floor of mouth and tongue, which were treated by laser resection using local anesthetic and intravenous sedation. Unfavorable airway incidents did not occur during surgery and no case required a change in anesthetic management to control the airway during surgery. In no case was it necessary to excessively deepen sedation to meet the needs of patient comfort. None of these patients required postoperative ICU for surgical site management and none of them required hospitalization for more than 48 hours.

CONSEQUENCES

Postoperatively there was a high level of patient acceptance. Objectively, they had much less edema and also resumed oral feedings more rapidly than did those patients with similar lesions who were treated by conventional surgery, particularly with electrocautery.

During follow-up examinations the use of postoperative analgesics was recorded. As noted in the literature[18,30] and confirmed in our own prospective and ongoing assessment of postoperative pain, the degree of pain to be anticipated is unpredictable.[31] Furthermore, approximately one third of patients will have less postoperative pain while another third will have more postoperative pain than do those patients having conventional surgery. Among those with less pain, a subgroup will experience a 2- or 3-day interval of suddenly increasing pain starting on postoperative day 4 or 5. Gaspar and Szabo[18] reported on 548 operations of different types in the oral cavity and found that only 31.2% of their patients required analgesics on the day of surgery. After day 5, only two patients required analgesics because of pain from exposed bone.

All of our patients were seen on a weekly basis until healing was complete. Independent of oral anatomic region, all patients were completely healed by the fifth postoperative week. This consistent epithelialization of the laser-induced wound in humans confirms the results of animal experiments in which reepithelialization from the peripheral border of a laser wound took place within 4 weeks.[30] These treatment areas in humans, as in dogs, were almost the same color and texture within 4 to 5 weeks, and after maturation were indistinguishable from normal mucosa. In addition, the healed oral mucosa preserves its elastic properties. This may be related to the minimal increase in mucosal thickness after CO_2 laser treatment compared with scalpel incisions[30] or it could be related to diminished activity of myofibroblasts in the healing wound.[32]

COMPLICATIONS

No split-thickness skin grafts were placed for any laser-treated cases. Postoperative scarring was minimal, although two patients from among 26 patients with floor of mouth or ventral tongue resection required scar release (7.7%) to improve tongue mobility and one patient with wide local excision of the tongue, floor of the mouth, and mandibular alveolus along with supraomohyoid neck dissection had a mild speech impediment for which he did not seek treatment.

Among the 106 patients treated by transoral resection with the free-beam CO_2 laser, postoperative bleeding while in hospital was limited to five events. Two occurred in patients with cirrhosis of the liver, who "oozed" for 2 to 3 days after surgery. There were two cases of delayed bleeding necessitating readmission to the operating room to control bleeding, both occurring on the first postoperative evening, and there was one patient who bled at the conclusion of surgery during emergence from anesthesia while still intubated, who required recoagulation of the floor of the mouth. There was also one case of delayed hematoma developing 10 days after resection of the ventral tongue and floor of mouth in a patient with cirrhosis of the liver. There were two cases of postoperative infection requiring treatment with systemic antibiotics, but there were no cases of significantly delayed healing. Similar findings have also been reported for use of the contact Nd:YAG (sapphire tip).[29] Strong et al.'s[24,25] original 1979 study of 57 oral cancers of unspecified stage removed using microscopic control by CW CO_2 laser did not report any postoperative infections.

Using these techniques to remove 106 cancers during the past 5 years, we have not had any patients stay in the hospital longer than 2 days. For larger T_2 lesions and those with posterior defects requiring insertion of a surgical pack, all stayed an average of 2 days. However, because of the consistent minimal postoperative edema, none of these 90 patients from whom 106 tumors were removed required overnight intubation or admission to an intensive care unit after surgery.

Although Panje et al.[3] reported swallowing difficulties in 21% of their cases treated by transoral resection with the CO_2 laser, we did not specifically monitor swallowing difficulties. All patients could eat a soft or normal diet by the time epithelial resurfacing was complete at 4 to 5 weeks. During this initial period none of these patients required intubation of the gastrointestinal tract to maintain their nutrition.

TIME AT OPERATION

Once the "learning curve" delay is overcome by clinical experience, laser cases go quite quickly. In fact, the average time during the past 5 years for resection of T_1 or T_2 oral lesions is less than 45 to 50 minutes including injection of local anesthetic, vital staining with toluidine blue, and a mandatory 5-minute (by the clock) hemostasis check prior to terminating the operation.

THE SUBMANDIBULAR DUCT

For anterior floor of mouth resection, no special care is taken in regard to Wharton's duct. In fact, they are completely ignored.[33] The laser is used to transect the duct if this is required to "clear the field" of cancer. Because of the known possibility of downgrowth into the duct of oral squamous cell cancer located over the duct,[34] it is wise to be quite liberal in regard to the indications for removing the duct as part of the en bloc resection. No sialodochoplasty of the part of the proximal duct remaining in situ is performed. Postoperatively the rate of significant submandibular gland enlargement secondary to obstruction requiring removal of the gland is 4% in our series.

SURGICAL CASES

General Comments: Free-Beam CO_2 vs. Contact Nd:YAG

Both the free-beam CO_2 laser and the contact Nd:YAG laser are applicable to the transoral resection of oral cancer. The major advantages for the use of lasers are minimal postoperative edema, which is usually but not always less than that encountered with electrosurgery; a dry operative field; and absence of muscular fasciculations, particularly of the tongue, which provides a "quiet" operative field. Most patients are discharged within 24 to 48 hours and patient acceptance is very high.

Surgery itself goes quickly, usually lasting less than 1 hour, and either general anesthesia or sedation techniques may be used along with local anesthesia. Blood loss is minimized. However, remember to rapidly clamp and tie or coagulate vessels if the laser does not stop the bleeding. The return rate to the operating theater to control delayed bleeding is about 4%.

Reconstruction after floor of mouth resection is particularly simplified by the lack of need for split-thickness skin grafts. Postoperative scar contraction is mild and persistent restricted oral opening following resection of posteriorly located lesions of the buccal mucosa, retromolar pad, or anterior tonsillar pillar is uncommon. Some patients will lose about 10 to 20% of their maximal incisal opening.

The free-beam CO_2 laser in chopped CW or RSP modes causes the least scarring because it causes the least heat damage. As a corollary it is also less hemostatic than either CW CO_2 or contact Nd:YAG. On the other hand, these latter two options create more unwanted heat effects both to the margin of the specimen and to the native tissue. The CO_2 laser does not provide tactile sensation to the operator, and for use in the area of the lingual anterior mandibular gingiva one must use a front surface dental mirror to change the beam direction. This requires a bit of practice for surgeons without dental training. The contact Nd:YAG provides tactile sensation and better hemostasis, but heat damage may exceed 3.6 mm whereas RSP CO_2 heat damage is usually less than 0.3 mm. Free-beam CO_2 wounds heal slightly faster but this is not clinically significant.

TRANSORAL CASE 1: FLOOR OF MOUTH

A 54-year-old African-American woman, with a 25-year history of daily smoking of two packs of cigarettes and of drinking four beers, presents with a 2-month history of an "irritation under my tongue." Examination, incisional biopsy, and systemic evaluation demonstrate a $T_1N_0M_0$ moderately well-differentiated squamous cell carcinoma of the anterior floor of mouth (FOM) that encroaches upon the terminus of Wharton's duct (Figs. 7–1 and 7–2). She is also noted to have mild von Willebrand's disease, chronic obstructive lung disease, stable coronary artery disease, and insulin-controlled diabetes mellitus. The free-beam CO_2 laser is chosen as the instrument of choice for removal of her tumor.

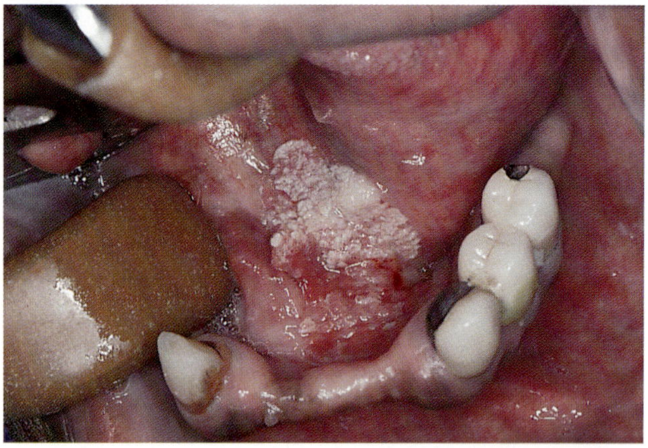

Figure 7–2. During operation, tongue properly retracted.

TECHNIQUE

After the completion of aerodigestive endoscopy with the patient receiving a general anesthetic, the airway is secured with a nasoendotracheal tube. The face is protected with moist saline eye patches and facial drapes, and the hypopharynx is packed with a wet throat pack. Local anesthetic solution containing 1:200,000 epinephrine and Pitressin 1.0 U/mL is injected along the planned lines of resection into the depth of the wound. While awaiting maximum vasoconstrictor effect, the oral mucosa is stained with toluidine blue. (See Chapter 4.) This is very helpful in assessing subclinical extent of spread of the mucosal tumor.

After washing the field with saline, the areas retaining the stain are noted (Fig. 7–3) and the peripheral resection margin is marked with the laser in the defocused mode (Fig. 7–4). The tip of the tongue is grasped with a towel clip to facilitate retraction. The handpiece for the free-beam CO_2 laser is now placed in contact (i.e., at the focal point) with the tissue to be excised to start the excision. The laser is adjusted so that in chopped CW or RSP mode an average power output of 20 to 30 W is delivered. By varying the handpiece distance from the tissue helium-neon (HeNe) guide beam spot size is varied from 0.3 to 3.0 mm. The true

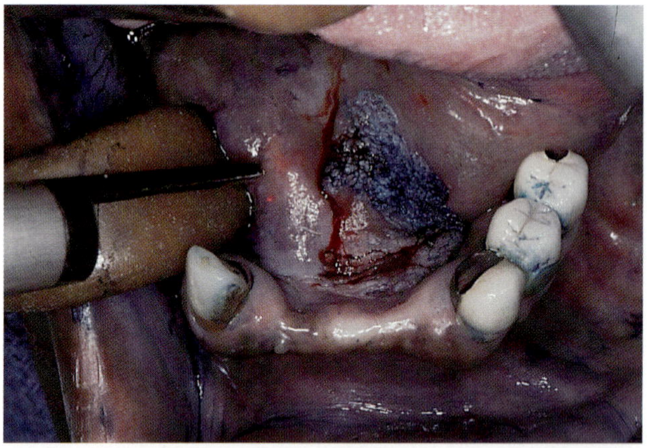

Figure 7–3. Lesion retains toluidine blue vital stain after acetic acid rinse. HeNe guide beam placed into contact with tissue at focal point of probe demonstrating 0.3-mm guide spot size for incision.

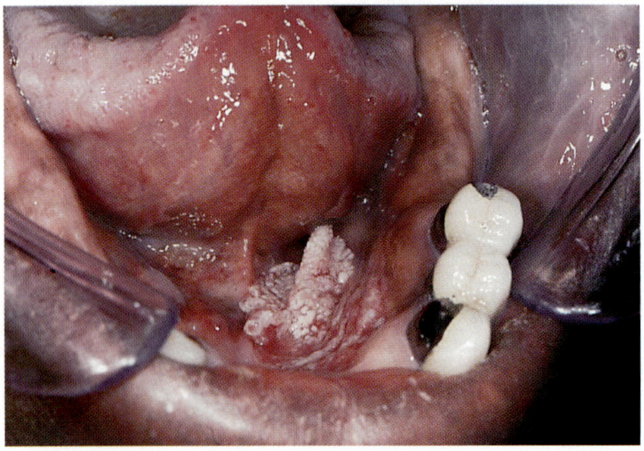

Figure 7–1. $T_1N_0M_0$ SCC of anterior floor of mouth.

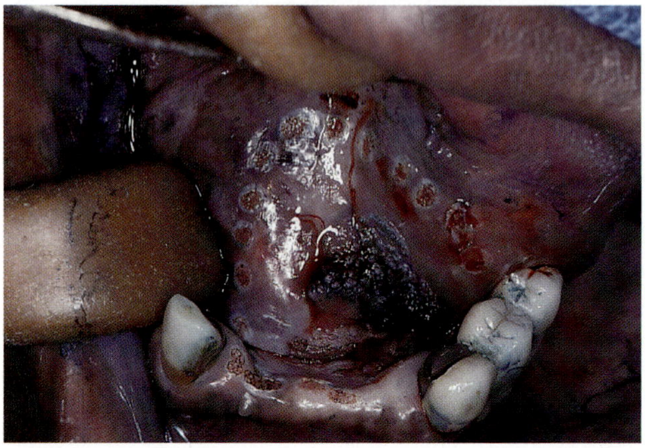

Figure 7–4. Defocused spots to mark resection margin. Handpiece is moved away from focal point until 2- to 3-mm spot size is obtained. Bloodless markings are made with single pulses (PD <500 W/cm^2).

vaporization spot size averages approximately 80% of the HeNe spot size. Therefore, the power density (PD) will range from 35,000 W/cm2 to 350 W/cm2 at 20-W output and from 52,000 W/cm2 to 525 W/cm2 at 30-W output. The former values are used for excision and the latter for coagulation.

Surgical principles of traction-countertraction are used to facilitate dissection (Fig. 7–5) and cautery or suture ligatures are used liberally to quickly stop bleeding. The submandibular ducts are transected at will at high PD in the pulsed mode, and no sialodochoplasties are performed. After determining the depth of resection anteriorly, dissection was continued posteriorly until an adequate margin was established. The posterior dissection was then made from the mucosa to the depth of the resection. The base of the resection was free of char except where deliberate coagulation was used (Fig. 7–6). The specimen was oriented and pinned on a wooden tongue blade to be sent to the pathology laboratory (Fig. 7–7). Note that the extent of the thermal damage on the deep side of the resection margin was only 0.16 mm (Fig. 7–8). Estimated blood loss was 5.0 mL and operating time was 40 minutes.

The patient was discharged in the morning with a prescription for a narcotic and a nonsteroidal anti-inflammatory analgesic. (If used, an oral pack is removed either at bedside prior to discharge, or in the office on the following day.) The day after surgery, the base of the wound was fibrin covered. The patient rinsed twice a day with chlorhexidine for the next 7 to 10 days. Progress of healing was checked approximately weekly (Figs. 7–9 to 7–14) until reepithelialization was complete, at which time postoperative observation was maintained according to the cancer surveillance protocol. At 1-year recall (Figs. 7–15 to 7–17) speech, swallowing, and range of motion of the tongue were all normal. There was no evidence of recurrent disease at 3 years.

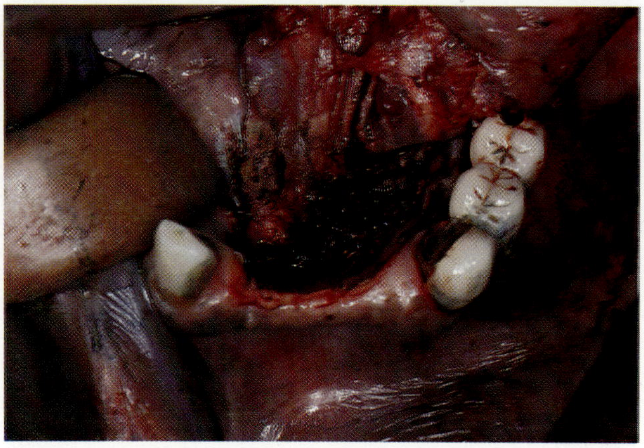

Figure 7–6. Base coagulated in CW mode at 30 to 40 W, defocused for maximum hemostasis. Note that both resection and coagulation violate the submandibular ducts.

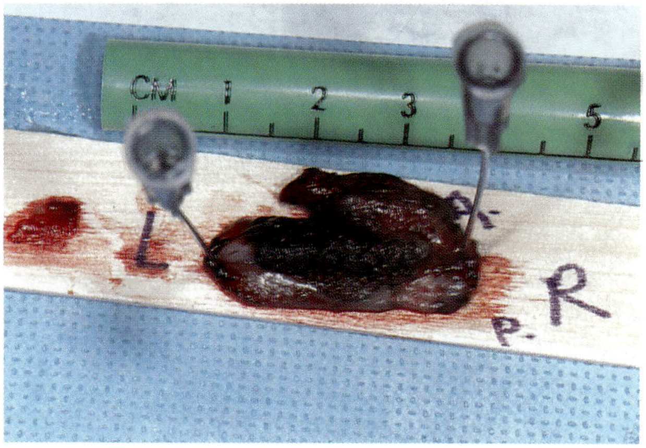

Figure 7–7. Specimen oriented and pinned for transfer to the pathologist.

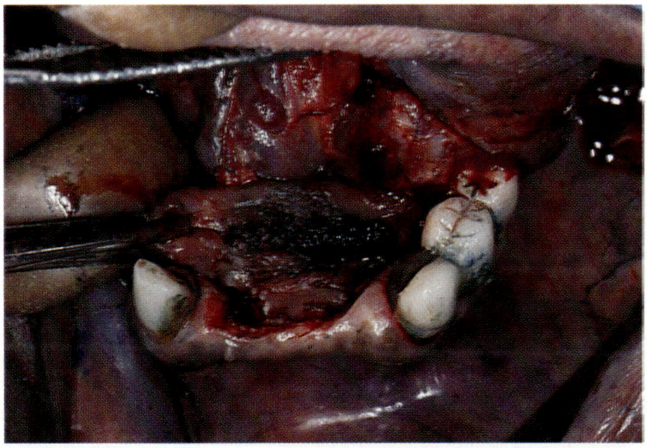

Figure 7–5. Specimen mobilized. Dissection made to base of deep resection margin. Note instruments retracting both tongue and specimen to provide traction-countertraction for good surgical exposure.

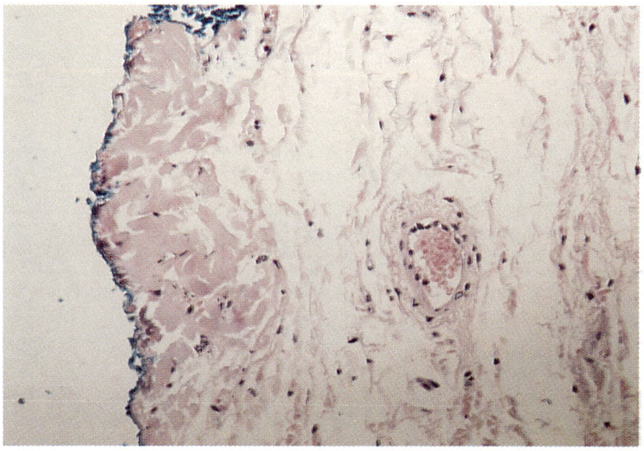

Figure 7–8. Histology: Note zone of thermal necrosis on base of specimen is only 0.16 mm (100×).

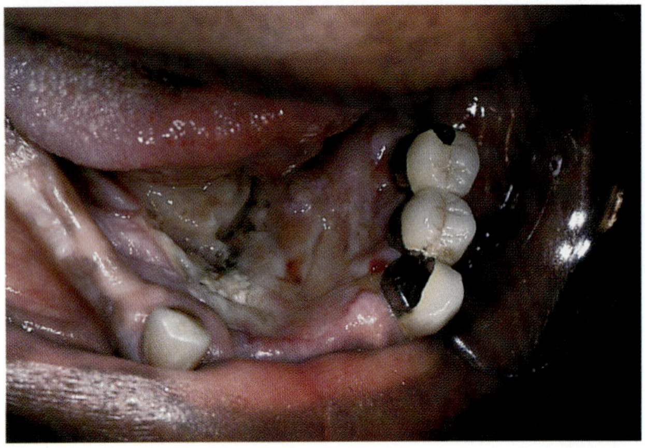

Figure 7–9. Fibrinous coagulum appears within the first 24 hours. Still present at 1 week.

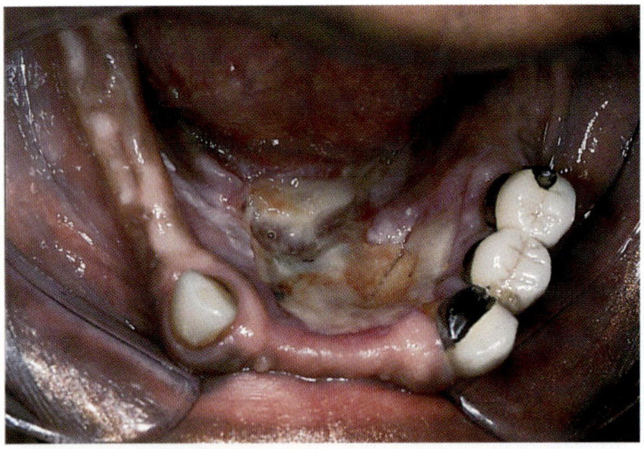

Figure 7–10. Two weeks. Note that reepithelialization occurs from the periphery. Note the exposed area of lingual plate of mandible on the patient's left side.

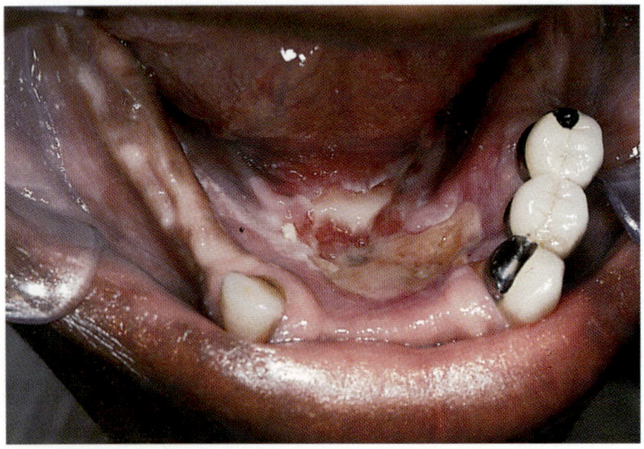

Figure 7–11. Twenty-two days. Note that most of oral floor is covered by new epithelium. Bone is still exposed.

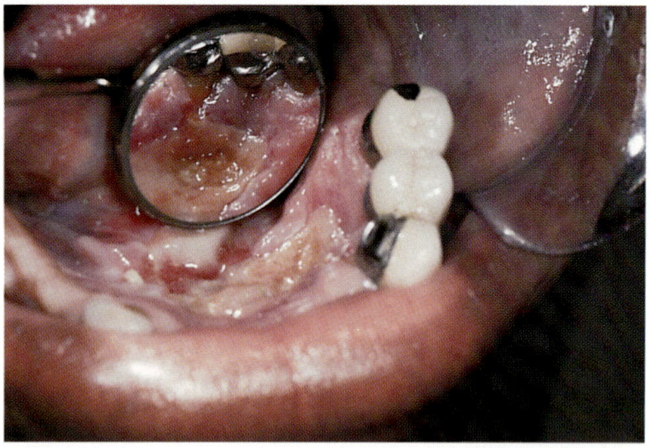

Figure 7–12. Twenty-two days. Mirror demonstrates area of exposed bone. One will expect a sequestrum, but not progressive osteomyelitis to develop. The patient has received no antibiotics.

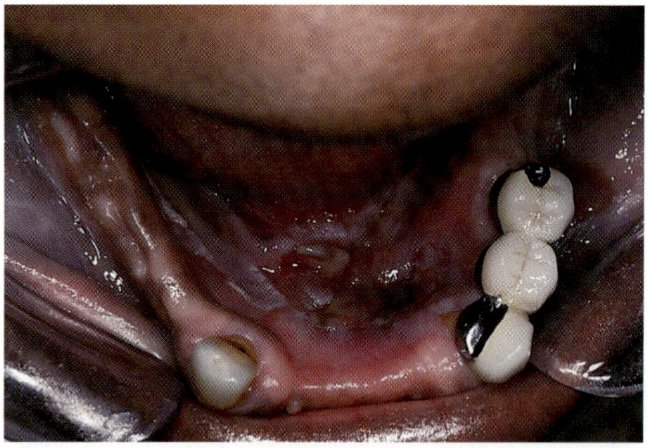

Figure 7–13. Thirty-two days. Most of the surgical site has reepithelialized.

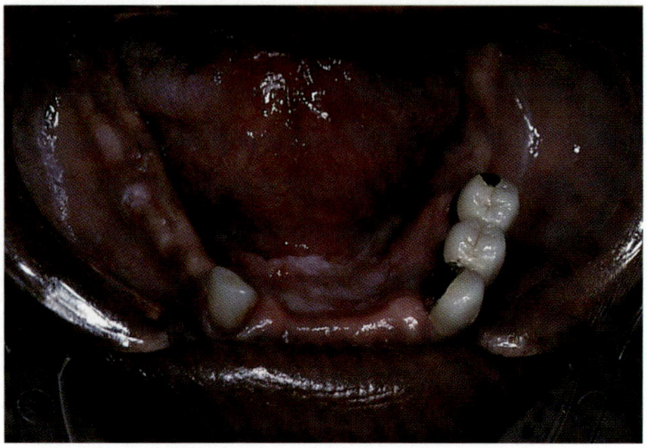

Figure 7–14. Forty-six days. Completely healed.

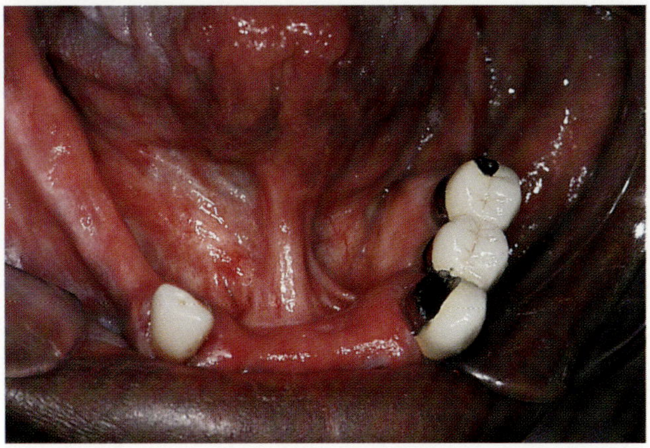

Figure 7–15. One year. Full range of motion of tongue. Speech is normal as it has been since the second postoperative month. Patient has been in regular cancer surveillance protocol since month 3.

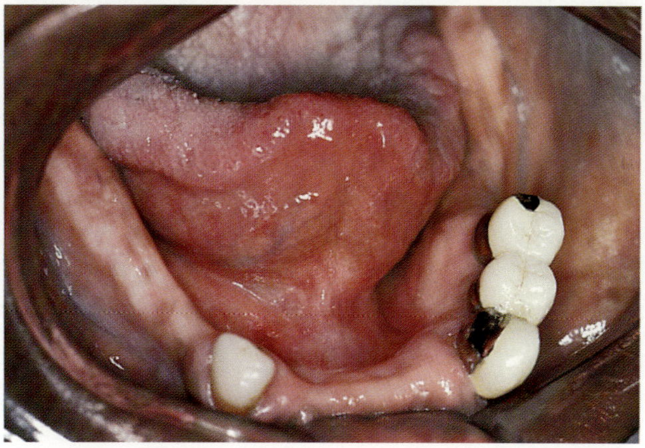

Figure 7–16. Note normal range of motion on tongue.

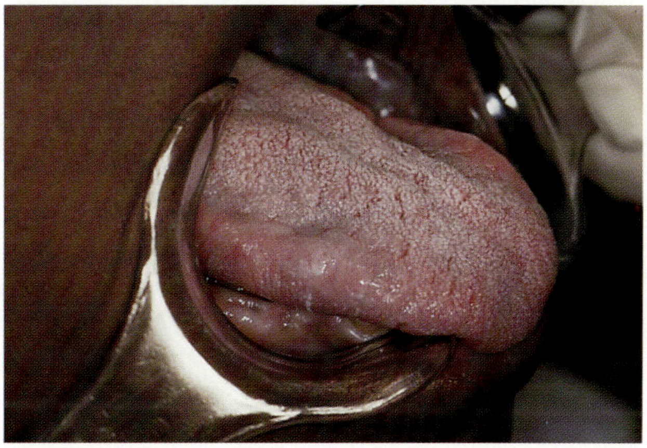

Figure 7–17. Speech and swallowing were normal. Patient had no evidence of disease at 3 years.

TRANSORAL CASE 2: FOM

A 56-year-old white man with a 25-year history of daily smoking of two packs of cigarettes and drinking four whiskey equivalents of beer per day presents with a 2-month history of an "irritation under my tongue." Examination, incisional biopsy, and systemic evaluation demonstrate a $T_1N_0M_0$ well-differentiated microinvasive squamous cell carcinoma of the anterior floor of mouth (FOM) that encroaches upon the terminus of Wharton's duct (Fig. 7–18). He is also noted to have chronic obstructive lung disease and coronary artery disease without recent anginal chest pain. The free-beam CO_2 laser is chosen as the instrument of choice for removal of his tumor.

TECHNIQUE

After inducing general anesthesia and securing the airway with an oral endotracheal tube, aerodigestive endoscopy is performed. The tube is then changed to a nasoendotracheal tube. The face is protected with moist saline eye patches and facial drapes, and the hypopharynx is packed with a wet throat pack. Local anesthetic solution of 0.5% bupivacaine containing 1:200,000 epinephrine and Pitressin 1.0 U/mL (1.0 mL of Pitressin added to 30 mL of bupivacaine) is injected along the planned lines of resection to the depth of the musculature of the oral floor. No preparation solution is used and neither prophylactic antibiotics nor steroids are given. While awaiting maximum vasoconstrictor effect, the oral mucosa is stained with toluidine blue (see Chapter 4) to assess any subclinical mucosal spread of the tumor.

The submandibular ducts are transected at will at high PD in the pulsed mode, and no sialodochoplasties are performed. After determining the depth of resection anteriorly, dissection continues posteriorly until an adequate margin guided by the initial marking out of the resection is established. The vertical component of the resection from mucosa to the depth of the resection is then completed. The base of the resection should be free of char except where deliberate coagulation was used. Estimated blood loss was 15 mL and operating time was 20 minutes. If hemostasis is satisfactory after 5 to 10 minutes of observation, the patient is brought to the recovery room. On the other hand, if hemostasis is imperfect, a bovine collagen pad is placed over the resection bed and an iodoform gauze pack is secured for overnight insertion. The patient is extubated in the recovery room when fully awake.

PROBLEM AREA: LINGUAL ANTERIOR MANDIBULAR GINGIVA

The most difficult area to adequately control is the region of the lingual gingiva, where it is often important to remove the soft tissue lining the lingual surface of the mandible in a supraperiosteal plane. This may be done in several ways. Either the scalpel is used to incise to bone, which unfortunately causes bleeding, or the laser must be redirected anteriorly so the incision can be carried down to the periosteum. This latter maneuver requires the use of an adjustable front surface mirror (Fig. 7–19) to redirect the beam. Alternatively, some of the supraperiosteal dissection may be performed with a periosteal elevator. Or, if using the laser, a contra-angle handpiece may be used instead of a front surface mirror depending on availability. The final incision of periosteum is best performed with a scalpel to avoid damaging the bone with the laser impacts. However, should the latter occur to a mild degree, epithelium will still completely cover laser damaged bone in about 4 weeks. It is not, however, uncommon for a small, thin sequestrum of part of the lingual plate of the mandible to be formed.

After removing the specimen (Fig. 7–20), margins were harvested from the patient for frozen section. The defect was packed with iodoform gauze and an antibacterial ointment. The patient was transferred to the recovery room where extubation was performed only when he was fully awake.

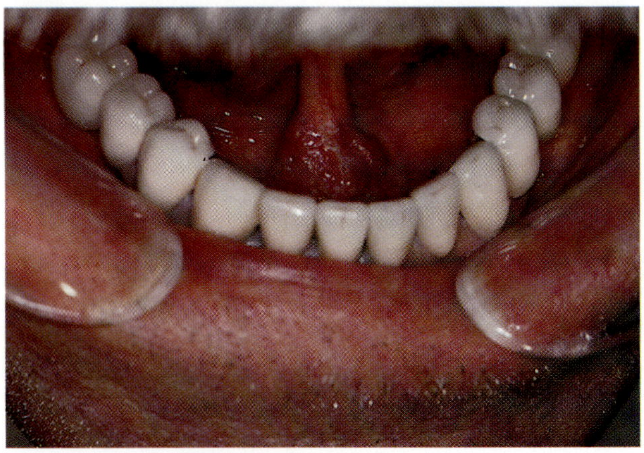

Figure 7–18. Microinvasive $T_1N_0M_0$ squamous cell carcinoma of anterior oral floor arising in proximity to Wharton's duct.

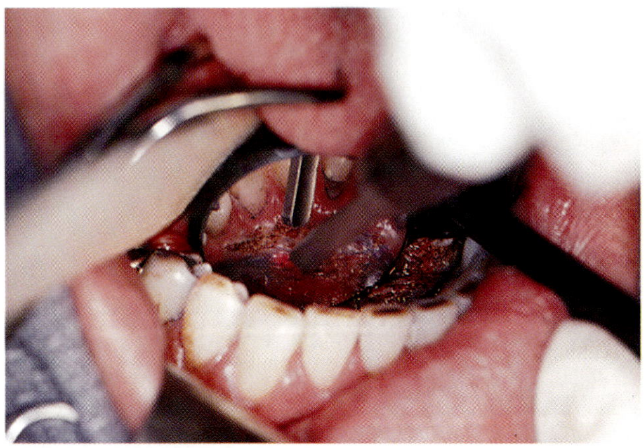

Figure 7–19. (From another patient) Note that a front surface mirror may be used to reflect the laser beam to reach the lingual aspect of the mucosa or gingiva lining the lingual surface of the mandible.

AFTERCARE

Oral fluids are administered that night and narcotics are prescribed intramuscularly or intravenously that night. The patient is discharged in the morning with a prescription for a narcotic and a nonsteroidal anti-inflammatory analgesic. The oral pack is removed either at bedside prior to discharge, or in the office on the following day. At this time, the base of the wound is fibrin covered (Fig. 7–21). The patient rinses twice a day with chlorhexidine for the next 7 to 10 days. Hydrogen peroxide/salt water rinses mixed 1:1 are used every few hours. Progress of healing is checked weekly until reepithelialization is complete (Figs. 7–22 and 7–23), at which time postoperative observation is maintained according to the cancer surveillance protocol. For anterior floor of mouth resections, there is no interference with normal swallowing. Speech usually returns to normal within 2 to 3 months and is accompanied by a normal range of motion of the tongue. Resections of the posterolateral floor of the mouth are more likely to be associated with minor speech impediments.

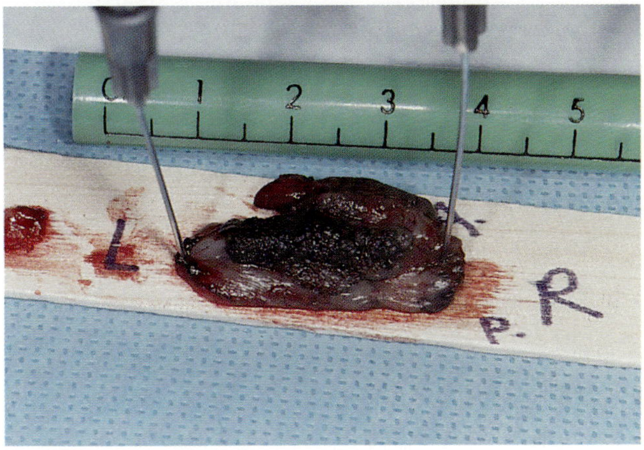

Figure 7–20. The specimen is pinned onto a wooden tongue blade, marked for orientation and demonstrated to the pathologist in the operating room. Frozen sections are obtained from the patient as required.

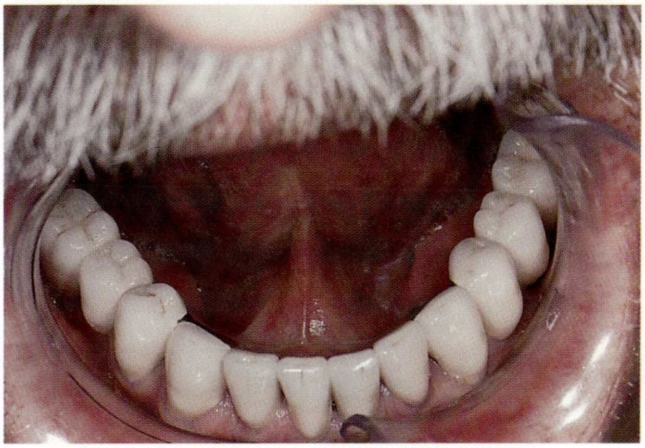

Figure 7–22. Oral floor well healed. Wound was reepithelialized in 25 days. Mature, pliable mucosa present (10 weeks).

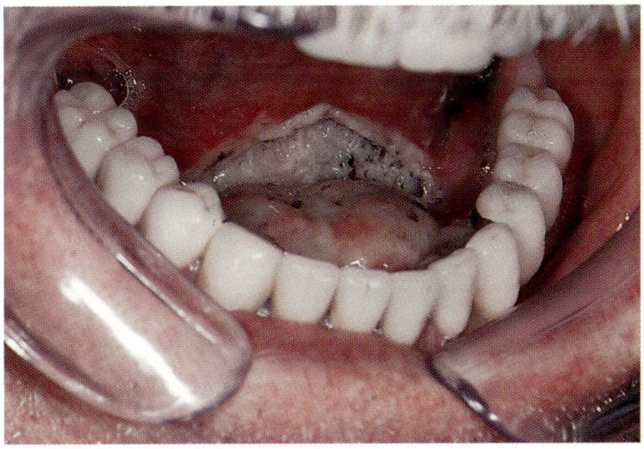

Figure 7–21. Fibrin coagulum still present at floor of resection, postoperative day 10.

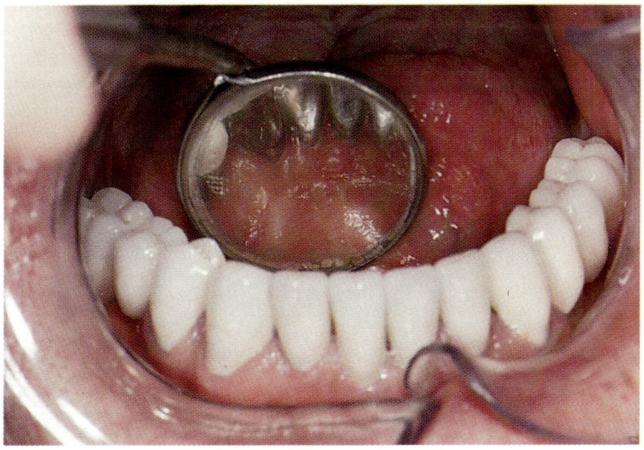

Figure 7–23. Lingual gingiva stripped at surgery has recovered completely (10 weeks). Recovery of tongue range of motion was complete.

CASE 3: TONGUE—FREE-BEAM CO_2

This 82-year-old white woman with hypertension and a 9-cm abdominal aortic aneurysm presented with a $T_2N_0M_0$ moderately well-differentiated carcinoma of the right lateral tongue (Fig. 7–24). After review by the head and neck cancer team, surgical removal of the tumor was recommended as the treatment of choice. Extensive preoperative counseling in regard to risks as well as the details of treatment secured her consent to remove the tumor using local anesthesia with supplemental intravenous sedation.

At surgery, after providing sedation, the tongue was anesthetized by lingual, inferior alveolar and long buccal blocks as well as by direct infiltration in the midline of the tongue and in the lateral oral floor with 0.5% bupivacaine with 1:200,000 epinephrine. This was given slowly over a period of 4 to 5 minutes to minimize the hypertensive effect of the epinephrine. Essentially, the entire right lower lip and oral cavity was anesthetized to provide comfort during retraction as well as pain prevention for the actual areas of incision.

The periphery of the planned resection was marked using the laser handpiece in the defocused mode at a PD of about 500 W/cm^2. After assessing for adequacy of margins, the resection commenced at an approximate PD of >50,000 W/cm^2 (Avg. P = 30W, pps = 118, HeNe spot = 0.3 mm, pulse width = 2.4 ms, interpulse distance = 9.9 ms, fluence = 290 mJ/pulse) starting lateral to the midline to preserve the maximum amount of usable tongue tip with the incision, then proceeding obliquely to reach the midline (Fig. 7–25). Now dissection was continued posteriorly in the relatively bloodless plane of the midline of the tongue.

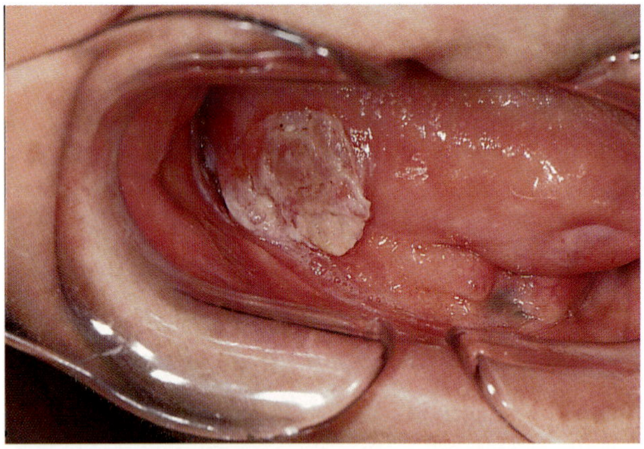

Figure 7–24. $T_2N_0M_0$ moderately well-differentiated squamous cell carcinoma of mobile tongue.

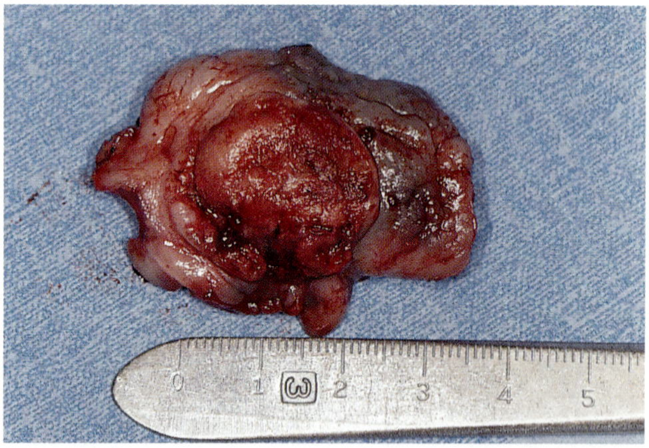

Figure 7–26. Oral side of specimen. Specimen measured 4.7 × 4.3 × 1.5 cm.

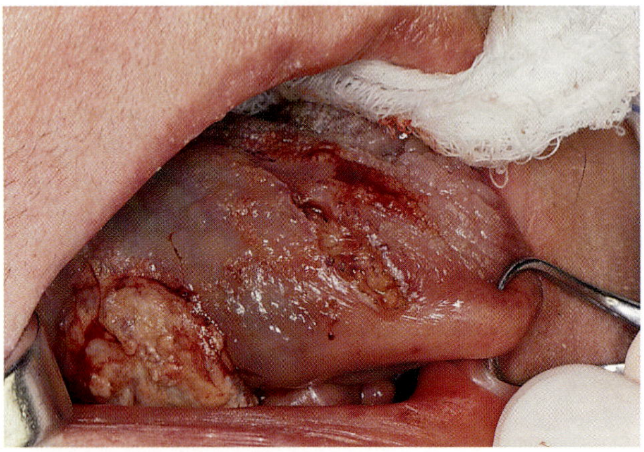

Figure 7–25. Margins marked. Superpulsed mode, defocused handpiece, PD = 450 W/cm^2.

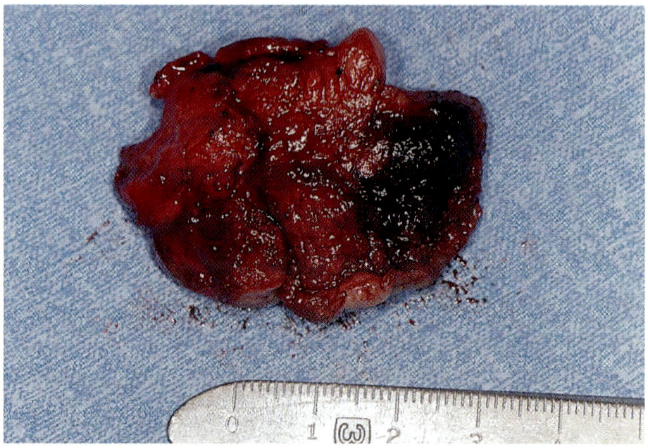

Figure 7–27. Deep resection margin of specimen. Note relative lack of charring. Approximately 5 mm of additional "marginal" tissue was vaporized at the depth of resection. (PD approximately 52,000 W/cm^2 for resection.)

At the posterior limit of the resection, the incision was extended laterally to join the line of resection at the oral floor. This latter was now joined by the anterior resection line at the level of the floor of the mouth and the specimen was delivered (Figs. 7–26 and 7–27). The base was coagulated at 30 W in CW mode with a 3-mm spot size, defocused to provide a PD = 425 W/cm^2. The base was deliberately left slightly charred to reduce the likelihood of postoperative bleeding (Fig. 7–28). Note the contrast to Figure 7–27 in which the deep surface of the specimen removed by the laser in superpulsed mode shows almost no char and therefore minimal heat effects. A simple gauze sponge was placed over the wound and the patient was asked to bite on it. Estimated blood loss was less than 50 mL, and operating time including administration of local anesthetic was 48 minutes.

Postoperatively, narcotic analgesics were required for 4 days. The patient started a clear liquid diet on the day of surgery and full liquids on the first postoperative day. There was no postoperative bleeding, and she was discharged on postoperative day 2. The sequence of healing from the first postoperative visit to complete reepithelialization is demonstrated in Figures 7–29 to 7–33. Functionally, speech and swallowing were completely normal within 9 weeks of the completion of surgery. There was no postoperative submandibular gland obstruction, and the patient remained disease free for 3 years until she died from a myocardial infarction.

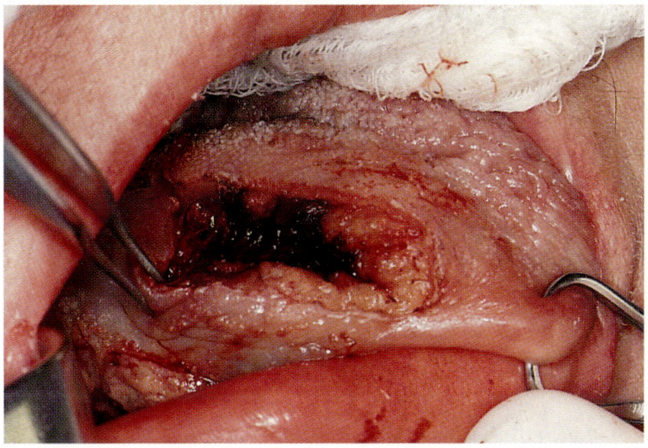

Figure 7–28. Base of resection. CW effect causing char left in situ to inhibit bleeding.

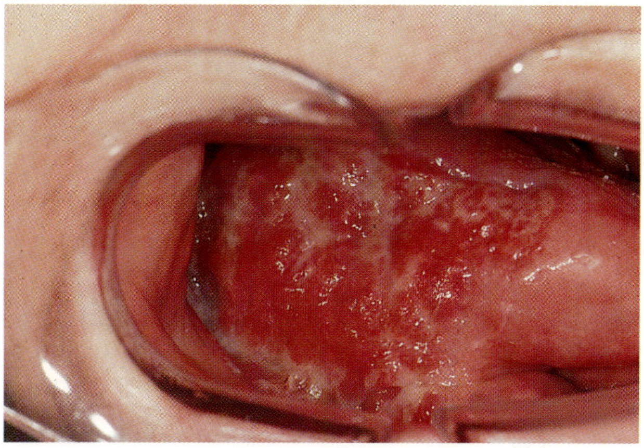

Figure 7–30. Day 10. Most of fibrin has been replaced by immature epithelium.

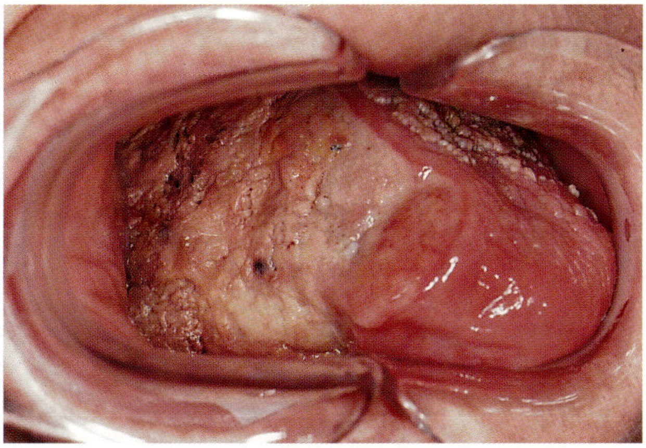

Figure 7–29. Day 4. Fibrin covering of laser wound left to heal by second intention. This forms during the first 24 to 48 hours after wounding and is gradually replaced by epithelial tissue.

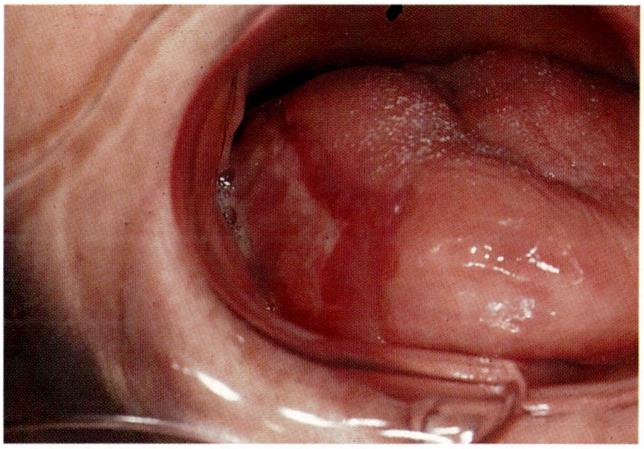

Figure 7–31. Day 18. Some wound contraction has occurred and most of wound is covered by new epithelium.

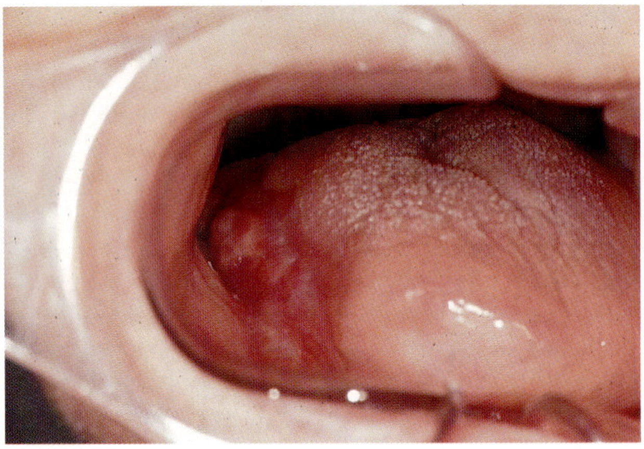

Figure 7–32. Day 25. All except one small area representing less than 10% of the total surface area of the wound has been replaced by new epithelium.

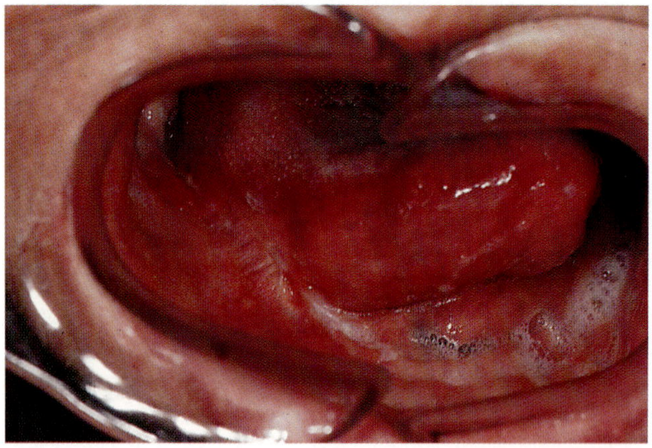

Figure 7–33. Eight weeks. Complete epithelialization occurred by day 31; 24 days later the surface is unchanged and the range of motion of the tongue is very good but slightly restricted.

CASE 4: TONGUE CANCER—PRIMARY CLOSURE

A 53-year-old white woman with a $T_1N_0M_0$ well-differentiated squamous cell carcinoma of the middle third of the lateral border of the mobile tongue (Figs. 7–34 to 7–37).

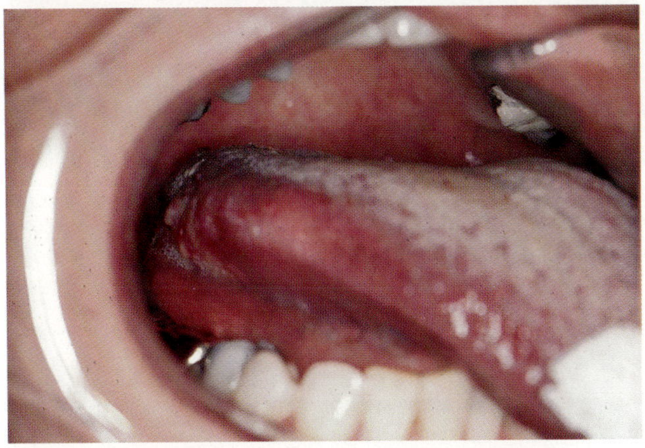

Figure 7–34. $T_1N_0M_0$ squamous cell carcinoma of mobile tongue.

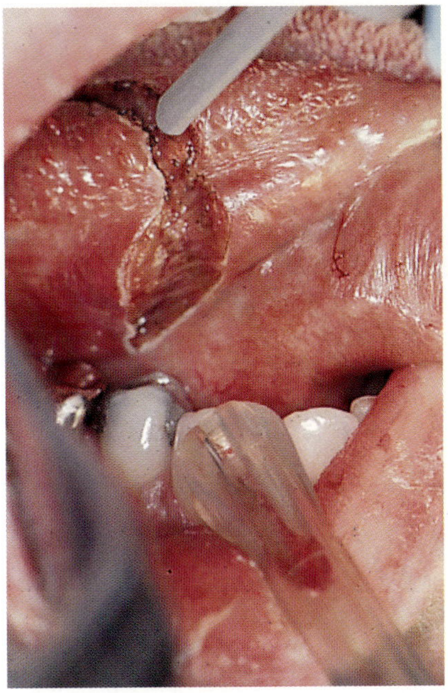

Figure 7–35. Starting the incision with the laser handpiece tip adjacent the tissue at the focal point. PD approximately 30,000 W, superpulsed mode. Note HeNe aiming beam just below tip within incision. Field is dry.

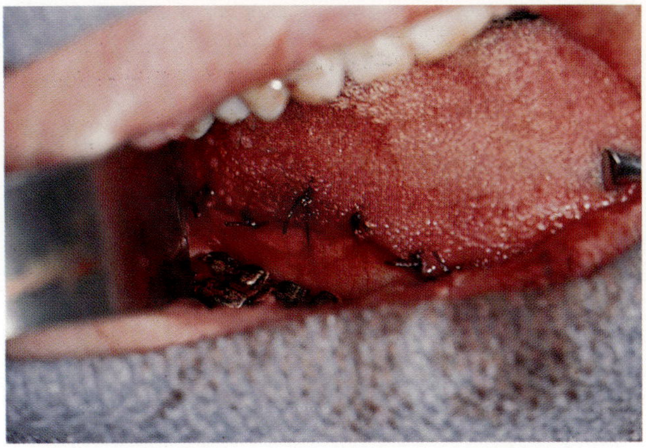

Figure 7–36. Primary closure of wound.

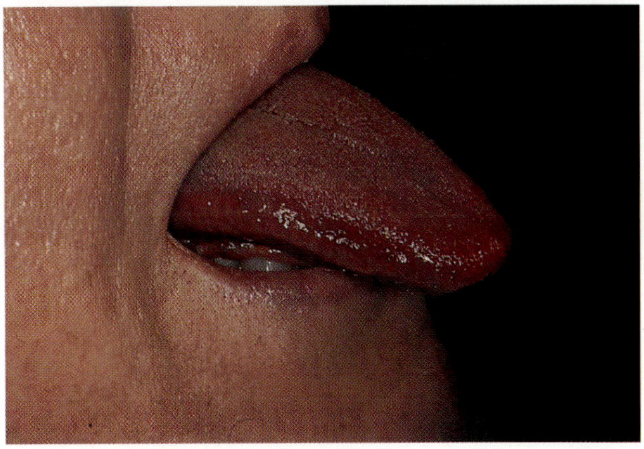

Figure 7–37. Normal tongue protrusion at 33 months. Patient had no evidence of disease at 8 years.

CASE 5: TONGUE—CONTACT ND:YAG LASER SCALPEL

This 83-year-old white man presented with a well-differentiated $T_1N_0M_0$ squamous cell carcinoma of the posterior third of the mobile tongue located along its ventrolateral surface. Seventeen years before he had had a wide local excision of the midportion of the left lateral tongue for a well-differentiated $T_1N_0M_0$ squamous cell carcinoma. He had discontinued smoking cigarettes after the treatment of his index cancer, but continued to consume four whiskey equivalents of gin per day. Liver function studies and quantitative platelet counts were normal. The collective recommendation of the head and neck tumor conference was to resect the tumor. The contact Nd:YAG laser (SLT) was chosen as the instrument of choice because of the need to extend the posterior limit of the resection along the lingual gutter into the upper hypopharynx, an area where control of the free-beam CO_2 becomes a bit difficult even with the use of a front surface mirror to alter the incident angle of the beam. In addition, the increased hemostasis of the contact YAG was considered to be of adequate benefit to accept the slight increase in thermal necrosis attendant to the contact laser compared with the free-beam CO_2. The silica contact scalpel probes (Fig. 7–38) were selected based upon their geometry for tissue excision in this highly vascular area.

At operation, general anesthesia with nasoendotracheal intubation to secure the airway was chosen. Bupivacaine 0.5% with epinephrine 1:200,000 was administered within the substance of the tongue both to enhance hemostasis and to provide postoperative analgesia. The field was stained with toluidine blue to assess for areas of subclinical neoplasia and/or areas of preneoplastic change (dysplasia). The hypopharynx was occluded with a wet gauze throat pack. An Allis clamp was placed in the left anterolateral tongue to facilitate retraction. With the contact YAG laser set at an

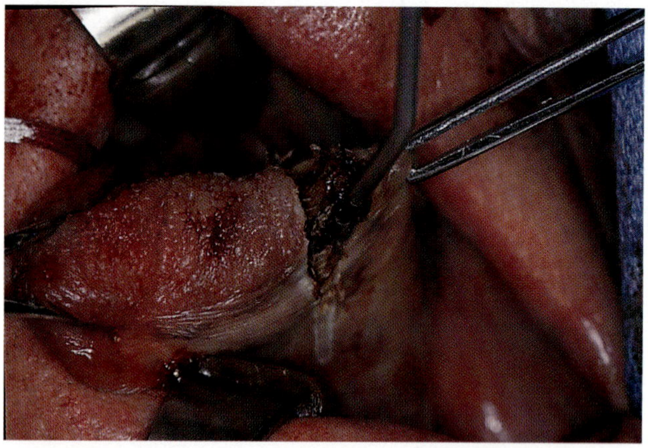

Figure 7–39. Laser is activated prior to touching probe against tissue. When probe tip reaches operating temperature, it is gently stroked along the path of incision. Tactile sense regulates rate and depth of incision. Dissection proceeding into depth of tongue. Note absence of bleeding.

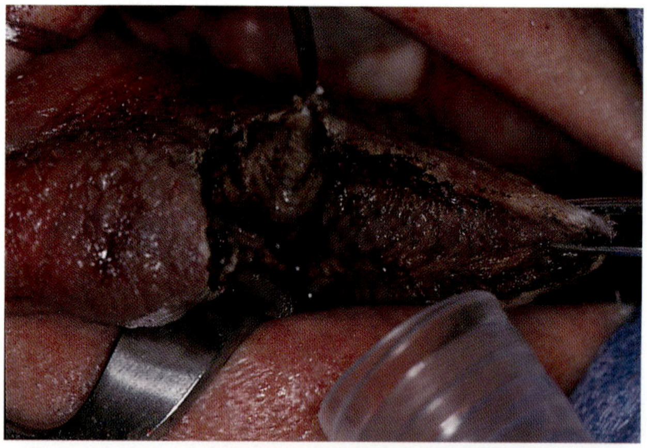

Figure 7–40. Posterolateral aspect of tongue adjacent to tongue base retracted laterally to demonstrate extent of posterior element of the excision. Note proximity of high-speed laser suction to laser probe tip.

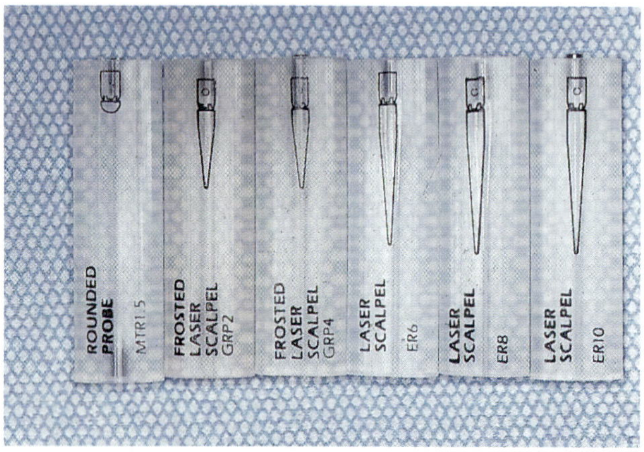

Figure 7–38. Silica scalpel tips for the contact Nd:YAG laser. (Scalpel tip number 6 used for incision at 15 W.)

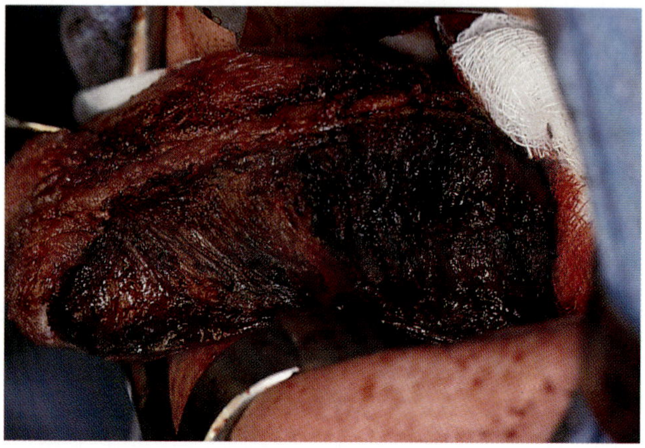

Figure 7–41. Depth of resection in residual mobile tongue.

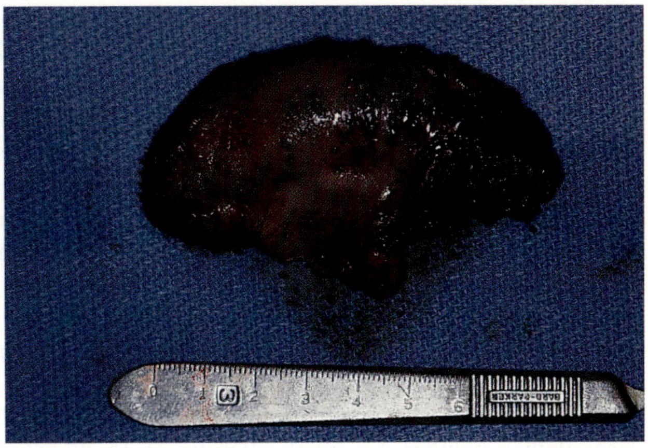

Figure 7–42. Specimen.

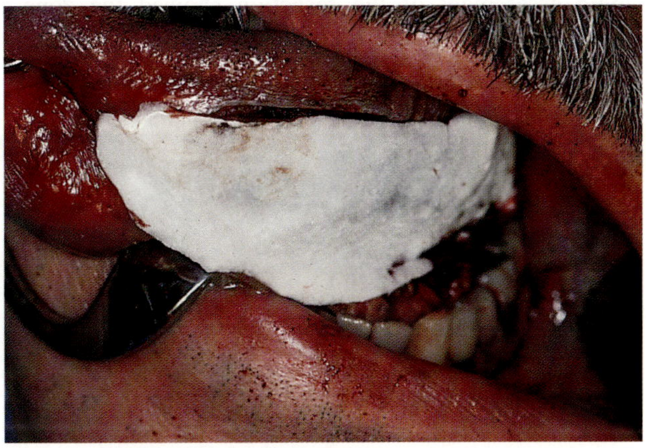

Figure 7–43. Bovine collagen dressing sutured in place to facilitate hemostasis (from a similar case).

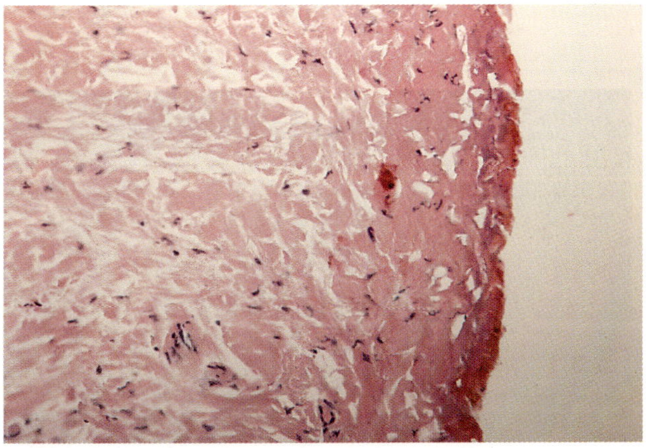

Figure 7–44. Histology of resection margin. Note that depth of coagulation necrosis from the contact YAG tip is only 0.22 mm. (Depending upon area examined it ranged from 0.22 mm to 0.67 mm.) (H&E 200×.)

output power of 15 W, and using the number 6 scalpel tip probe, the prospective margin was gently scribed approximately 1 cm beyond the visible and/or palpable tumor edge. Now, the probe tip was changed to a number 8 scalpel tip, the laser turned on, and the pedal was depressed to permit heating of the probe tip, which was only then inserted into the tissue to begin the excision. With slight charring of the tip occurring, heat transfer was now kept constant by periodically wiping the probe tip to maintain a consistent level of carbonization. In this way, the dissection was completed (Figs. 7–39 to 7–41) using tactile cues very similar to those used for electrocautery in "cut" mode. Gentle pressure on the hand probe permitted unforced penetration of the tissues. This prevented excessive buildup of charred tissue on the probe tip, which would otherwise have changed the output power (heat) and beam geometry.

At the conclusion of this subtotal posterolateral glossectomy, estimated blood loss was 125 mL and operation time was 40 minutes. The specimen (Fig. 7–42) was reviewed with the pathologist in the operating room. The entire tongue wound was left to heal by secondary intention, and postoperative hemostasis was enhanced by applying a bovine collagen patch to the surface of the tongue, which was sutured along its periphery (Fig. 7–43). The histologic specimen (Fig. 7–44) showed thermal necrosis limited to 0.3 to 0.7 mm. After surgery, the patient applied pressure until the following morning. He resumed oral intake the next morning, and he was discharged the following day. His speech was intelligible on the day after surgery, and it returned to normal during postoperative week 5 (Fig. 7–44). Postoperative narcotic analgesics were required for 6 days after surgery. However, there was minimal postoperative edema and there was no postoperative bleeding. Swallowing was normal by week 8. At 18 weeks the range of motion of the tongue was normal, as was swallowing (Fig. 7–45). Metastatic disease appeared in the ipsilateral neck during the fifth month after surgery.

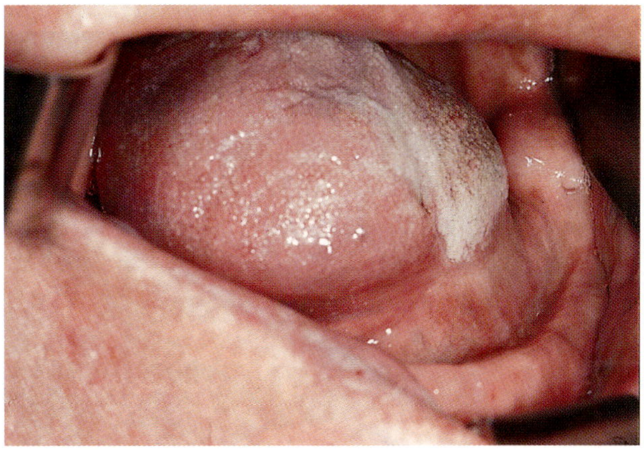

Figure 7–45. At 18 weeks. Range of motion of tongue good. Mild speech impediment. Normal swallowing.

COMPLICATIONS

Case 7: Palate—Postoperative Tonsillar Hypertrophy

This 49-year-old white man presented with his second primary squamous cell carcinoma. The index lesion was a $T_1N_0M_0$ moderately well-differentiated squamous cell carcinoma of the left ventrolateral tongue treated by free-beam laser excision 12 months previously. He continued to smoke one and a half packs of cigarettes per day, and to drink two or three beers per day. A second primary tumor, a $T_1N_0M_0$ well-differentiated squamous cell carcinoma, developed on the left soft palate and a new leukoplakia developed on the right soft palate. The treatment plan called for wide local excision of the new primary cancer and evaporative ablation of the leukoplakia after directed biopsy guided by vital staining with toluidine blue.

There were no unexpected extensions of the palatal cancer. Resection commenced with the SLT contact Nd:YAG laser silica probe tip. Output power was 12 to 20 W. Dissection was carried full thickness through the levator veli palatini muscle after first marking the periphery for margins with the number 4 scalpel tip used at 20 W. Now using the number 8 scalpel tip at 15 W, the tip was angled to maintain proper position in the depth of the resection. In this case some palatal muscle was preserved and there was no perforation of the nasopharyngeal mucosa. Histopathologic assessment of the specimen confirmed adequacy of resection. The margins were somewhat affected by heat artifact from the YAG contact laser with the deep margin showing 1.6 mm of thermal necrosis. However, hemostasis was excellent and the more extensive heat damage was not clinically significant.

An unexpectedly exuberant host response to the palatal resection occurred during the second month of observation.

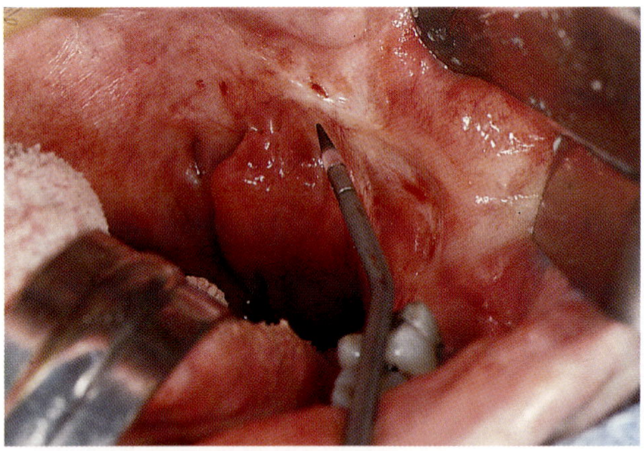

Figure 7–50. Outlining the mass: SLT contact YAG: number 6 scalpel tip at 15 W.

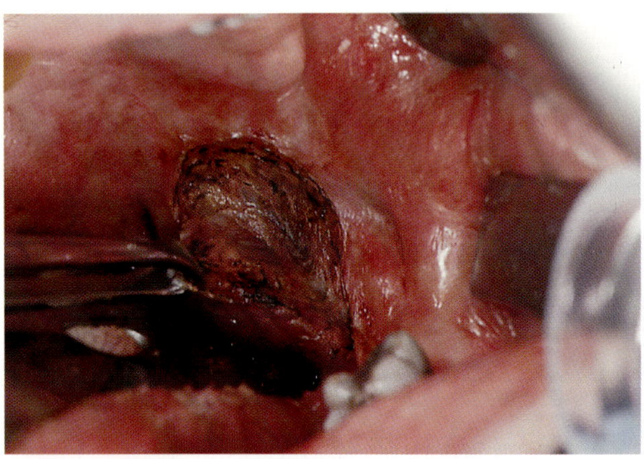

Figure 7–51. Traction as dissection reaches depth of tonsillar crypt. No bleeding. Note smoke generation. The high-speed laser smoke evacuation system still must be used, just as it is for the free-beam CO_2 laser.

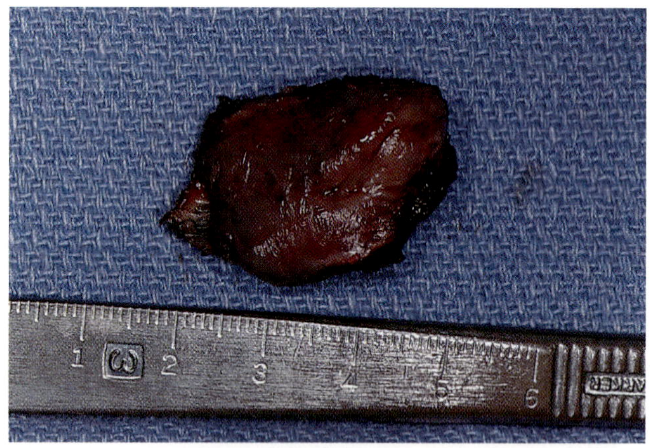

Figure 7–52. Specimen.

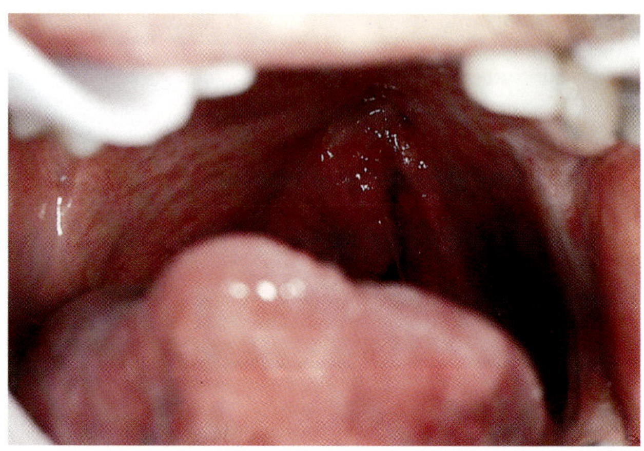

Figure 7–53. Complete reepithelialization and healing at 3 weeks.

Unilateral hypertophy of tonsillar tissue developed adjacent to the resection site (Fig. 7–50). This was removed for histopathologic assessment using the bloodless technique of the contact:YAG laser. The contact:YAG provided the security of tactile feedback while performing surgery at the depth of the tonsillar fossa. The lesion was easily delivered from a bloodless field (Figs. 7–51 and 7–52). Significant laser smoke was generated by the YAG tip in contact with the tissue. As always it was mandatory to use the high-speed laser suction.

The tonsillar fossa was not bleeding at the conclusion of surgery and raw surface area was reduced by partially closing the fossa. The surgical site was reepithelialized and completely healed in 3 weeks (Fig. 7–53). Postoperatively, speech and swallowing were completely normal within 6 weeks after surgery.

CASE 8: FOM COMPLICATION—RESTRICTED TONGUE MOTION

A 72-year-old white woman with $T_1N_0M_0$ moderately well differentiated squamous cell carcinoma. Anterior floor of mouth. Limitation of range of motion of tongue occurred requiring scar release (Figs. 7–54 and 7–55).

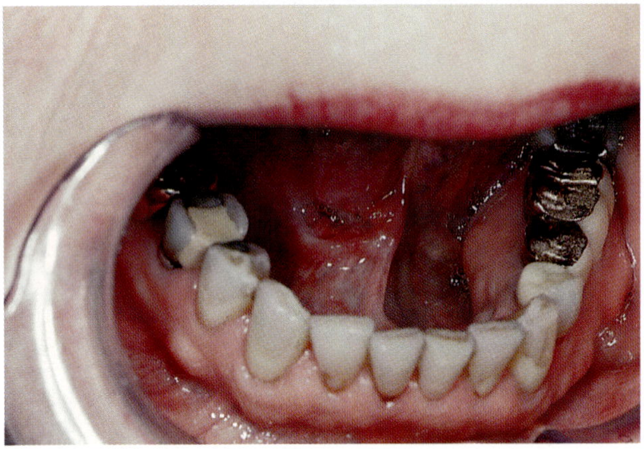

Figure 7–54. $T_1N_0M_0$ squamous cell carcinoma of anterior floor of mouth.

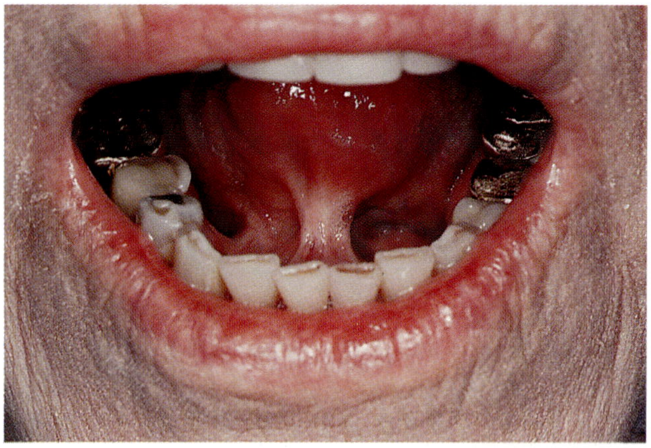

Figure 7–55. Restricting scar band: Pseudoankyloglossia at 19 months. Release of wide and thick scar band causing pseudoankyloglossia. RSP, 118 pps, PD approximately 500 to 600 W/cm^2.

CASE 9: BUCCAL MUCOSA WITH PROLIFERATIVE GRANULATION TISSUE

A 58-year-old woman with a verrucous carcinoma, $T_2N_0M_0$ of the right buccal mucosa, was treated by wide local excision with the free-beam RSP CO_2 laser at an average power of 25 W, 0.3-mm spot size for incision, defocused spot size of 2.0 to 2.5 mm for coagulation at 86 pps, 290 mJ/pulse (Figs. 7–56 to 7–59). Although, most of the treated area reepithelialized normally, a 1.5-cm-diameter mass of granulation tissue persisted at the proximal edge of the resection margin. Trauma from her molars occluding into the proliferative scar prevented its resolution. After an additional 2 months of maturation the lesion persisted. It was, therefore, excised using the same parameters described above. A maxillary acrylic prosthesis with a buccal flange was worn for 1 month to prevent occlusal trauma to any granulation tissue that might have proliferated at the treatment site. Within 1 month of excision, the buccal mucosa had healed completely and maximum incisal opening was normal. She has been cancer free and the proliferative lesion has not returned.

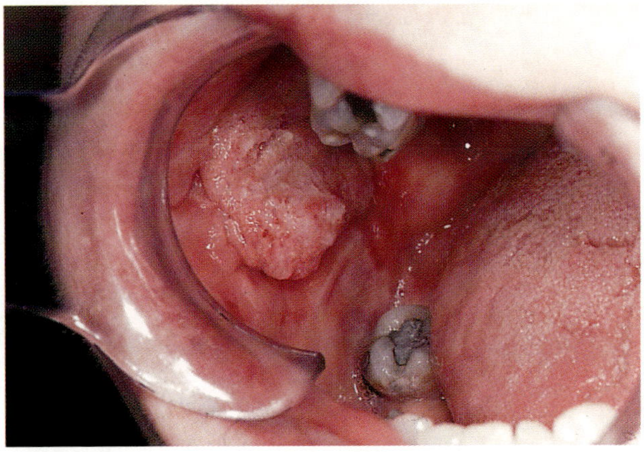

Figure 7–56. $T_2N_0M_0$ verrucous carcinoma of right buccal mucosa.

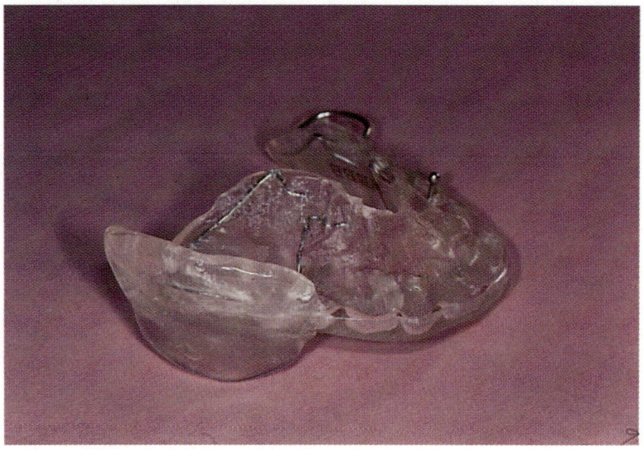

Figure 7–58. Maxillary prosthesis to protect cheek.

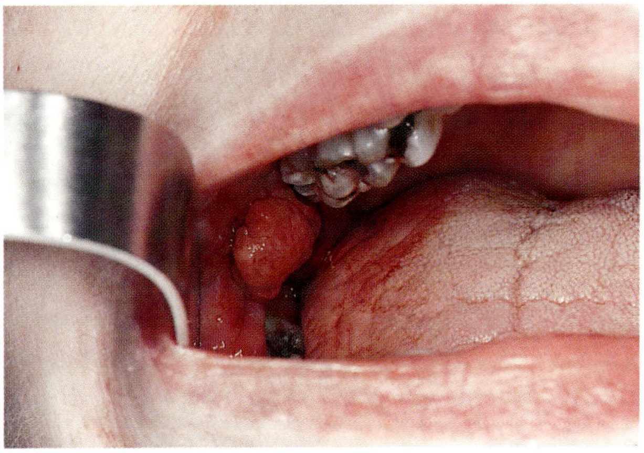

Figure 7–57. Proliferative granulation tissue arose, at proximal edge of resection margin. Matured lesion now appeared as a large pedunculated polyp. Excised with the RSP CO_2 laser.

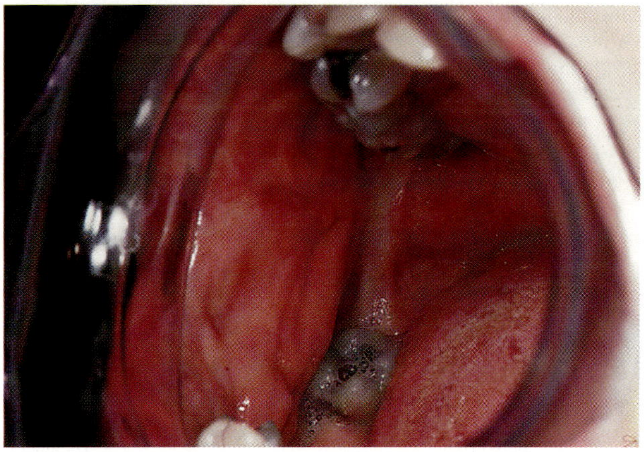

Figure 7–59. Buccal mucosa, 9 months after excision of polyp. Three years later there is still no recurrence of the polyp or the cancer; mouth opening and buccal mucosa are both normal.

CASE 10: ADJUNCTIVE USE OF THE CO_2 LASER—TUMOR DEBULKING

When treating patients with head and neck cancer who have failed definitive therapy, one is confronted with the problem of designing compassionate palliative treatment to debulk recurrence at the primary site. Satisfactory palliation should provide pain relief, create a wound that is easy to clean, and reduce the smell of necrotic tissue, and the palliative procedure should be brief. The high-powered free-beam CO_2 laser serves this purpose well.

A 68-year-old man developed recurrent squamous cell carcinoma under his pectoralis major myocutaneous flap that extended into the submental triangle (Figs. 7–60 to 7–63). The original tumor was a stage IV, $T_3N_3M_0$ squamous cell carcinoma of the tongue and his recurrence developed 27 months after treatment of the index tumor by a combined regimen of chemotherapy, radiotherapy, and surgical resection with immediate soft tissue reconstruction. The CO_2 laser with a handheld probe was used in the defocused mode at an output power of 90 W CW with a spot size of 2.0 to 3.0 mm giving an average PD of 3500 W/cm^2 to 1560 W/cm^2. This provided adequate hemostasis while permitting debulking of the tumor. General anesthesia was used and the operation required less than 30 minutes. A collagen hemostatic dressing was applied to the depth of the wound to aid in hemostasis. The wound remained clean and without an offensive odor until the patient's death 3 months later.

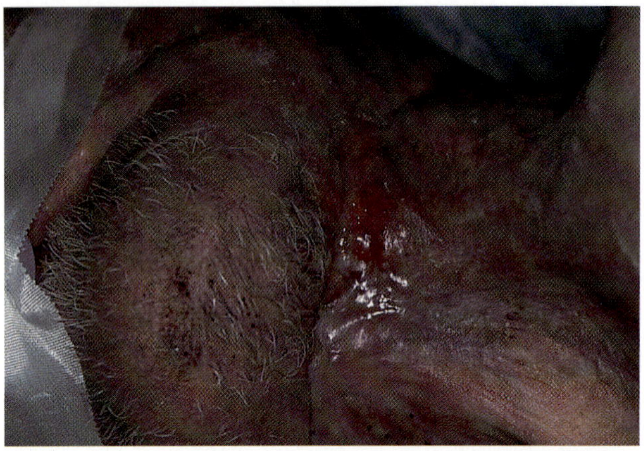

Figure 7–60. Recurrent carcinoma of anterior neck and floor of mouth occurring inferior to a myocutaneous flap 27 months after resection of a $T_3N_3M_0$ squamous cell carcinoma of the tongue.

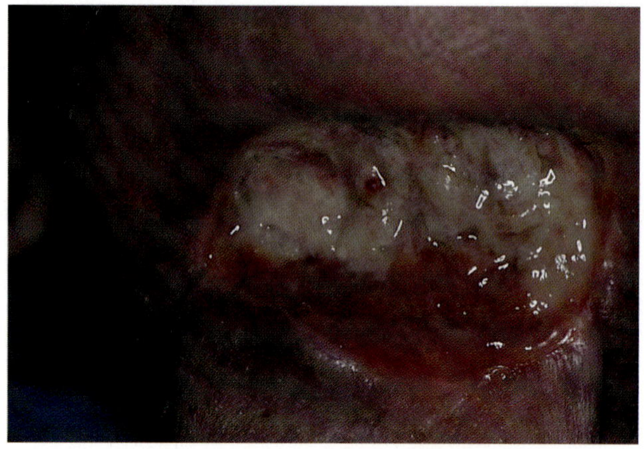

Figure 7–62. Tumor bed is clean 3 weeks after treatment.

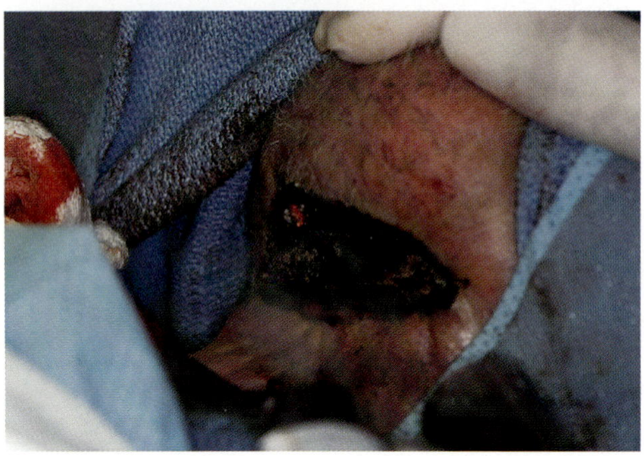

Figure 7–61. Ablation of recurrent tumor. Free-beam CO_2, 90 W, 2- to 3-mm spot size. Note HeNe aiming beam in upper left corner of wound. Significant plume production occurred at this power density.

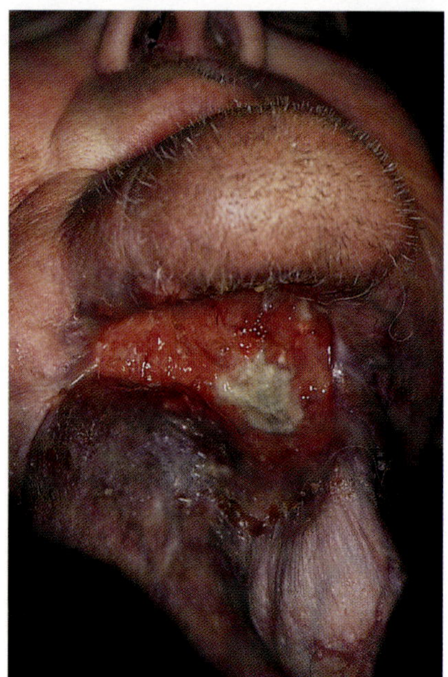

Figure 7–63. Three months after treatment just before death. The treated area remains quite clean.

REFERENCES

1. Ries LAG, Miller BA, Hankey BF, Kosary CL, Harras A, Edwards BK, eds. *SEER Cancer Statistics Review 1973–1991.* Table and Graphs. NIH Pub. No. 94-2789. Bethesda: National Cancer Institute; 1994.
2. Examinations for oral cancer—United States, 1992. *MMWR* 1994;43:198–200.
3. Panje WR, Scher N, Karnell M. Transoral carbon dioxide laser ablation for cancer, tumors and other diseases. *Arch Otolaryngol Head Neck Surg* 1989;115:681–688.
4. Carruth JAS. Resection of the tongue with the carbon dioxide laser: 100 cases. *J Laryngol Otol* 1985;99:887–889.
5. Nagorsky MJ, Sessions DJ. Laser resection for early oral cavity cancer results and complications. *Ann Otol Rhinol Laryngol* 1987;96:556–560.
6. Guerry TL, Silverman S Jr, Dedo HH. Carbon dioxide laser resection of superficial oral carcinoma: indications, technique and results. *Ann Otol Rhinol Laryngol* 1986;99:547–555.
7. Clayman L. Transoral resection of oral squamous cell cancer (abstract). Annual Meeting of the American Society for Lasers in Medicine and Surgery, April 1995, San Diego.
8. Davis RK, Steiner W. Transoral CO_2 laser excision of stage II glottic cancer: current indications and results in 84 patients. Abstract No. 181. American Society for Lasers in Surgery and Medicine, Annual Meeting, 1994, Toronto.
9. MacLean AB, Murray EL, Sharof, More IAR. Residual cervical intraepithelial neoplasia after laser ablation. *Lasers Surg Med* 1987;7:278–279.
10. Spiro RH, Spiro JD, Strong EW. Surgical approach to squamous carcinoma confined to the tongue and the floor of the mouth. *Head Neck Surg* 1986;9:27–30.
11. Panje WR, Smith B, McCabe BFG. Epidermoid carcinoma of the floor of the mouth. Surgical therapy vs. combined therapy vs. radiation therapy. *Otolaryngol Head Neck Surg* 1989;88:714–720.
12. Rodgers LW, Stringer SP, Mendenhall WM, Parsons JT, Cassisi NJ, Million RR. Management of squamous cell carcinoma of the floor of the mouth. *Head Neck* 1993;15:16–19.
13. Ildstad St, Bigelow ME, Remensnyder JP. Intra-oral cancer at the Massachussetts General Hospital: squamous cell carcinoma of the floor of the mouth. *Ann Surg* 1983;197:34–41.
14. Lydiatt DD, Robbins KT, Byers RM, Wolf PF. Treatment of stage I and stage II oral tongue cancer. *Head Neck* 1993;15:308–312.
15. Feldman M, Vemakli A, Strong MS, et al. Applications of carbon dioxide laser surgery and radiation. *Arch Otolaryngol Head Neck Surg* 1983;109:240–242.
16. McDonald GA, Simpson GT. Transoral resection of lesions of the oral cavity with the carbon dioxide laser. *Otolaryngol Clin North Am* 1983;16:839–847.
17. Mihashi S, Jako CJ, Incze J, Strong MS, Vaughan CW. Laser surgery in otolaryngology. Interactions of CO_2 laser and soft tissue. *Ann NY Acad Sci* 1976;267:263–294.
18. Gaspar L, Szabo G. Manifestation of the advantages and disadvantages of using the CO_2 laser in oral surgery. *J Clin Laser Med Surg* 1990; Feb: 39–43.
19. Verschueren RJ. *The CO_2 Laser in Tumor Surgery.* Assen, Van Gorcum; 1976.
20. Braun R, Liebow C. Clinical evaluation of tumor promotion by CO_2 laser. *Lasers Orthop Dental Veterinary Med* 1991;1424:138–140.
21. Oosterhuis JW. Tumor surgery with the CO_2 laser, studies with the Cloudman S91 mouse melanoma. PhD thesis, Rijksuniversitet Groningen, 1977.
22. Ammirati M, Rao LN, Murty MS, Buchmann T, Goldschmidt RA, Scanlon EF. Partial nephrectomy in mice with milliwatt carbon dioxide laser and its influence on experimental metastasis. *J Surg Oncol* 1989;41:153–159.
23. Maker VJ, Elseth KM, Radosevich JA. Reduced in vivo local recurrence with contact neodymium:yttrium-aluminum-garnet (Nd:YAG) laser scalpels. *Lasers Surg Med* 1995;17:370–374.
24. Strong MS, Vaughan CW, Jako GJ, Polanyl T. Transoral management of localized carcinomas of the oral cavity using the CO_2 laser. *Otolaryngol Clin North Am* 1979;12:207–218.
25. Strong MS, Vaughan CW, Healy GB, Shapshay SM, Jako GJ. Transoral management of localized carcinoma of the oral cavity using the CO_2 laser. *Laryngoscope* 1979;89:897–905.
26. Walsh JT, Flotte TJ, Anderson RR, Deutsch TF. Pulsed CO_2 laser tissue ablation: effect of tissue type and pulse duration on thermal damage. *Lasers Surg Med* 1988;8:108–118.
27. Fuller TA. *Thermal Surgical Lasers.* Surgical Laser Technologies; 1991.
28. Royston DD, Torres JH, Thomsen S, Sriram PS, Welch AJ. Comparison of the thermal tissue effects produced by the aged sapphire and silica hemispherical tips. *Lasers Surg Med* 1994;14:47–58.
29. Gallucci JG, Zeltsman D, Slotman G. Nd:YAG laser scalpel compared with conventional techniques in head and neck surgery. *Lasers Surg Med* 1994;14:139–144.
30. Roodenburg JLN, tenBosch JJ, Borsboom PCF. Measurement of the uniaxial elasticity of oral mucosa in vivo after CO_2-laser evaporation and surgical excision. *Int J Oral Maxillofac Surg* 1990;19:181–183.
31. Clayman L. Management of mucosal premalignant lesions. *Oral Maxillofac Clin North Am* 1994;6:431–443.
32. Loumanen M, Lehto VP, Meurman JH. Myofibroblasts in healing laser wounds of rat tongue mucosa. *Arch Oral Biol* 1988;33(1):17–23.
33. Fisher SE, Frame JW. The effects of the carbon dioxide surgical laser on oral tissues. *Br J Oral Maxillofac Surg* 1984;22:414–425.
34. Browne RM, Potts AJC. Dysplasia in salivary gland ducts in sublingual leukoplakia and erythroplakia. *Oral Surg Oral Med Oral Path* 1986;64:44–48.

8 *Section 1:* Outpatient Treatment of Snoring and Sleep Apnea Syndrome with CO_2 Laser: Laser-Assisted Uvulopalatoplasty

Yves-Victor Kamami

The laser-assisted uvulopalatoplasty (LAUP) is a surgical technique designed to correct breathing abnormalities during sleep that result in snoring or mild to moderate obstructive sleep apnea syndrome (OSAS).[1,2] This is a short operation, performed in the office using local anesthesia and a surgical laser. The objective is to reduce pharyngeal airway obstruction by reducing tissue volume in the uvula, the velum, and the superior part of the posterior pharyngeal pillars.

INDICATIONS

It has been demonstrated that the majority of snorers benefit from LAUP[1] as do many patients with OSAS whose respiratory distress index (RDI) is less than 50. For those with severe OSAS (RDI >75), who have severe mandibular retrognathia or nasal tract obstruction, other treatment methods, particularly continuous positive airway pressure (CPAP) or mandibular advancement osteotomy, are required. However, even in some cases of severe OSAS with obstruction at the pharyngeal level who do not respond to CPAP, LAUP may be of limited benefit in increasing pharyngeal airway compliance.

Further contraindications to LAUP are severe macroglossia and morbid obesity with hypopharyngeal obstruction at the tongue base. In the rare condition of floppy epiglottis, LAUP is also not of benefit.

COMPARISON TO UVULOPALATOPHARYNGOPLASTY (UPPP)

The proper use of the thermal properties of the CO_2 laser provides technical advantages over scalpel techniques for the surgical treatment of snoring. The accessibility of the velum, uvula, and posterior tonsillar pillar to direct sculpting by the laser allows the operator to selectively regulate tissue removal. After treatment, postoperative edema and pain are minimal and healing is rapid, predictable, and free of uncontrolled scar formation. Because of the hemostatic action of the laser, the procedure may be performed using local anesthesia with minimal bleeding despite the highly vascular tissue of the oral mucosa. Unlike UPPP, the LAUP is a limited operation with low morbidity that does not require general anesthesia and may be performed in an office or day surgery center. The lack of morbidity from LAUP allows patients to return to work immediately after surgery. The LAUP allows more precise tissue removal, less tissue loss, and better overall control of surgery. It is more attractive to surgeons who question traditional UPPP because of its anesthetic risk and increased postoperative pain, swelling, and potential risk of developing velopharyngeal incompetence (VPI).

LAUP may also be useful when UPPP has failed due to obstruction of the hypopharynx from fatty and redundant tissue on the posterolateral pharyngeal walls. It is also a good alternative for patients who present with major surgical and anesthesia-related risks. In all cases, the healing of the laser-induced wounds is faster than after standard UPPP, except in the cases of alcohol or tobacco use. In these cases, the duration of postoperative pain is prolonged.

As is the case for UPPP, snoring and OSAS may also recur after LAUP. This is due to velopharyngeal hypotonia secondary to age, obesity, tobacco and alcohol use, excessive consumption of sedative-hypnotic drugs or tranquilizers, or untreated hypothyroidism. If symptoms of snoring or OSAS recur, a second treatment directed at the palate may induce remission. The CO_2 laser or contact neodymium:yttrium-aluminum-garnet (Nd:YAG) laser is preferred to the use of the Nd:YAG fiber-delivered laser in this procedure because of the low volume of absorption of the CO_2 laser beam or contact Nd:YAG in tissue. This property prevents excessive thermal necrosis of the target tissue. The YAG laser also does not have a backstop, although this problem is eliminated for contact YAG lasers. An additional advantage of the CO_2 laser is its use as a "no-touch" technique, thereby eliminating contact with the palate and pharyngeal walls. This property reduces gagging, especially for the hypersensitive individual whose gagging occurs on a psychological basis despite having adequate anesthesia at the surgical site.

DESCRIPTION OF THE PROCEDURE

LAUP is performed with a free-beam CO_2 laser with a backstop. Beam guidance is provided by a coaxial helium-neon (HeNe) laser. Standard CO_2 laser safety precautions have to be followed. The output power is set at 20 to 30 W average power in a pulsed mode, depending on the thickness of tissue that is to be incised. A specific snoring handpiece is used with a variable spot size of 0.6 to 3.51 mm at a focal length of 300 mm. This handpiece has a focus-defocus ring: focus to cut, and defocus to coagulate.

The patient is premedicated with an oral analgesic and antiemetic. Blood pressure is monitored during the operation. At the time of the session, the patient is placed in a seated position with the mouth open. The eyes are protected with goggles or wet gauze sponges. The patient then is given breathing instructions: to take a deep breath and very slowly let it out. Local anesthesia is then administered using a lidocaine 15% spray followed by an injection of 2% lidocaine with epinephrine (1.25 mg in 2.0 g of lidocaine) into the base of the uvula on both sides. Between 1 and 2 mL are infiltrated on each side.

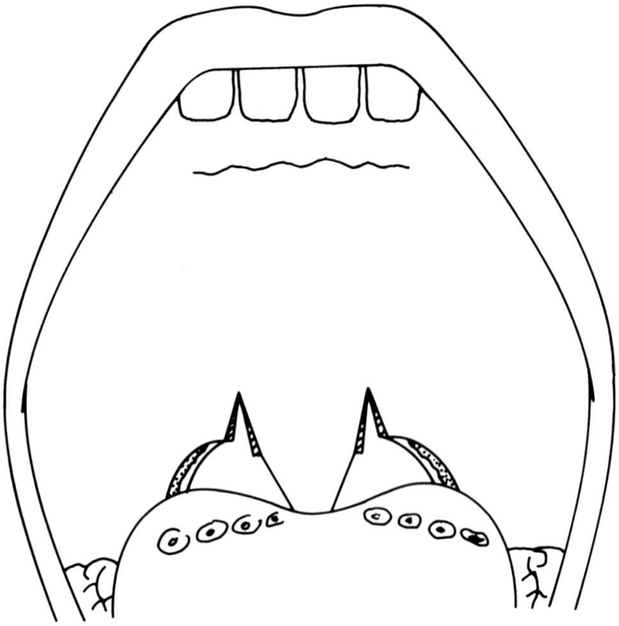

Figure 8–1. Laser-assisted UPPP (LAUP) in four to five sessions. Illustration demonstrates the vertical and horizontal incision cutting of the soft palate, laterally to the root of the uvula, at the left, then at the right side of the uvula.

The "Multiple-Stage" Technique

This procedure is designed to remove the minimal amount of tissue consistent with the reduction of snoring. Usually the surgery is repeated a second or a third time. This conservative approach to tissue removal essentially eliminates the development of VPI as a complication of LAUP. Bilateral vertical incisions are made lateral to the uvula, sparing the uvula itself. These are full-thickness "trenches" on either side of the uvula (Fig. 8–1). The uvula is then shortened by approximately 50% of its length and "reshaped." A "neo-uvula" is created, with further debulking of the inferior and lateral sides of the uvula. Its anterior and posterior sides must be preserved, leaving the mucosa intact to prevent granuloma formation and facilitate reepithelialization. This is done by vaporization at the point of focus (0.6 mm) using a pulsed mode "Swiftlase" attachment for the Shaplan laser, which produces minimal char while ablating the tissue rapidly and bloodlessly. The slightly defocused beam when applied to the area of incision adequately controls bleeding from any discrete area that still bleeds after making the incision. No sutures are required. At each of the planned sessions, about 5 to 8 mm of the velum is removed. Extending the incisions much higher onto the soft palate will usually result in increased postoperative pain. In this way the neo-uvula will gradually assume a more superior position following each treatment until it reaches the level of Passavant's ridge (Figs. 8–2 and 8–3).

A handpiece specifically designed for this procedure incorporates a backstop and a smoke evacuator. The backstop protects the posterior pharyngeal wall and the smoke evacuator maintains clear visibility in the operative field.

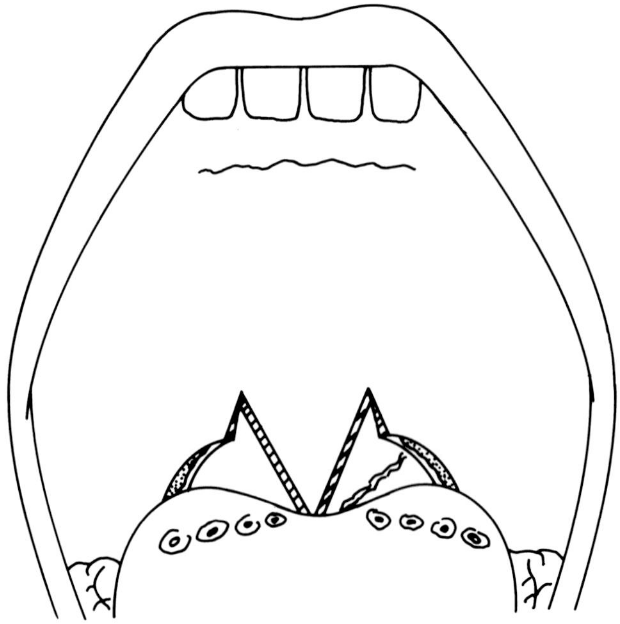

Figure 8–2. LAUP in multiple sessions: reducing lateral aspect of uvula.

Subsequent sessions are basically the same as the first one. The end point is determined when the patient or bed partner stops complaining about snoring. In patients with a narrow nasopharyngeal orifice, a horizontal section is performed on the upper part of the posterior tonsillar pillars, to enlarge the aperture. This removal of the upper part of the

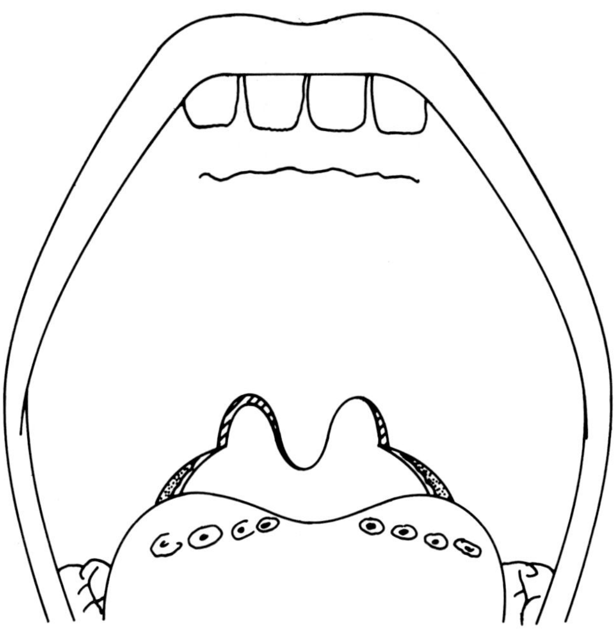

Figure 8–3. LAUP: multiple sessions. Creation of a "neo-uvula," by debulking of the inferior and the lateral sides of the uvula. Repeat sessions will gradually result in the "neo-uvula" assuming a more superior and dorsal position, closer to Passavant's ridge.

tonsillar pillar is usually done in the last session, causing an anterior and superior motion of the neo-uvula, as retraction occurs.

In the OSAS patients, the uvula is usually thicker and longer than in patients with simple snoring. The operations are therefore longer for apneic snorers than for nonapneic snorers because of the longer time needed to transfix and trim the uvula. If there is hypertrophy of the lingual tonsils, it is possible to perform a tonsil ablation with either a fixed 90° or an adjustable front surface mirror handpiece, which permits one to redirect the laser beam to the posterior third of the tongue.

Five watts of continuous power and a local anesthetic spray are used. Bleeding is usually minimal or more likely nonexistent. When there is bleeding, it is controlled with the defocused beam, which coagulates vessels less than 0.5 mm in diameter. If bleeding continues, it is controlled with bipolar electrocautery. Smoke is evacuated by a high-speed dedicated laser evacuation system, which is connected to the laser handpiece.

Palatine or lingual tonsillar hypertrophy is treated by laser-assisted tonsil ablation (LATA) with the "Swiftlase" if tonsillar size is contributing to the OSAS by obstructing the oropharynx. In cases of nasal obstruction caused by turbinate hypertrophy or septal deviation, a CO_2 laser–assisted partial inferior turbinectomy (LAPT) or a septoplasty may have to be performed. Actually, most patients may have a LAPT about 1 month after the completion of the LAUP procedure to ensure better nasopharyngeal air flow.

In the multistage technique, three to four sessions of 5 minutes each are performed, generally spaced at monthly intervals. The length and number of the sessions will vary according to the thickness of the arch and soft palate and the hypertrophy of the tonsils. The average number of sessions is 3.77 in nonapneic snorers and 4.3 in OSAS patients.

The "Single-Stage" Technique

To facilitate rapidity of the correction of snoring, a "single-stage" technique has now been developed. This should only be performed by surgeons experienced in the multistage technique. Two paramedian vertical incisions or transfixing "trenches" are made to a height of 2 to 3 cm. These incisions are lateral to the root of the uvula and extend superiorly up to the junction of the soft and hard palate at the "dimple point." The base of the uvula is then held with a Kocher clamp to pull it laterally to facilitate a horizontal incision just under the base of the uvula (Fig. 8–4). Reshaping of the uvula at the apex of the soft palate is carried out, resulting in a small "neo-uvula." This neo-uvula hangs from the rear of the hard palate, preventing centripetal scar fibrosis, because of the specific makeup of its muscle fibers (which seems to be different from non-snorers) (Fig. 8–5). In addition, the upper part of the posterior pillars are debulked and both the superior portion of the vertical incisions and the neo-uvula are made into a U shape using the Swiftlase attachment (Fig. 8–5). It contains a portion of the azygos muscle that can still contract and prevent VPI from occurring, like a mainmast supporting the palatine arch, a

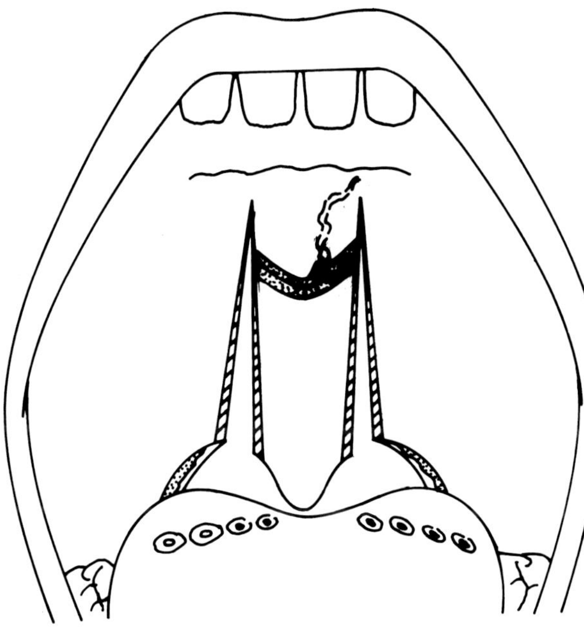

Figure 8–4. LAUP: one-stage vertical incisions and creation of neo-uvula.

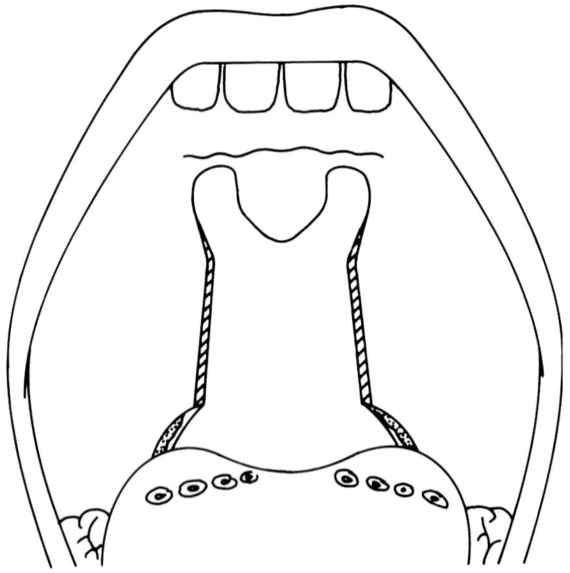

Figure 8–5. LAUP: one stage. Debulking the superior part of the posterior pillars to create a U shape.

stub middle pillar similar to those of the ribbed vault of a church, flanked by the two lateral posterior pillars. The mainmast of the uvula is made by the palatostaphylinus or uvula azygos muscle. This small, spindle-shaped, vertical muscle is entirely enclosed in the velum; its main action is to raise the uvula, and this muscle is only attached to the posterior side of the hard palate at its upper edge. So it is very important to partially preserve this mainmast as a support of the middle of the velum.[3]

OPERATIVE OUTCOME

After the procedure, the patients are given a prescription including mild analgesics, peroxide and water gargles, topical anesthetic throat lozenges, anesthetic mouth sprays, and viscous lidocaine to relieve throat pain. They are instructed to avoid drinking alcohol, eating food with vinegar, lemon, or spices and taking aspirin and nonsteroidal anti-inflammatory drugs (NSAIDs) for 10 days after the operation.

Patients complain only of a moderate to severe "swallowing pain" similar to a "sore throat" for about 10 days. Pain intensity reaches its peak 3 to 5 days postoperatively, but doesn't inhibit eating food or drinking, speaking, or working immediately afterward. Rarely, spitting of blood may occur either during the first 48 hours or approximately 8 days after the session, but can easily be stopped in minutes with peroxide and water gargles.

Usually, no serious complications occur during the operation or during the immediate postoperative phase after LAUP. Postoperative observation in a medical care unit is unnecessary. There are no clinically identifiable changes in speech or velopharyngeal function. No fibrosis causing narrowing of the nasopharyngeal aperture has been observed as sometimes has been seen after UPPP. Nasal regurgitation has not been reported after the laser surgery. Infections were rare except for occasional oral candidiasis.

OSAS PATIENTS

To ensure physiologic night ventilation in severe OSAS patients, nasal continuous positive airway pressure (N-CPAP) is utilized for the duration of the laser treatment. Following completion of the LAUP treatment, polysomnography is repeated. CPAP is discontinued when the polysomnogram becomes normal.

RESULTS OF A PERSONAL SERIES

Nonapneic Snorers

From December 1988 to July 1994, 856 patients were treated with LAUP by the author. There were 715 men and 141 women, with a mean age of 49.2 years (range: 25 to 80). The mean body mass index (BMI) was 25.9 (range: 17.1 to 45). No recordings of snoring were carried out, as the diagnosing and treatment indications were based on the spouse's complaint and not on a measured level or character of noise.

After treatment, 70.4% of patients (603 patients) had a complete or near elimination of snoring, with no long-term recurrence; 24.4% (209 patients) had improvement in their snoring, without disturbing the spouse, and 5.1% (44 patients) showed no response after LAUP. In these "failures" there was always a diminution of snoring but the bed partner was still unhappy about the intensity of snoring. Of the 644 patients treated with the multistage technique, results showed clinical improvement by the second or third LAUP session. A clear decrease of snoring was seen, and the mean session number was 3.77. Among the 212 patients cured with the one-stage technique, there were only seven patients who needed a second session, 1 month later. The mean duration time of postoperative pain was 11.2 days.

Early postoperative results were better than for the classic UPPP, but longer follow-up showed reduced success. After several months, snoring had reappeared in a few cases, but with much less disturbance than before. A further study of long-term results by telephone interview is currently in progress to determine the exact percentage of snoring recurrence several years after LAUP. Levin and Becker[4] have shown that snoring recurred in most patients 6 to 12 months after UPPP; 28% of patients with initial complete abolition of snoring had returned to preoperative levels (after UPPP). Usually, after LAUP, the rare patients who came back again for another session because of snoring recurrence have been cured of their discomfort. The most frequent cause of recurrence is tobacco smoking. Of the 25 cases of conventional UPPP failures treated by LAUP, there were 14 complete cures, 10 were improved, and 1 failed. In the majority of the patients, there was also a significant reduction of daytime somnolence, sleep awakenings, morning tiredness, morning headaches, and sexual problems (erectile dysfunction).

Obstructive Sleep Apnea Syndrome

From December 1988 to May 1994, 70 adult patients were included in this study as "OSAS snorers," 64 men and 6 women, with a mean age of 53.9 (range: 23–72). The mean BMI was 29.2 (range: 22.3–40) and the BMI was found to be more than 30 in 23 cases. All had pre- and postoperative evaluation by polysomnography and demonstrated evidence of repeated obstructive respiratory events during sleep on presurgical polysomnography.

For severe OSAS, CPAP was initiated before LAUP. Polysomnography was carried out before and after LAUP. After LAUP, there was an improvement of sleep efficiency as measured by nocturnal EEG, which demonstrated longer periods spent in stages III to IV and REM sleep. In 56 patients (80%), there was complete or near-complete elimination of snoring, with no recurrence. In 11 patients (15.7%), there was improvement of snoring, but still a small amount of occasional noise persisted. In three patients (4.3%) there was a decrease in snoring, but the noise was still disturbing to the spouse. Daytime sleepiness disappeared in 82% of cases, decreased in 15% of cases, and was unchanged in 3% of cases. Morning tiredness disappeared in 94% of cases and decreased in 6% of cases. Among the 26 patients who suffered from morning headaches, this symptom disappeared in 25 cases, and remained unchanged in one case. Among the 56 patients with frequent sleep awakenings, this symptom disappeared in 30 cases, decreased in 18 cases, and remained as before LAUP in eight cases. Among the 27 patients who suffered sexual problems (erectile dysfunction, loss of libido), 23 said that their sex life was improved after LAUP.

Sleep efficiency (total sleep time × 100/total sleep period) was improved in 63% of patients among patients with pre- and postoperative nocturnal EEG studies. Also shown was an increase in deep sleep time (stages III to IV and REM), in 63% of patients confirmed by nocturnal EEG studies. Furthermore, 44 patients noticed a reappearance of dreaming. A complete cure of OSAS was achieved in 36 patients (51.4%), and a clear improvement of OSAS in 26 patients (37.1%), with at least a 50% reduction in both the preoperative oxygen desaturation index and of the duration of the apneas. Eight patients (11.4%) were unimproved. However, these patients had better long-term acceptance of CPAP because of the reduction of the upper respiratory tract obstruction.

As for UPPP, high RDI and sleep apnea indices and morbid obesity also predicted a poor response to LAUP.

Among 62 patients classified as successful responders, the respiratory disturbance index (RDI) was reduced by more than 50%. The reduction of apnea length and of preoperative oxygen desaturation index was greater than 50%. The mean responder RDI decreased from 37.6 to 15.9, and the mean apnea index from 23.3 to 6.2, while the mean apnea index for the nonresponders decreased from 23.8 to 17.5. There were no complications reported. For all 70 patients, the mean RDI decreased from 37.8 to 19. Their mean apnea index decreased from 23.3 to 7.7. One very significant result is that the apneas have been transformed to hypopneas, which are less dangerous for these patients. The mean SaO_2 for the 70 patients improved from 93.1% preoperatively to 93.9% postoperatively. The mean lowest SaO_2 changed from 77.3% to 80.5% postoperatively.

Four patients were surgical UPPP failures corrected by LAUP. After LAUP, the results were two complete recoveries and two failures. Thirteen patients were also cured of nasal obstruction by laser-assisted partial turbinectomy combined with the LAUP. It is essential to convince our treated patients to maintain long-term follow-up examination and to repeat a full sleep study several months after surgery to confirm the efficacy of the LAUP operation.

CASE 1

A 55-year-old obese (102 kg, or 225 lbs) man, 1.73 m (5 feet, 8 inches) tall, presented with a 30-year history of snoring and moderate sleep apnea. Examination revealed that the tip of the soft palate extended to the inferior base of the tongue, predisposing to pharyngeal collapse. No maxillofacial abnormality was found. His initial polysomnography confirmed the diagnosis of OSAS, with an RDI of 62.8/hour and a sleep apnea index of 46.6/hour, and a total duration time of apneas of 126 minutes 14 seconds; 48% of sleep registering time occurred in association with a SaO_2 of less than 95%. Nasal CPAP was initiated 10 days later at a pressure of +11 cm of H_2O, resulting in REM positive sleep. A strict weight reduction diet was started. The patient wanted to discontinue the N-CPAP and agreed to undergo LAUP in several sessions. The first and second sessions performed 2 months apart still required continued use of N-CPAP. Polysomnography was repeated 3 weeks later, which found significant improvement of the OSAS, with an RDI of 22.6 and an apnea index of 12.5, a mean SaO_2 of 93.9, and a lowest SaO_2 of 61.6%. The total duration of apneas was 41 minutes 12 seconds. The patient noticed a clear improvement of clinical symptoms, including a reduction of weight to 98 kg (216 pounds).

Four months after the initial LAUP, a third operation was performed. This was followed 3 weeks later by polysomnography showing an RDI of 13/hour, and an apnea index of 7.3/hour. The mean SaO_2 was 92.9% and the lowest SaO_2 was 72.5%. The N-CPAP was decreased to 7 cm H_2O. A fourth and fifth session was done, respectively, 7 and 8 months after initial treatment. A repeat polysomnogram 9 months after initial treatment confirmed the elimination of OSAS and the CPAP was stopped. The patient later complained of nasal obstruction, and a laser-assisted partial turbinectomy of the left inferior and middle turbinate was performed 14 months after initial treatment. The right turbinates were treated by LAPT 3 weeks later. The patient returned for examination 4 months later with no more morning tiredness or daytime somnolence, improvement of sexual problems and of sleep efficiency, and only occasional soft snoring, still a bit disturbing to his wife.

CASE 2

A 50-year-old medical doctor presented with a 1-year history of snoring, morning tiredness, sexual problems, no daytime somnolence, and a BMI of 24.6. He underwent a one-stage LAUP and returned for reexamination 1 month later at which time there was cessation of snoring, although he complained of chronic nasal obstruction. Examination of his nose demonstrated a mild septal deviation and hypertrophy of the turbinates. Laser-assisted turbinectomy of the left inferior and middle turbinates, was carried out in two sessions. When reevaluated 4 months later, he had no more morning tiredness and there was improvement of his sexual dysfunction and of sleep efficiency with the reappearance of dreaming. There was no more snoring.

CONCLUSION

LAUP can lift the drooping soft palate on both sides of the uvula, similar to the way a theater curtain rises. After 5 years of experience with LAUP, this technique has improved or eliminated OSAS in most cases and probably shall be routinely used in OSAS surgery in a few years if the results are confirmed by other investigators. It would become a valuable alternative technique to conventional UPPP, with its great potential to reduce morbidity and cost to patients.

Popularization of the LAUP will require serious training of surgeons and further study with special emphasis on long-term assessment, especially in surgery for OSAS, which is more difficult to treat because of the thickness of the soft palate. In these patients, long-term polysomnographic controls are necessary to study long-term results.

REFERENCES

1. Kamami YV. Laser CO_2 for snoring, preliminary results. *Acta Otorhinolaryngol Belg* 1990;44:451–456.
2. Kamami YV. Outpatient treatment of sleep apnea syndrome with CO_2 laser, LAUP: laser-assisted UPPP results on 46 patients. *J Clin Laser Med Surg* 1994;12:215–219.

8 *Section 2:* Further Comments on the Laser-Assisted Uvulopalatoplasty

James W. Wooten

The laser-assisted uvulopalatoplasty (LAUP) to eliminate snoring first described by Kamami,[1] has become a low morbidity operation that may safely be performed in an ambulatory setting (office or surgicenter). The operation is conducted using local anesthesia with optional sedation in a series of one to five surgeries staged 3 to 5 weeks apart. Recovery is relatively uneventful. Long-term success rates are high with elimination of snoring being rated as complete in 70.4% of cases, satisfactory in 24.4%, and unimproved in 5.2%.[2]

Procedure[1,2,5–7]

Vertical full-thickness incisions are made bilaterally adjacent to the uvula extending from the free edge of the soft palate superiorly for approximately 1 to 2 cm (Fig. 8–6a). The superior extent of the incision length is marked by the attachment of the levator veli palatini muscles. The superior extent of the incision is limited by an imaginary line located at the posterior/inferior border of the levator's insertion. The position of its attachment is in the midline, anterior and superior to the base of the uvula. It is recognized by having the patient forcefully say, "Ha!, Ha!" A dimple will briefly appear on the oral surface of the soft palate. This dimple is marked by either silver nitrate ($AgNO_3$) or by a laser etching of the mucosa (Fig. 8–6b).

WARNING: Extension of the vertical incisions above the level of the dimple may cause velopharyngeal incompetence (VPI), resulting in nasal reflux of fluids and hypernasal speech. This must be avoided. After the vertical incisions are performed bilaterally, the uvula is generally reduced by one half (Fig. 8–6c). This will vary according to the length of the uvula.

In most cases the laser is next used to create a 2 mm deep and 4 mm wide trench on the anterior mucosal surface of the posterior tonsillar pillars bilaterally. This incision extends from the start of the initial vertical palatal incision and extends laterally and inferiorly to the base of the posterior tonsillar pillar (Fig. 8–6d). These are generally less than 3 cm in length.

Second Procedure

Three to five weeks postoperatively the patient's snoring status should be reevaluated. If snoring persists or if the patient can still snort, then the procedure can be repeated. Ordinarily a less extensive procedure is accomplished on repeat LAUPs. If low palatal webbing persists, thereby giving a constricted appearance to the velopharyngeal ring, an additional vertical release of 3 to 5 mm is placed laterally to the original vertical incisions.

One procedure is successful approximately 75% of the time. More than two procedures are seldom required.

Case Report

A 39-year-old man was referred from the sleep laboratory for evaluation of snoring and hypoxemia. He is 6 feet tall,

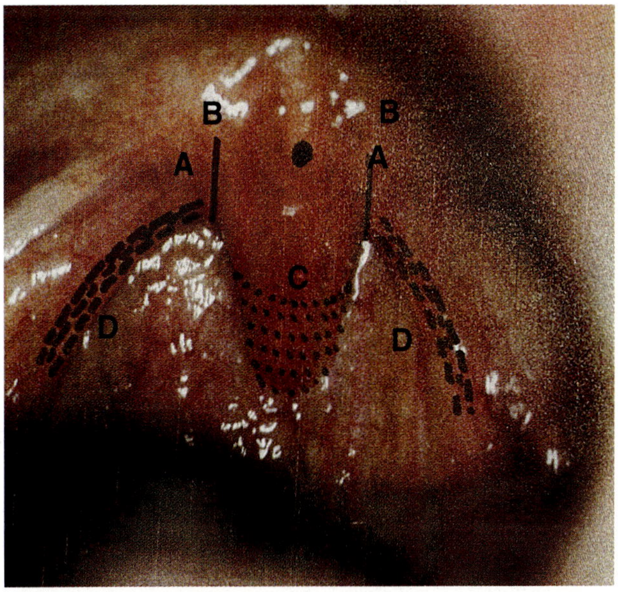

Figure 8–6. **(A)** Vertical incisions are made on each side of the uvula. **(B)** Superior extension of incision is determined by the position of attachment of the levator palati. **(C)** The uvula is generally reduced the same length as the vertical incisions. **(D)** Lateral trenches are created on the anterior surface of the posterior pharyngeal pillars.

weighs 245 lbs. (114 kg) and has a history of severe continuous snoring. Sleep studies indicated an apnea index of 1 and an oxygen desaturation index of 31. During 18% of his sleep time, oxygen saturation was less than 80%. A lateral cephalometric radiograph showed adequate posterior airway space in the hypopharyngeal region. A nasopharyngoscopy demonstrated a narrowing of the airway from each side and a closure of the retropalatal area during Müller's maneuver.[8] Oral examination revealed a low webbed soft palate and a long uvula. The lateral pharyngeal walls were thickened (Fig. 8–7). The sleep laboratory workup included recommendations to use CPAP and lose weight, but the patient was unwilling to do either. Therefore, the LAUP was recommended as a conservative surgical treatment because the nasopharyngoscopy demonstrated a retropalatal closure. After counseling and obtaining informed consent, the patient agreed to have the operations.

Topical anesthesia of the nasal and oropharyngeal tissues was accomplished by nasal insufflation of 2% lidocaine/2% Neo-Synephrine solution and by spraying of the oropharynx with Cetacaine. Sedation was initiated and maintained with 3 mg midazolam, which was eventually supplemented by three additional 1-mg increments. Local anesthesia was obtained with 0.5% bupivacaine using 0.2 to 0.3 mL to the right and left sides of the attachment of the levator palatini, into the center of the uvula and then bilaterally into the midposition of the posterior pharyngeal pillars. The dimple was then marked with the laser using 10-W pulses to etch the mucosal surface lying directly over the dimple marking the attachment of the levator palatini (Fig. 8–8). Using a CO_2 laser adjusted to 15 W output power with a backstopped handpiece, 13-mm through-and-through vertical incisions were made on each side of the uvula. The inferior aspect of the uvula was shortened 13 mm by excising it with a nonbackstopped handpiece. During the procedure the uvula was stabilized with a wet wooden tongue blade. With the same handpiece, a 4 mm wide, 2 mm deep, and 15 mm long trench was created on both the right and left sides extending laterally and inferiorly on the anterior surface of the posterior pharyngeal pillar (Fig. 8–8). This was all accomplished without difficulty and without physical discomfort to the patient.

Postoperative medications were ketorolac trimethamine (Toradol) 60 mg i.m. and liquid oxycodone 5 mg/acetaminophen 500 mg. A topical anesthetic solution containing a mixture of 90% diphenhydramine HCl syrup, 9% tetracycline or doxycycline suspension, and 1% of a 1% betamethasone lotion to be gargled and expectorated four times a day and p.r.n. was given. A nystatin suspension was prescribed with 1 mL to be gargled and expectorated q.i.d.

The postoperative course was benign and the mucosae were well healed at 3 weeks (Fig. 8–9). The patient returned to his normal work on an offshore oil rig 2 days after surgery. At 4 weeks the patient stated that his dormitory mates commented that his snoring was much less severe, although it still persisted. Upon retesting, the patient could still snort and the second stage was then planned.

Seven weeks after the initial surgery, a second procedure was done to completely stop the snoring. Using the same i.v. sedation and anesthesia protocol, the patient was anxiety and pain-free yet awake and cooperative. The dimple was marked and vertical incisions were made on the right and left sides of the uvula extending vertically 6 to 7 mm

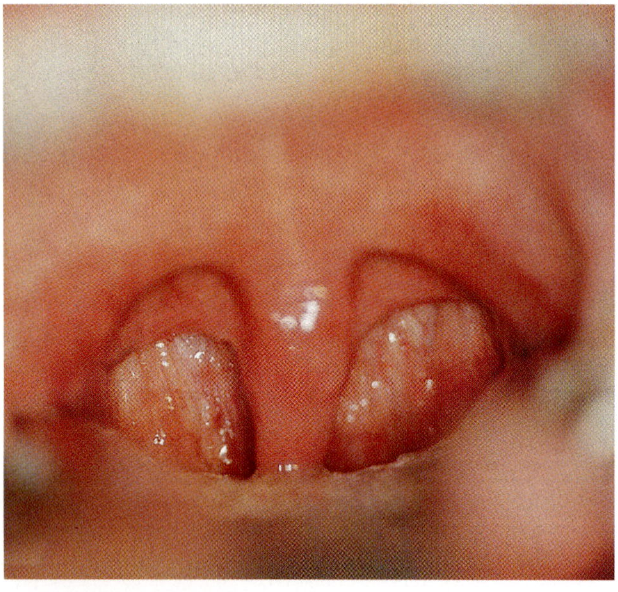

Figure 8–7. Preoperatively the patient has a long uvula and a low webbed soft palate.

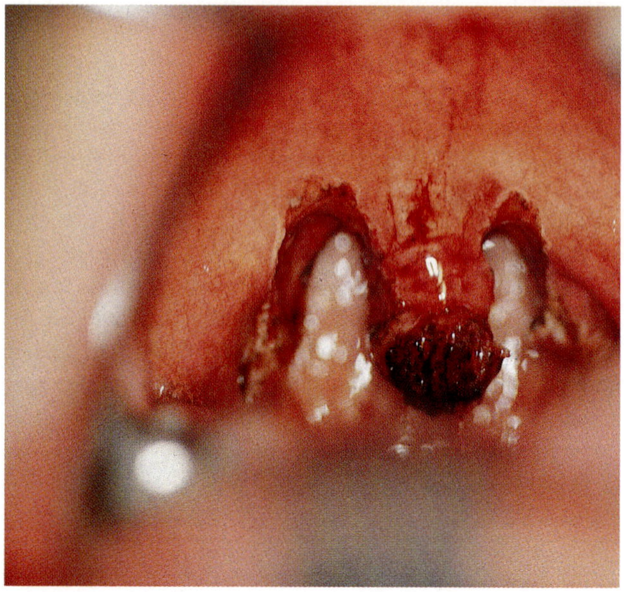

Figure 8–8. Vertical incisions of 13 mm length were placed on each side of the uvula. The uvula was shortened the same distance. Lateral trenches 4 mm wide, 2 mm deep, and 15 mm long were created on the anterior surface of the posterior pharyngeal pillar.

using 15 W output power. Additional vertical incisions of 4 to 5 mm in length were placed 3 to 4 mm lateral to the original cuts. The uvula was then shortened 4 mm and lateral trenches 1 cm long, 4 mm wide, and 2 mm deep were created on the anterior surface of the posterior pharyngeal arch (Fig. 8–10). The postoperative regime was the same as for the first procedure and the recovery was uncomplicated.

Three months after the original surgery, a repeat sleep study demonstrated an apnea index of 1 and an oxygen desaturation index of 23. Most impressively, the patient's lowest oxygen saturation was 72% and only 1.7% of his sleep time was associated with an oxygen saturation of less than 80%. His dormitory mates reported complete cessation of snoring.

Four months after the initial surgery, the palate has good form with a less constrictive velopharyngeal ring and a shorter uvula (Fig. 8–11). The patient is very satisfied. Instructions to lose 15 to 20% body weight were once again given to the patient.

CONTACT ND:YAG

An alternative technique for LAUP is to use a contact Nd:YAG laser instead of the free-beam CO_2. Preoperative assessment and the technique for adequately anesthetizing the operative site remain the same. With the patient seated and the mouth open, a black (nonreflective) metal tongue blade is used to depress the tongue. The patient's mouth is conveniently held open by a bite block or side action mouth prop. The long contra-angle handpiece is used to provide a clear line of sight along the handpiece. After positioning the high volume smoke evacuator at the corner of the mouth the operation commences. A scalpel-type probe tip (see Fig. 7–38) is chosen for the incisions that are made as recommended by Kamami earlier in this chapter. After creating the general U-shaped form for the neo-uvula as illustrated by Kamami and Wooten in Figs. 8–4, 8–6 and 8–10), final adjustments of contour as well as deepening of the superior part of the incisions may be performed with the rounded

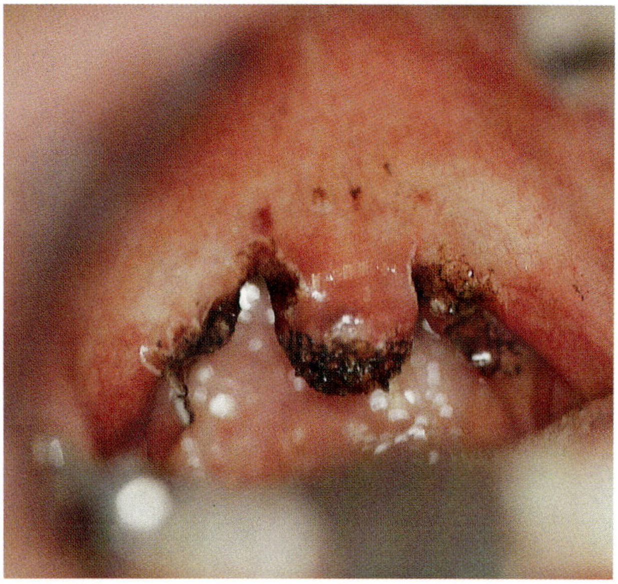

Figure 8–10. The secondary procedure was less extensive when performed at 7 weeks after initial surgery.

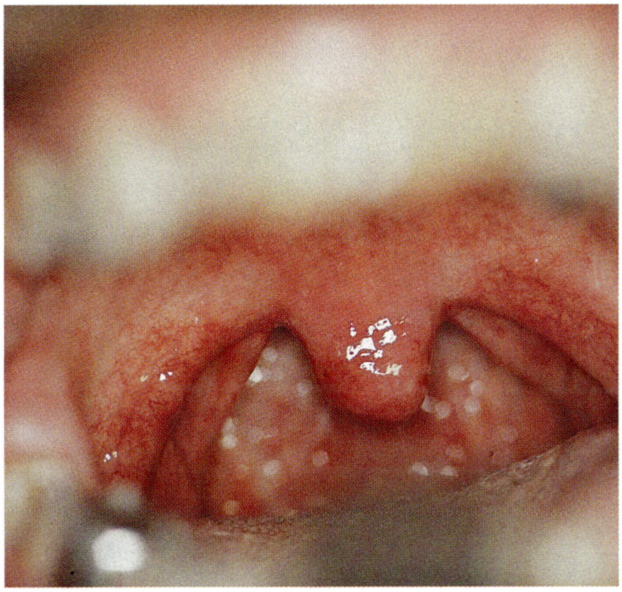

Figure 8–9. At 3 weeks the mucosa was healed but, some snoring persisted.

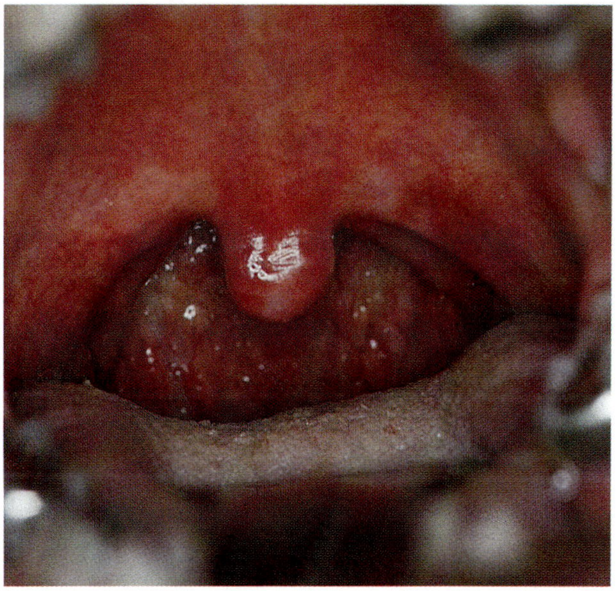

Figure 8–11. Four months after original surgery, the patient has a well-contoured soft palate and is sleeping without snoring.

tips that, by delivering a flatter beam profile, permit subtle contouring with only minor thermal damage to native tissue. Any bleeding points are easily coagulated with the probe.

Output power of the Nd:YAG should be in the range of 12 to 15 W using a number 6 SLT contact probe for rapid operating time, excellent hemostasis, and predictable results.

REFERENCES

1. Kamami YV. Laser CO_2 for snoring, preliminary results. *Acta Otorhinolaryngol Belg* 1990;44:451–456.
2. Kamami YV. Outpatient treatment of sleep apnea syndrome with CO_2 laser, LAUP: laser-assisted UPPP results on 46 patients. *J Clin Laser Med Surg* 1994;12:215–219.
3. Couly G. *Anatomie Maxillo-faciale 25 questions pour la préparation des examens et concours.* Paris: Prélat J; 1974.
4. Levin BC, Becker GD. Uvulopalatopharyngoplasty for snoring: long term results. *Laryngoscope* 1994;104(9):1150–1152.
5. Krespi Y, et al. The efficacy of laser assisted uvulopalatoplasty in the management of obstructive sleep apnea and upper airway resistance syndrome. *Operative Tech Otolayrngol Head Neck Surg* 1994;5(4):235–243.
6. Cornay WJ III. Personal communication.
7. Krespi YP, Keidar A. Laser-assisted uvulopalatoplasty for the treatment of snoring. *Operative Tech Otolaryngol Head Neck Surg* 1994;5(4):228–234.
8. Sher AE, Thorpy MJ, Sphrintzen RJ, Spielman AJ, et al. Predictive value of Muller's maneuver in selection of patient for uvulopalatopharyngoplasty. *Laryngoscope* 1985;95(12):1483–1487.

9 The Carbon Dioxide Laser in Laryngeal Surgery

Robert J. Meleca

Coupling the operating microscope with the CO_2 laser launched a new era in the field of laryngeal microsurgery. With the development of microsurgical instrumentation and a micromanipulator laser attachment that produces a reduced spot size diameter of 0.25 mm at a 400-mm working distance, the CO_2 laser combines surgical microprecision with capillary hemostatic capability and has become the instrument of choice for a number of laryngeal pathologies. The glottis is an ideal structure for the use of a CO_2 laser because of its high tissue water content, especially in Reinke's space, allowing for diffusion of thermal energy away from the impact site of the beam and resulting in less surrounding tissue injury.[1] The benefit of minimal thermal damage from CO_2 laser surgery results in less postoperative tissue edema, minimal scarring, and rapid wound healing.[2] It is ideally suited for removal of recurrent laryngeal papillomas, vascular lesions of the larynx such as hemangiomas and hemorrhagic polyps, laryngeal cysts, granulomas, and early glottic carcinomas. The CO_2 laser may also be utilized alone or in combination with conventional surgical techniques for removal of vocal fold cysts or treatment of Reinke's edema.

When used properly the CO_2 laser is an effective and safe instrument for laryngeal surgery, but despite meticulous safety precautions complications will occur. These may include cuff rupture, endotracheal tube ignition, ignition of pledgets or drapes, burns to the skin or mucosa of the patient or operating room personnel, corneal injury, pneumothorax, subcutaneous emphysema, and hemorrhage (see Chapter 2 for more details).

Several experimental studies have demonstrated delayed healing and increased scarring when the CO_2 laser is used.[2–4] However, the development of new microsurgical instrumentation, reduced beam spot size, and better operator techniques have led to equivalent, or improved, vocal fold mucosal healing and voice quality.[5]

Laser parameters and laryngeal surgical techniques that will decrease surrounding soft tissue thermal injury include (1) using a micromanipulator that produces a spot size of 0.25 mm with a 400 mm focal length lens; (2) utilizing low power settings (0.5 to 6 W); (3) using short pulse durations in a superpulse mode to decrease the time over which thermal energy buildup occurs in the tissues (0.1 to 1.0 seconds in a 10% duty cycle); (4) suctioning the vapor plume from the operative field, which will limit the amount of heat buildup and decrease thermal injury to surrounding tissues; (5) frequently removing carbonaceous debris (char) from the soft tissue laser excision site with laryngeal suction to decrease heat transfer; and (6) keeping tension at the laser excision line by stretching the tissues with microsurgical forceps; this produces a cleaner incision by minimizing char formation, thus preventing heat-induced soft tissue damage.[6]

The following sections describe the pathophysiology of specific laryngeal lesions, indications for their removal, and CO_2 laser techniques. Generally, for all procedures described below the patient is intubated with a small (6.0 to 6.5 mm inner diameter) laser-resistant endotracheal tube (jet ventilation may be used to avoid placement of an endotracheal tube). The endotracheal tube cuff is filled with methylene blue to allow for rapid detection of a cuff leak from a misdirected laser "hit." Use of oxygen concentrations between 30 and 40% will decrease the chance of endotracheal tube ignition. Suspension microlaryngoscopy is performed using a large-bore laryngoscope with 10× to 25× magnification, a moisturized pledget is placed over the cuff to protect the cuff and distal tissues, and the eyes and face are protected with dampened eyepads and a head drape, respectively (Figs. 9–1 and 9–2).

LARYNGEAL PAPILLOMAS

Laryngeal papillomas are cauliflower-like lesions caused by infection with the human papilloma virus (HPV) (Figs. 9–3 and 9–4). This lesion is the most common benign neoplasm of the larynx. During infancy or adulthood its presenting symptoms are hoarseness or airway obstruction. The natural history of this disease is one of multiple recurrences, especially with the juvenile onset type; therefore, CO_2 laser vaporization of these lesions, although the accepted procedure of choice today, is thought to be only palliative in most cases. Multiple recurrences are thought to be caused by persistent growth of HPV in subclinically infected normal-appearing tissue bordering the area of treatment.[7] The goal of laser va-

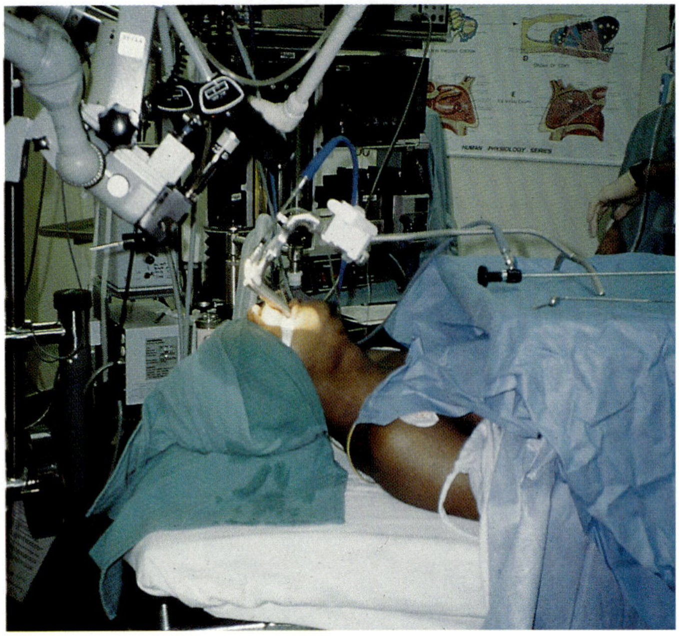

Figure 9–1. Intraoperative view demonstrating the equipment used for a patient undergoing suspension microlaryngoscopy and CO_2 laser excision of subglottic granulation tissue. The microscope is coupled to a CO_2 laser micromanipulator. This allows for a magnified and binocular view of the lesion, which is exposed using a laryngoscope placed in suspension. Note that a 400-mm lens on the microscope provides adequate working distance between the microscope and the laryngoscope.

porization is to eradicate this lesion and establish an adequate airway and functional voice without causing submucosal damage that may result in vocal fold scarring and fibrosis. Simultaneous removal of papillomas from both sides of the anterior or posterior commissure should be avoided, as this maneuver often results in commissure web formation.[8] Typical CO_2 laser settings for such a procedure include using a 0.25-mm spot size at a working distance of 400 mm, 2- to 3-W power, and 0.5- to 1.0-second pulse durations.

LARYNGEAL AND SUBGLOTTIC HEMANGIOMAS

Hemangiomas are uncommon neoplasms that may occur anywhere in the larynx and histologically are capillary, cavernous, or mixed capillary/cavernous lesions. They may present in a pediatric or adult form; the pediatric form is predominantly capillary in nature and the adult form more often mixed or cavernous.[6] The pediatric hemangioma char-

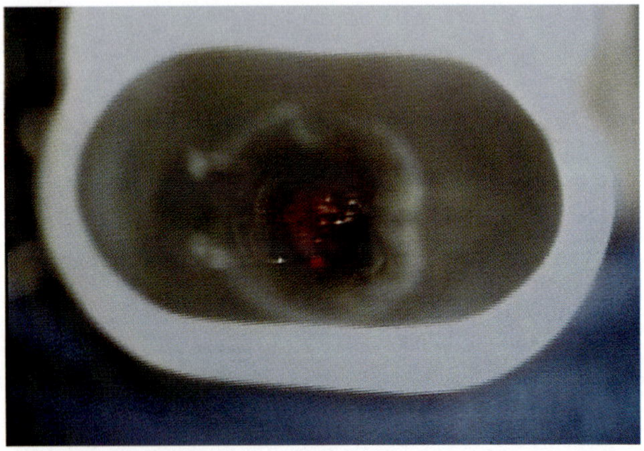

Figure 9–2. Example of the view obtained through the subglottiscope used for the patient in Fig. 9–1. Note the red beam of the CO_2 laser located at the inferior boundary of the lesion.

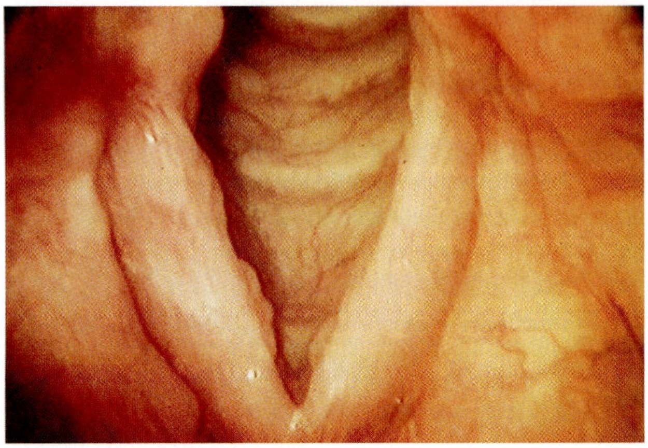

Figure 9–3. Preoperative view of a 27-year-old patient with laryngeal papillomas involving both true vocal folds and the anterior false fold on the right. (Photo courtesy of Robert W. Bastian, M.D., Loyola University, Chicago.)

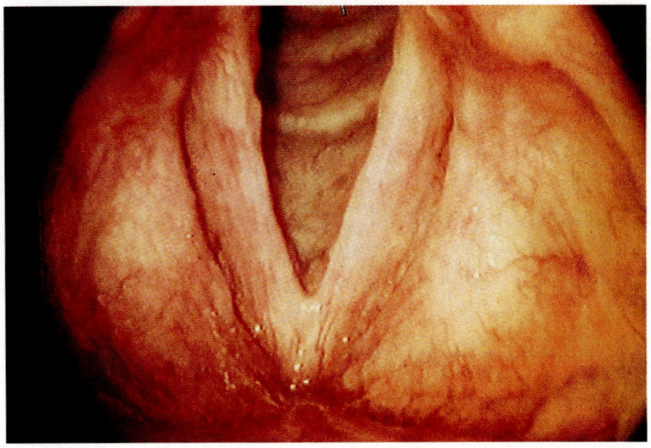

Figure 9–4. Two-week postoperative view demonstrating mild vocal fold edema, but the voice is significantly improved. (Photo courtesy of Robert W. Bastian, M.D., Loyola University, Chicago.)

acteristically presents shortly after birth, has a proliferative phase that may last up to 1 year followed by an involutional phase occurring from 1 to 7 years of age. These lesions often occur subglottically and may progress in size, resulting in airway obstruction. CO_2 laser treatment may be used safely to remove these lesions while simultaneously maintaining a patent airway and thereby avoiding need for a tracheotomy.[9] With the use of a subglottoscope and a laser with increased pulse duration settings to allow for more thermal diffusion and better coagulation of small vessels, capillary hemangiomas may be effectively treated.[6] These lesions can be managed using a laser with a 0.25-mm spot size at a 400-mm focal distance, 2- to 3-W power, and 0.5- to 1.0-second pulse durations. Cavernous lesions often present bleeding problems during removal that are not effectively controlled using the CO_2 laser, thereby requiring the use of other forms of therapy.

REINKE'S EDEMA AND VOCAL FOLD POLYPS

Reinke's edema and vocal fold polyps represent a disease process induced by chronic irritation to the vocal folds with resultant fluid accumulation in the superficial layer of the lamina propria. This fluid accumulation usually occurs bilaterally and may be diffuse (Reinke's edema) or localized (vocal fold polyp). Polyps may be fusiform, pedunculated, hemorrhagic, or generalized. The irritating stimuli producing these pathologic changes include vocal abuse, chronic throat clearing or cough, cigarette smoke, or gastric acid associated with gastroesophageal reflux. Surgical intervention is recommended for immature, soft lesions failing conservative therapy, or for polyps demonstrating fusiform, pedunculated, or hemorrhagic characteristics.[6] The CO_2 laser is particularly useful for removal of pedunculated, hemorrhagic polyps. Vessels leading to the polyp are coagulated, and the incision site is then carefully outlined with the CO_2 laser. Using microsurgical instrumentation the lesion is retracted medially, thus placing the area to be incised under tension. This allows for less char formation and decreased peripheral thermal tissue damage. The lesion is removed at its base with care taken not to induce thermal damage deep to the superficial lamina propria. Appropriate laser settings for such a procedure might include using a 0.25-mm spot size with a 400-mm lens, 0.5- to 2-W power, and pulse durations of 0.1 to 0.5 second.

LARYNGEAL CYSTS

Mucus-retention cysts may occur in the supraglottis where mucus-secreting glands exist in abundance. Congenital saccular cysts or laryngoceles are rare and may present with voice change or airway compromise. The CO_2 laser is ideal for complete removal of these lesions endoscopically. Marsupialization and ablation of the cysts lining may be attempted;[10] however, recurrence is not uncommon. Laser settings for such a procedure include a 0.25-mm spot size, 0.5 to 2 W, and a 0.1- to 0.5-second pulse duration.

GRANULOMA

Laryngeal granulomas typically arise in the posterior glottis, over the medial aspect of the vocal process. Etiologies include previous trauma from endotracheal intubation, gastroesophageal reflux, or vocal abuse. These lesions often begin as ulcerations with progression toward granulation formation. They characteristically present with symptoms of hoarseness, chronic throat clearing, sore throat, or a globus sensation. Effective treatment usually includes removal of the irritating source, administering antibiotics and antireflux medications, as well as speech therapy. With long-term conservative therapy most granulomas will resolve in an orderly fashion by progressing from an ulcerative state to a broad-based granuloma, and finally to a pedunculated mass that will eventually fall off. When conservative treatment fails, the CO_2 laser is ideal for surgical excision. The laser is used to precisely excise the granuloma without exposing underlying cartilage.[6] Any remaining granulation tissue can be spot vaporized. Typical laser settings for removal of such lesions include using a 0.25-mm spot size with a 400-mm lens, 0.5- to 2-W power, and a 0.1- to 0.5-second pulse duration.

MALIGNANT NEOPLASMS

Vocal fold hyperkeratosis, erythroplasia, carcinoma in situ, or early invasive carcinoma can all be effectively treated using the CO_2 laser (Figs. 9–5 to 9–9).[2] When comparing CO_2 laser resection with irradiation for T_1 carcinomas of the glottis, the cure rates are equivalent.[11–13] Voice quality in select patients with T_1 carcinomas treated with CO_2 laser resection equals that for similarly staged patients treated with radiation therapy, but when more than 50% of the vocal fold width is resected using the laser, voice quality deteriorates.[14] Suggested criteria for CO_2 laser removal of a glottic carcinoma include T_1 lesions involving the midcord, without involvement of the anterior commissure or vocal process of the arytenoid. CO_2 laser excision is an excellent alternative to irradiation because it allows for a simultaneous staging excisional biopsy and definitive therapy, all in an outpatient setting. Typical settings used for laser excision of T_1 glottic carcinomas include a 0.25-mm spot size at a working distance of 400 mm, 4- to 6-W power, with a 0.5- to 1.0-second pulse duration.

In summary, the CO_2 laser combines surgical microprecision with hemostasis of capillary size blood vessels. These qualities result in less postoperative tissue edema, minimal scarring, and rapid wound healing when compared with other surgical techniques. The laser may be used to treat a number of benign, premalignant, and malignant lesions of the larynx, including laryngeal papillomas, hemangiomas and cysts, vocal fold polyps and granulomas, as well as vocal fold hyperkeratosis, erythroplasia, carcinoma in situ, and invasive squamous cell carcinoma. With the development of more sophisticated instrumentation, combined with operator expertise, the field of microlaryngeal surgery will continue to evolve at an accelerated pace.

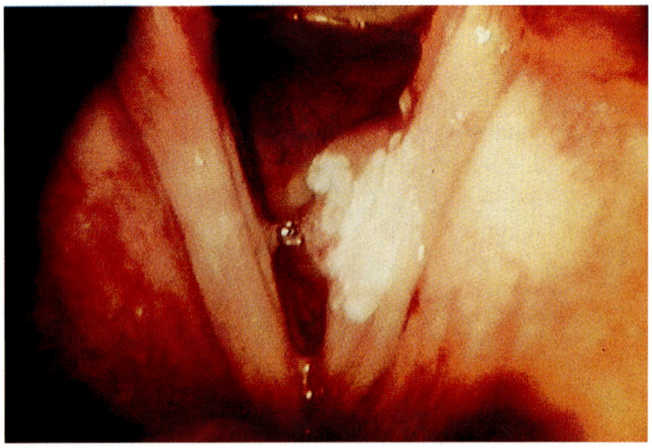

Figure 9–5. Preoperative view of a 57-year-old patient with a T_1 squamous cell carcinoma involving the left true vocal fold after biopsy at an outside institute. This lesion is ideal for laser removal because of its position on the midcord, without involvement of the anterior commissure or vocal process. (Photo courtesy of Robert W. Bastian, M.D., Loyola University, Chicago.)

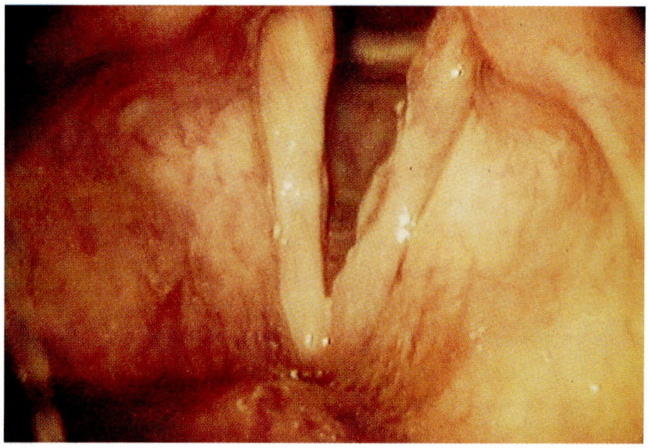

Figure 9–7. Six-week postoperative view with near complete healing of the left vocal fold. (Photo courtesy of Robert W. Bastian, M.D., Loyola University, Chicago.)

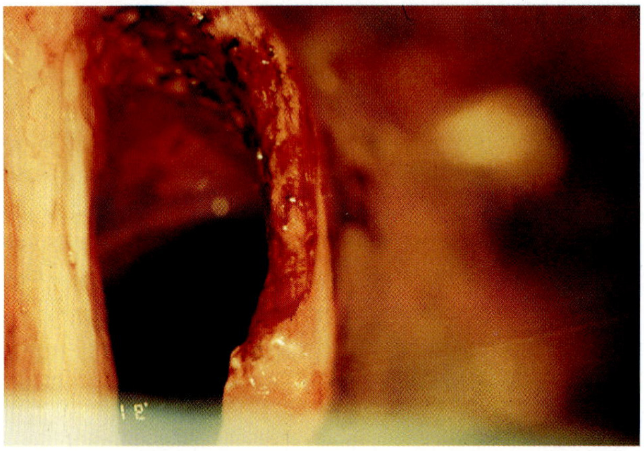

Figure 9–6. Intraoperative view after removal of the lesion. The laser was used to outline the carcinoma with a 2- to 3-mm margin. After frozen section confirmation of clear margins the final defect included removal of the medial one third of the vocalis muscle. (Photo courtesy of Robert W. Bastian, M.D., Loyola University, Chicago.)

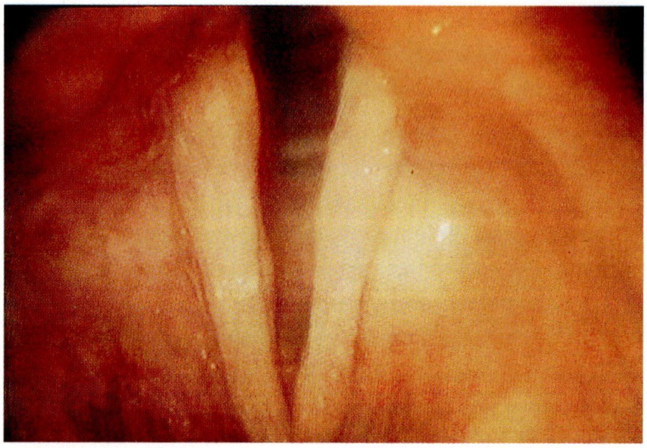

Figure 9–8. Six-month postoperative view with a mucosalized scar band extending across the original excision site. (Photo courtesy of Robert W. Bastian, M.D., Loyola University, Chicago.)

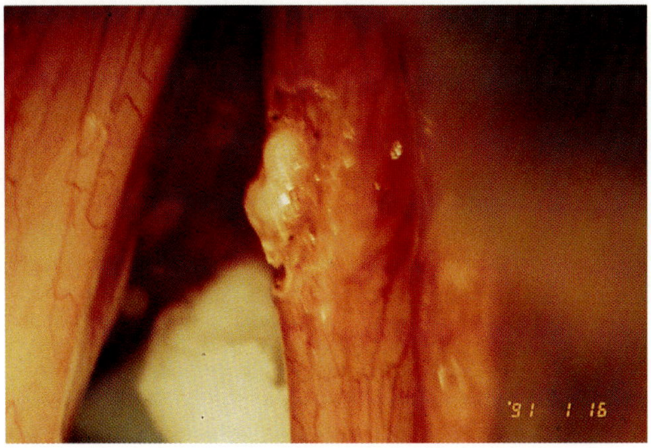

Figure 9–9. Example of how the laser is utilized to outline a small glottic carcinoma prior to removal. (Photo courtesy of Robert W. Bastian, M.D., Loyola University, Chicago.)

CASE PRESENTATIONS

The following case presentations have been selected because they represent lesions that are ideally suited for CO_2 laser excision. The cases presented include laryngeal papilloma and T_1 glottic carcinoma.

Laryngeal Papilloma

HISTORY

This 27-year-old patient without a smoking history presented with 4 months of progressive hoarseness (Figs. 9–3 and 9–4).

EXAMINATION FINDINGS

Papillomas involving the true vocal folds bilaterally with involvement of the anterior false vocal fold on the right (Fig. 9–3). The arytenoid and anterior commissure regions are free of disease.

TREATMENT

Laser Type Carbon dioxide laser with micromanipulator coupled to an operating microscope at 10× magnification. A 400-mm lens on the microscope provides enough working distance for microlaryngeal instrumentation.

Parameters A 0.25-mm spot size, 2-W average power, 0.5- to 1.0-second pulse duration in a 10% duty cycle (superpulse mode).

COMMENTS

Laryngeal papillomas grow superficially and should be ablated at the mucosa or submucosa level without penetration into the vocal ligament or vocalis muscle. Close postoperative follow-up is important as the natural history of this disease is one of multiple recurrences.

HEALING SEQUENCE

Two weeks postoperatively (Fig. 9–4) this patient has mild true vocal fold edema, but the voice is significantly improved, both subjectively and objectively. Note small focus of residual disease just anterior to the right vocal process.

T_1 Glottic Carcinoma

HISTORY

This is a 57-year-old man with a significant history of smoking and ethanol use who presented with a 3-month history of progressive hoarseness and an episode of hemoptysis (Figs. 9–5 to 9–8).

EXAMINATION FINDINGS

This is a biopsy-proven squamous cell carcinoma of the left true vocal fold involving the midcord region (Fig. 9–5). The left vocal fold moves freely and the anterior commissure, vocal process, ventricle, and subglottic regions are free of disease.

TREATMENT

Laser Type Carbon dioxide laser with micromanipulator coupled to an operating microscope at 10× magnification, containing a 400-mm lens.

Parameters A 0.25-mm spot size, 4-W average power, 0.5-second pulse duration in a 10% duty cycle (superpulse mode).

COMMENTS

The lesion is carefully outlined (Fig. 9–9) with the laser, a small cuff of normal tissue is taken with the tumor, and frozen section confirmation of free margins is obtained (Fig. 9–6). Patients with glottic carcinoma should be seen once a month for the first postoperative year, every 2 months for the next year, and regularly thereafter for a total of 5 years so that recurrent disease can be detected early and further therapy instituted promptly.

HEALING SEQUENCE

After resection of a midcord carcinoma a mucosalized scar band forms across the area of excision (Figs. 9–7 and 9–8).

ACKNOWLEDGMENT

The author would like to thank Robert W. Bastian, M.D., from Loyola University, Chicago, for use of the case illustrations.

REFERENCES

1. Freche C, Jakobowitz M, Bastian RW. The carbon dioxide laser in laryngeal surgery. Ear Nose Throat J 1988;67:436–445.
2. Crockett DM, Reynolds BN. Laryngeal laser surgery. Otolaryngol Clin North Am 1990;23(1):49–66.

3. Cochrane JP, Beacon JP, Creasey GH, et al. Wound healing after laser surgery: an experimental study. Br J Surg 1980;67:740–743.
4. Mihashi S, Jako GJ, Incze J, et al. Laser surgery in otolaryngology: interaction of the CO_2 laser and soft tissue. Ann NY Acad Sci 1976;267:263–294.
5. Shapshay SM, Rebeiz EE, Bohigian RK, et al. Benign lesions of the larynx: should the laser be used? Laryngoscope 1990;100:953–957.
6. Werkhaven J, Ossoff RH. Surgery for benign lesions of the glottis. Otolaryngol Clin North Am 1991;24(5):1179–1199.
7. Strong MS, Vaughn CW, Healy GB, et al. Recurrent respiratory papillomatosis: management with the CO_2 laser. Ann Otol Rhinol Laryngol 1976;85:508–516.
8. Saleh EM. Complications of treatment of recurrent laryngeal papillomatosis with the carbon dioxide laser in children. J Laryngol Otol 1992;106:715–718.
9. Healy GB, McGill T, Friedman EM. Carbon dioxide laser in subglottic hemangioma: an update. Ann Otol Rhinol Laryngol 1984;93(4 Pt 1):370–373.
10. Komisar A. Laser laryngoscopic management of internal laryngocele. Laryngoscope 1987;97:368–369.
11. Mcguirt WF, Koufman JA. Endoscopic laser surgery: an alternative in laryngeal cancer treatment. Arch Otolaryngol Head Neck Surg 1987;113:501–505.
12. Ossoff RH, Sisson GA, Shapshay SM. Endoscopic management of selected early vocal cord carcinoma. Ann Otol Rhinol Laryngol 1985;94:560–564.
13. Shapshay SM, Hybels RL, Bohigian RK. Laser excision of early vocal cord carcinoma: indications, limitations, and precautions. Ann Otol Rhinol Laryngol 1990;99:46–50.
14. Mcguirt WF, Blalock D, Koufman JA, et al. Comparative voice results after laser resection or irradiation of T_1 vocal cord carcinoma. Arch Otolaryngol Head Neck Surg 1994;120:951–955.

10 Uses of Lasers in Dentistry

Harvey Wigdor

The concept of using lasers in dentistry is as old as the first laser developed by Maiman in 1960. Soon afterward Stern and Sognnaes[1,2] became the first to study potential dental hard tissue applications and reported their results in 1964. They evaluated the possible use of the ruby laser to fuse the caries susceptible occlusal pits on the chewing surface of teeth. They also investigated the use of these lasers to alter the smooth surfaces of teeth to reduce their susceptibility to decay. Progress was slow in developing laser applications in cutting dental hard tissues because of the thermal damage caused by the laser wavelengths available at the time. Although investigational activity was sparse there were some published research papers that evaluated the effect of lasers on hard dental tissues.[3–6] Adrian et al.[7] examined the effects of the ruby laser on the dental pulp and found that thermal damage was significant. However, it was the development of the CO_2 laser that stimulated an increase in activity investigating the tissue-altering effects of lasers on enamel and dentin.

Recent years have seen the development of lasers whose manufacturers have suggested their use to cut hard dental tissues. Unfortunately, marketing efforts outstripped research activity and the training manuals of some of the neodymium:yttrium-aluminum-garnet (Nd:YAG) laser manufacturers suggested uses including removal of small carious lesions of enamel, removal of subgingival calculus, apicoectomy, and treatment of small carious cervical lesions in teeth. All of these published suggested applications were advocated prior to the Food and Drug Administration's (FDA) clearance of hard tissue applications in dentistry. Regrettably these recommendations are largely unwarranted because thermal damage to the treated tissues continues to be problematic.[8]

LASER HARD DENTAL TISSUE ABLATION RESEARCH

During the last few years research performed by Hibst and Keller[9,10] has shed some light on the use of an erbium (Er):YAG laser with a wavelength of 2.94 μm for cutting hard dental tissues. They showed that this laser could effectively cut teeth to make cavity preparations for simple dental restorations. Their thermal studies showed little or no effect on teeth including dental pulp when this laser was used.

As with any light source irrespective of wavelength the material that is being irradiated may either absorb, transmit, scatter, or reflect the light energy. The summation of the light-tissue interaction will determine the effect of the laser (see Chapter 1).

Clinical effects are predominantly the result of the absorption of the laser light in the tissues being treated. Some of the unabsorbed light can also scatter causing a more diffuse effect in the tissue. The desired clinical effects in surgery are mostly controlled by the absorption and somewhat by the scatter of the light in the tissue. The power of the laser used and the time that the energy is in contact with the tissue being treated are very important parameters that determine the observed clinical effect.

After understanding the effects lasers may have on any material including dental hard tissues an understanding of the optical properties of dental hard tissues is in order. Fried et al.[11,12] determined the absorption and scattering coefficients, using wavelengths of 543,632 and 1053 nm. These coefficients are the quantifiable amounts of absorption and scatter in enamel and dentin. At these wavelengths their results showed that light in the visible (543,632 nm) and the near infrared (1053 nm) are only negligibly absorbed by enamel and dentin. Visible light is scattered somewhat but the near infrared is strongly transmitted straight through these tissues and only weakly scattered.

Fried et al. placed the enamel sample, as well as dentin, in an optically matched solution. The sample was then subjected to spectroscopic analysis. Using an integrating sphere of a spectrophotometer the light from the sample was collected and a determination was made that quantified the amount of light absorbed by the sample. Integrating spheres are totally enclosed detectors that receive and contain the light from the sample for evaluation. The internal surface of the spheres are highly reflective, allowing the light to remain in the sphere until hitting the detector. The optically matched solution, which has the same optical properties as the samples, allowed uniformity between the light and the sample. If it had not been used, the air-sample interface that the light would pass through would act as two different optical materials. This would cause the sample to reflect some of the incident light, thereby reducing the transmitted light detected in the integrating sphere. The optically matched solution gives more accurate values of the true optical properties of these tissues when it is used.

When dentin samples in an optically matched solution

were studied using the same wavelengths as in the enamel there was some variability in the scattering coefficient based on tubule density and orientation. It was found that even though the absorption coefficient was low, if enough energy is deposited on the tissue over the visible and near infrared spectra it is absorbed by dentin. Unfortunately, the high amount of energy necessary at these wavelengths to cause clinical effects can also cause very damaging thermal side effects. However, if lower energy levels are used, most of the light is transmitted and/or scattered, being absorbed as it passes into deeper regions of the dentin. Clinically this is significant, for if a laser were used that has the potential for deeper penetration, the underlying tissues beneath the area of treatment may be adversely affected by the laser.

It seems that at the present moment the optimal laser for oral hard tissue ablation is one that has high absorption within the volume of tissue being treated, thereby reducing both the depth of penetration (ablation) and thermal injury. Both of these characteristics are essential when considering that tissues being treated by dentists are usually thin and very susceptible to thermal damage.

The most efficient ablation with the lowest thermal effect occurs when the laser energy is highly absorbed in a small volume of tissue. This requires close matching of the wavelength of the incident beam to the target chromophore. Simultaneously, the energy density must be adequate to induce the desired tissue effect during an application time short enough to preclude lateral thermal conduction (see Chapter 3). The inverse effect occurs if the laser wavelength is not well absorbed, which requires a longer time of exposure on the tissue. This longer exposure would cause a deeper zone of damage and more thermal effect. From Fried et al.'s[11,12] research, laser light from the noncontact Nd:YAG laser (1.06 μm) causes significant heating in hard tissue (dentin, enamel, and bone), while the contact Nd:YAG has less heat effect.

For hard tissue ablation a laser that is highly absorbed by one or more of the components in the hard tissue would be most advantageous. The recent interest in the suitability of the Er:YAG laser's effects on hard dental tissues is based upon the characteristic of its 2.94-nm wavelength. It is very highly absorbed by water and moderately well absorbed by hydroxyapatite, a major constituent of both dentin and enamel. Because of the high absorption characteristic of this laser in both dentin and enamel, it can ablate these hard tissues efficiently with very little heat production, thereby avoiding damage to the dental pulp, which has very little heat tolerance. It must be the goal of any laser that is to be used in dentistry to produce minimal heat as it cuts through the hard dental tissues.

The precise mechanism of the ablation of hard tissues with the Er:YAG laser remains unclear. One theory suggests that when the laser interacts with the hard tissue it is absorbed by the water and hydroxyapatite. The laser heats the water causing it to become steam. This expansion during the change of state of water causes cracking of the tissue. As the steam expands it also forces the cracked material away from the ablation zone. Because this is a very rapid action, it is explosive in nature. The effect of this laser is somewhat different in enamel compared with dentin. As discussed by Hibst and Keller[9] the Er:YAG laser energy is absorbed about twice as intensely in dentin as in enamel. They suggest that the relative ratio of water to hydroxyapatite is the reason for this difference. They calculated the absorption of the Er:YAG laser in dentin to be in the order of 2000 cm^{-1} and in enamel to be 1000 cm^{-1}. Further work by Hibst and Keller[13] using ultrashort flash photography to evaluate the plume arising from the ablation of dental hard tissues was published in 1993. Their results substantiate the theory of the Er:YAG laser mechanism observed on dental hard tissues. They further suggest that the glow observed in front of the tissue surface is caused by the particles being heated after ejection from the tissue (see Fig. 10–16). This heating causes a considerable energy loss, which prevents the expected linear increase in crater depth with time of exposure. In addition the velocity of the ejection plume for enamel is less than that for dentin. The differential ratio of the water and hydroxyapatite content in these two tissues appears to be the reason for this difference.

Recent studies included histologic and scanning electron microscopic (SEM) evaluation of the effect of Er:YAG lasers on teeth. Wigdor et al.[14] evaluated the effect of the Er:YAG laser on dog teeth in vivo and in vitro (extracted teeth). Er:YAG holes were made in the teeth. The output power of the laser was 1.5 W with an energy of 500 mJ per pulse at 3 Hz. Amalgam restorations were then placed in the ablation holes. After 4 days the teeth were extracted and decalcified. Figure 10–1 is a photograph of the holes created by the laser in the canine teeth. After decalcification the teeth were sectioned and stained with hematoxalin and eosin. Figure 10–2 is a photomicrograph of an untreated control tooth. Note the loose connective tissue in the pulp and the normal appearance of the odontoblasts lining the dentin. Figure 10–3 is a photomicrograph of a tooth that had been irradiated by the Er:YAG laser. The laser defect can be seen as a depression in the dentin. Note that the pulp-

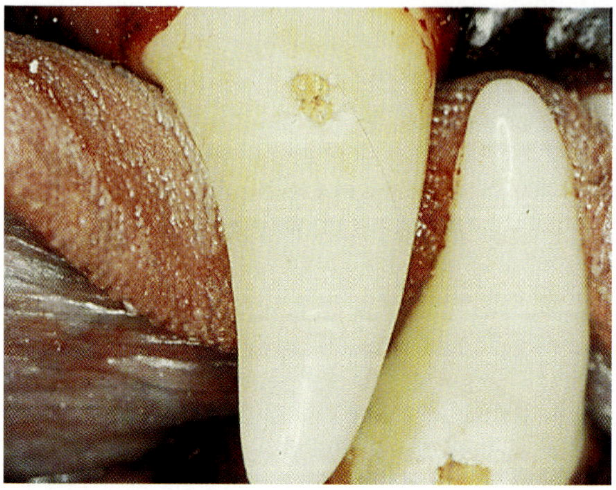

Figure 10–1. Er:YAG laser holes on dog canine teeth.

al tissue appears normal. Higher magnification failed to demonstrate any harmful effects of the Er:YAG laser on the pulpal tissue. The lack of increased vascularity or of inflammatory cells and the absence of disruption of the odontoblastic layer suggests no harm to the pulp in this tooth.

Another tooth treated with the Er:YAG laser showed a thickening of the dentin beneath the laser defect. Figure 10–4 shows a photomicrograph of the pulp just beneath the Er:YAG laser–induced defect. Note that there appears to be an increase in the dentin adjacent to the defect. After just 4 days this change would not be expected. The cause of this increased layer of dentin is not known.

The death of one dog from anesthetic complications just after the teeth were irradiated permitted the assessment of the acute effects of this laser on teeth. The teeth were removed just after the dog died and decalcified and stained. On a high-power view (Fig. 10–5) the predentin layer just beneath the laser defect shows dark inclusions that are probably cellular components of odontoblasts. These inclusions can also be seen in the dentinal tubules just above the predentin layer. Figure 10–6 is a view distant from the laser ablation in the same tooth showing normal predentin and dentin where no inclusions are present. The exact cause of these changes is unknown but one consideration is that the pressure from the Er:YAG ablation explosion may be traveling down the dentinal tubules causing these changes.

Extracted human teeth stored in 5% sodium hypochlorate solution were also irradiated by the Er:YAG laser using the same parameters as above in the dog study and evaluated with SEM. Figure 10–7 is an SEM photomicrograph of the surface of dentin that was cut with a high-speed dental handpiece: note the patent dentinal tubules. A representative selection showing a typical zone of Er:YAG irradiation can be seen in Figure 10–8. It is evident that the dentinal tubules have retained their patency after the Er:YAG laser irradiation. The similarity of the SEM's photomicrographs

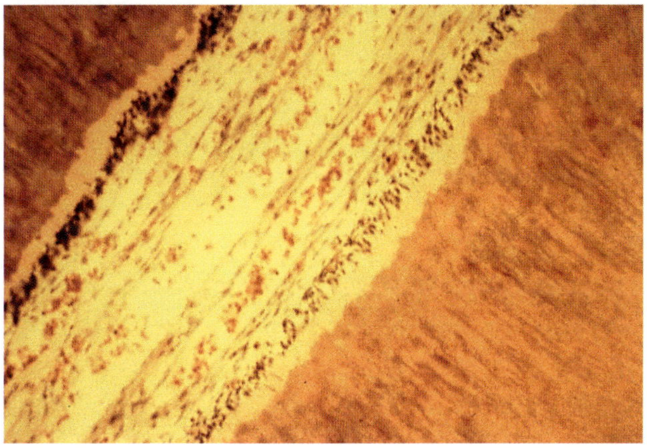

Figure 10–2. Normal pulpal and dentin histology. (×100 H&E stain.)

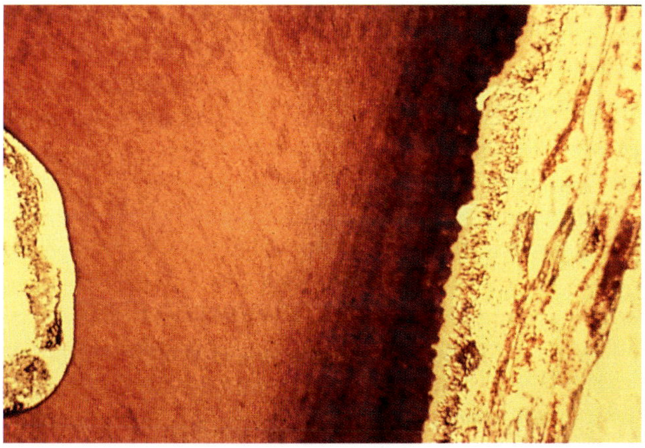

Figure 10–3. Pulpal histology beneath an Er:YAG laser hole (right). (×100 H&E.)

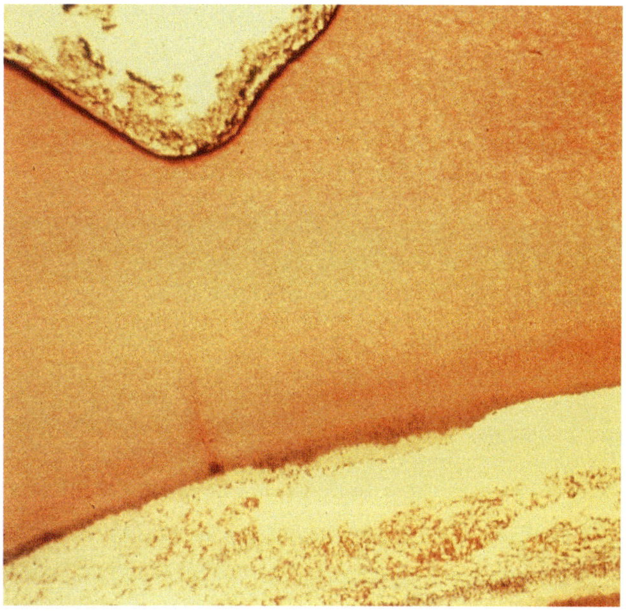

Figure 10–4. Photomicrograph of the dentin just beneath the Er:YAG laser hole. Note the increased dentin in the area beneath the laser hole. (×100 H&E.)

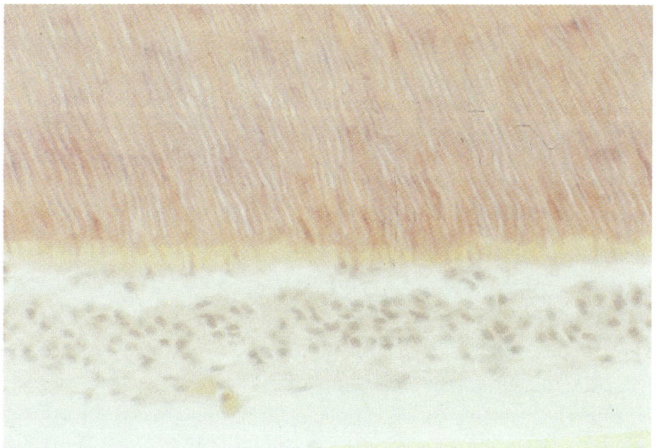

Figure 10–5. Higher power view of the predentin layer just beneath the laser hole. Note the dark inclusions in the predentin. (×400 H&E.)

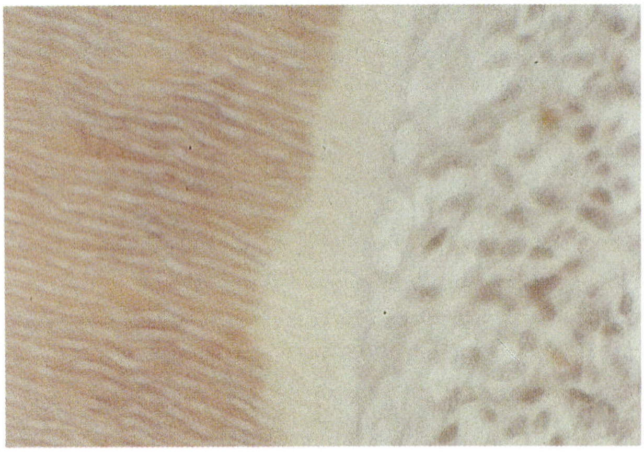

Figure 10–6. Higher power view of the predentin layer in an area not affected by the laser. (×400 H&E.)

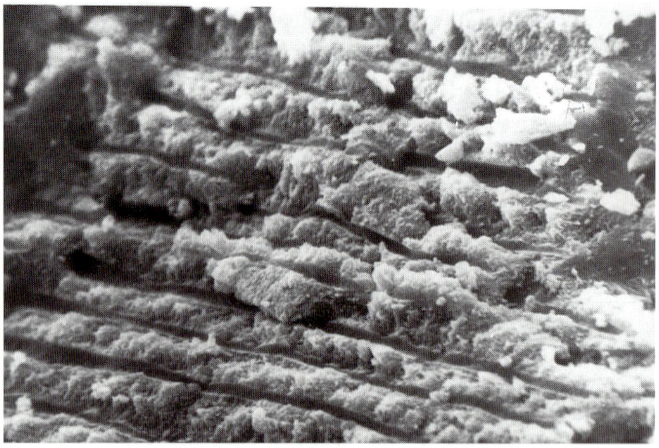

Figure 10–8. SEM photomicrograph of dentin ablated with an Er:YAG laser (×1200 longitudinal section).

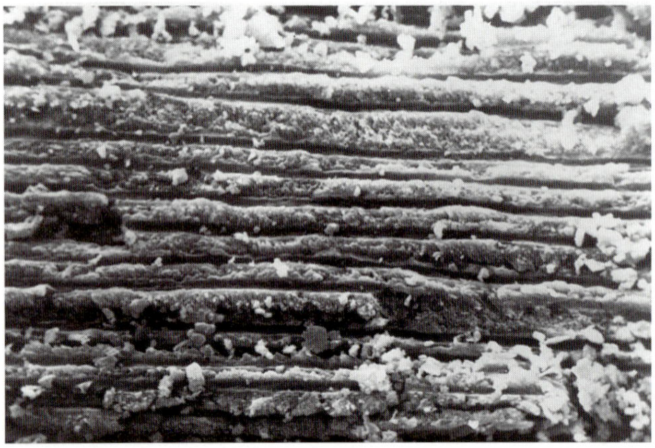

Figure 10–7. SEM photomicrograph of dentin cut with a high-speed dental drill (×1000 longitudinal section). (All SEM photographs are courtesy of Dr. S. Ashrafi.)

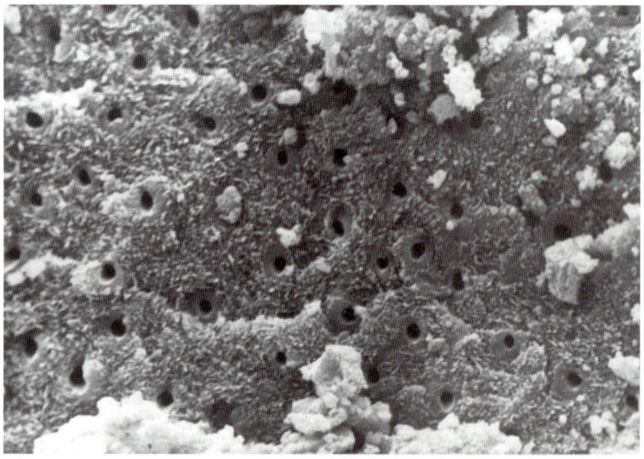

Figure 10–9. SEM photomicrograph of dentin ablated with an Er:YAG laser (×500 cross section).

of the dental handpiece and laser-treated dentin may suggest that the laser affects dentin in a way similar to conventional high-speed turbine tissue removal. Figure 10–9 is a cross section of dentin treated with the Er:YAG laser. Again, the patent dentinal tubules are obvious. Research performed by Visuri et al. from Northwestern University (Evanston, Il) and the author have repeated some of the projects performed by Hibst and Keller with water added as a coolant.[15–18] Our studies showed that at the power necessary for effective ablation of teeth and dental materials (150–650 mJ/pulse) some heat is produced by the Er:YAG laser. To prevent this increase in temperature, water was used as a coolant. Because water absorbs the 2940-nm wavelength very efficiently, there was concern about how the water might affect ablation efficiency.

The first series of studies was designed to evaluate the ablation efficiency of the Er:YAG laser. To accomplish this holes were created with the Er:YAG laser and then dental impressions were taken of these holes. The silhouettes of these impressions were then projected on a grid for quantification. Extracted molar teeth were used and the buccal surfaces were irradiated with the beam perpendicular to the surface. The energy per pulse was varied and a pulse width of 250 μs with an 800-μm spot size was used. Figure 10–10 is a photograph of the ablation holes created in the enamel of the buccal surface of an extracted molar tooth. The lack of char is evident. A photomicrograph of the SEM (Fig. 10–11) of similar holes shows well-defined holes in the enamel. Figure 10–12 is an impression of the ablation holes and Figure 10–13 is the projected image of the impressions of these holes. The results showed that the amount of material removal is directly proportional to the energy deposited on the tooth. As noted in the graph (Fig. 10–14) at high energy (626 mJ/pulse) 115 μm of material was removed per pulse. At lower energy (187 mJ/pulse) 22 μm of material was removed. The next study evaluated the ablation efficiency and temperature changes of the Er:YAG laser on dental hard tissues. Sections of extracted human teeth were cut into known thicknesses and ablated with the Er:YAG laser. A thermocouple was placed on the side opposite the

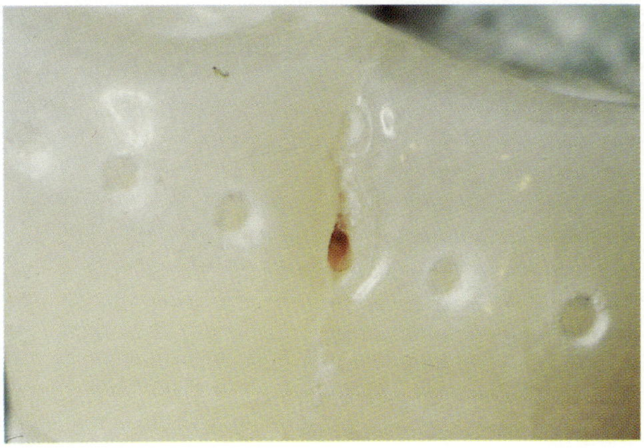

Figure 10–10. Ablation holes from an extracted tooth. Note the lack of char.

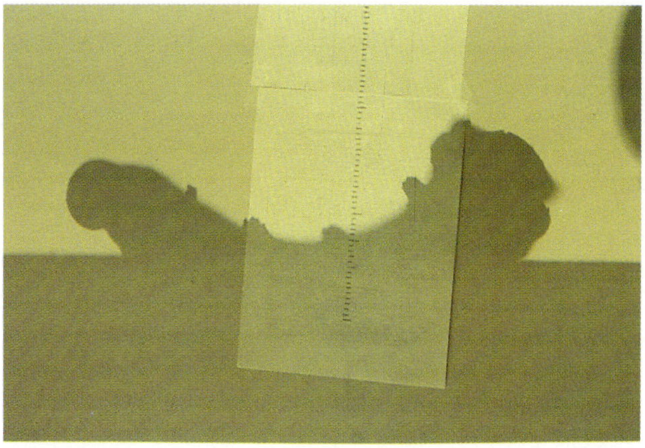

Figure 10–13. Projected image of the impression from Figure 10–12.

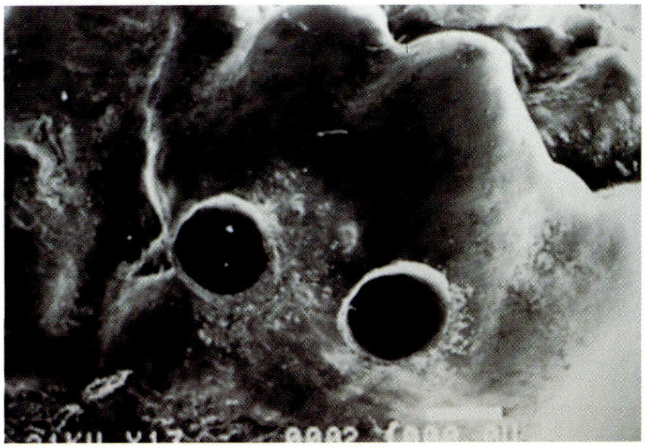

Figure 10–11. SEM photomicrograph of Er:YAG laser holes in the buccal surface of an extracted tooth.

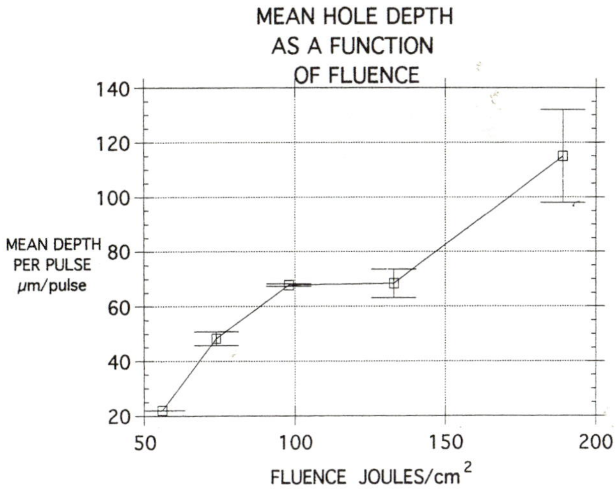

Figure 10–14. Table of ablation efficiency from the impression method in Figure 10–13.

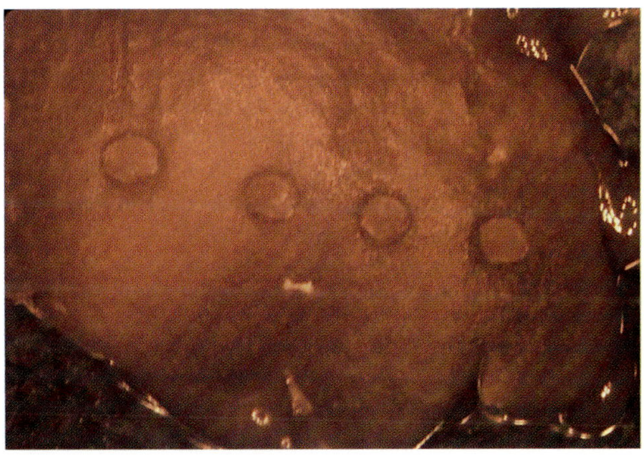

Figure 10–12. Dental impression from a tooth after Er:YAG ablation holes.

ablation surface. Figure 10–15 is a photograph of the setup design of the experiment. A stream of water was directed to the area of the laser beam and the flow rate of water volume was controlled. During the ablation process the temperature of the tooth was determined without water flow and then with water directed at the spot of the ablation. Figure 10–16 is a photograph of the ablation plume during the ablation of dentin with the laser beam coming from the left and Figure 10–17 is a photograph of the holes that were created by the laser in the cross-sectional slice of dentin.

In our studies the effect of the Er:YAG laser on dental amalgam and composite materials was also studied. Dental amalgam is a mixture of a number of metals, including silver, zinc, copper, and tin, that are mixed with mercury to form a material that hardens a short time after mixing.

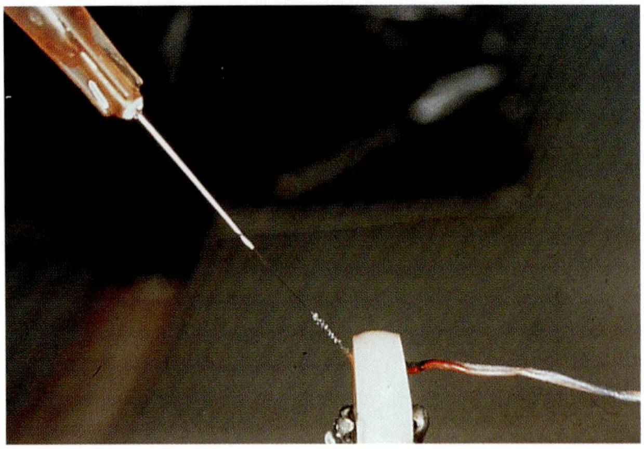

Figure 10–15. Laboratory setup for the study of dentin ablation.

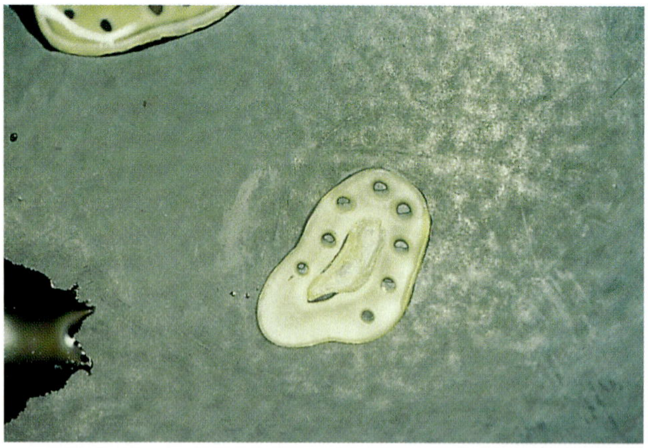

Figure 10–17. Ablation holes created in dentin sections from extracted teeth with the Er:YAG laser.

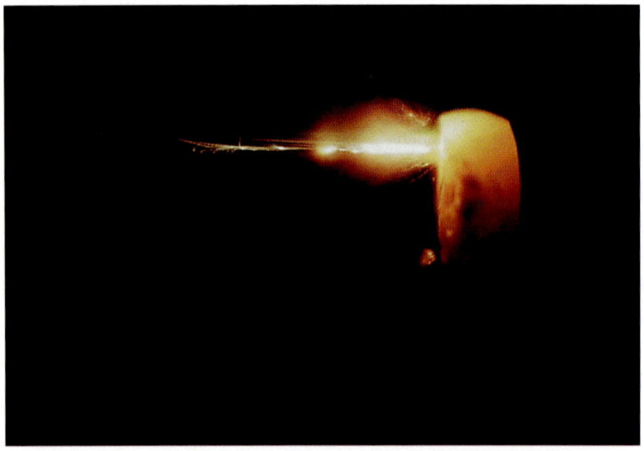

Figure 10–16. Plume from dentin ablation with the Er:YAG laser.

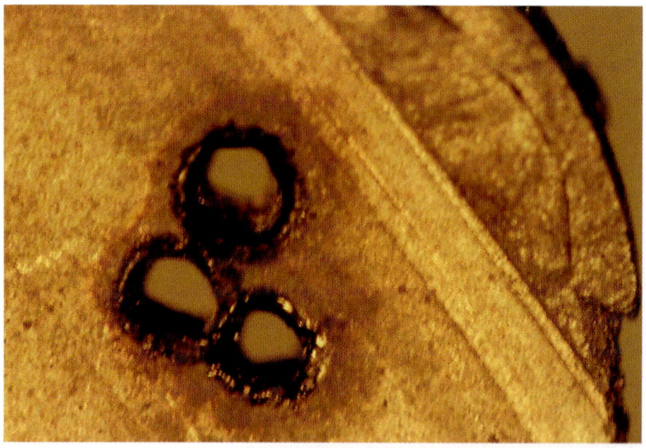

Figure 10–18. Ablation holes created in amalgam sections with the Er:YAG laser.

Composites are tooth-colored dental materials that are used as restorative materials for dental restorations when aesthetics are a concern. They are a blend of acrylic and quartz particles that are placed in cavity preparations in teeth to restore defects caused by dental decay. Any laser that will be used to cut dental hard tissues must also remove the existing materials in teeth being prepared for restorations.

For this study cores of these materials were ablated by an Er:YAG laser. The ablation efficiency of the laser was determined with and without water. The method used was similar to that for the dentin ablation study shown in Figure 10–15. The amalgam ablation plume was rather large and similar in size with and without water. Of great interest for study are the products created when amalgam is ablated. Studies are now under way to analyze the plume by-products and to evaluate their possible toxic effect to patient and treatment team members. Figure 10–18 is a photograph of the ablation holes created by the Er:YAG laser. The three holes were created at different powers and the effect was not influenced by the water coolant.

Figure 10–19 is a photograph of the ablation holes created in dental composite restorative material with and without water coolant. The hole on the right was cut without water. Note the char that was caused by the laser. The hole on the left was created with the laser using water as a coolant. It has a well-defined border and no char is evident. It is apparent that the water made a dramatic difference when it was used in the composite ablation studies.

The results of the ablation efficiency and the thermal effects on the different materials tested (dentin, enamel, amalgam, and composite) were very similar. Therefore, the composite ablation results are presented here as a summary of the laser effects on the materials tested. Figure 10–20 is a graph of the temperature changes that occurred as the ablation progressed through the sample. As the ablation progressed the hole became deeper and closer to the thermocouple. Two energy levels were used with and without water. The results show that as the ablation hole deepens the temperature rises when water is not used. The rate of this rise is almost the same for the two energy levels. The

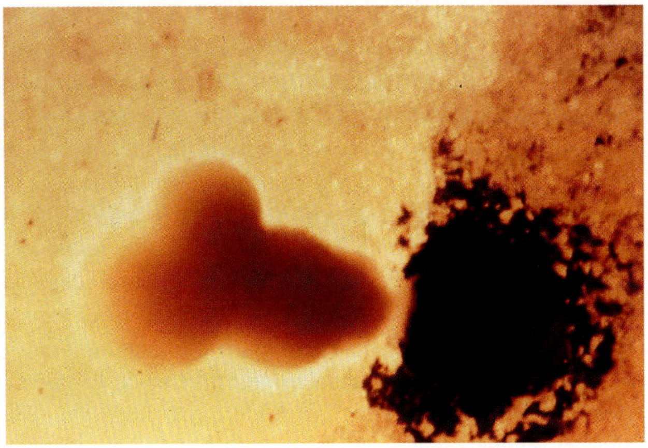

Figure 10–19. Ablation holes created in composite sections with the Er:YAG laser. With water (L); without water (R).

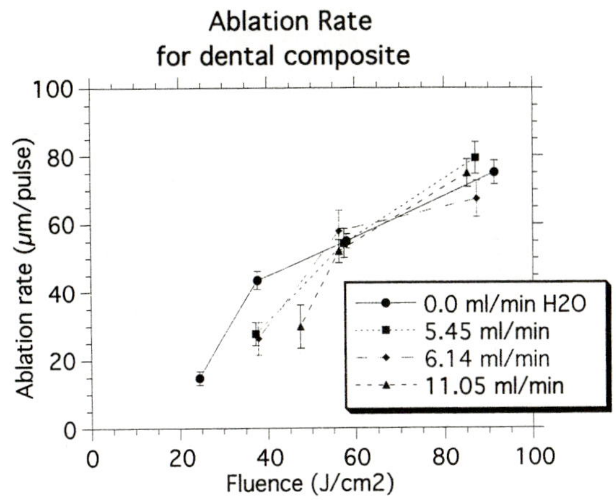

Figure 10–21. Graph of the ablation rate as the fluence and water are varied.

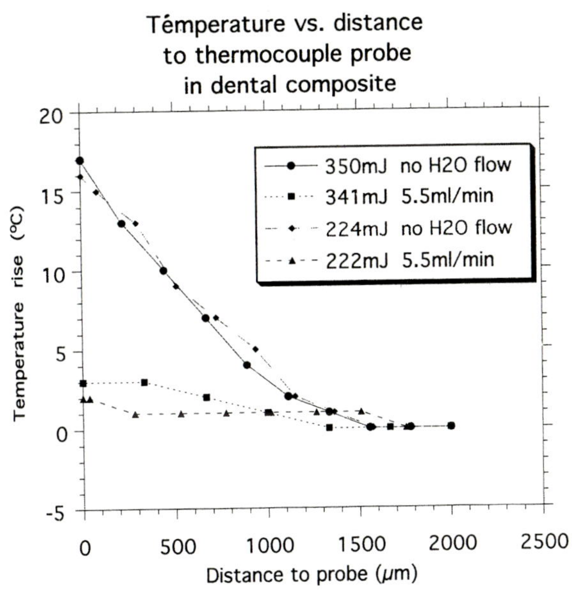

Figure 10–20. Graph of the temperature changes as the ablation progressed through the sample with and without water.

maximum temperature of about 17°C occurred just as the laser penetrates through the sample. Work by Zach and Cohen[19] has shown that if the temperature of the tooth rises more than 5°C the pulp may be harmed. When water was used during ablation the temperature did not rise by more that 3°C.

Figure 10–21 is a graph of the ablation rate as the energy (fluence) and water flow were varied. The amount of ablation was recorded as the increase in depth of the hole per pulse. As can be seen in the graph, water slightly reduces the composite ablation efficiency at lower fluences. The graph shows that at higher flow rates more energy was necessary for equal ablation. However, after reaching a fluence of 60 J/cm^2 there is a convergence of the water flow lines on the graph and they appear to be superimposed over each other, suggesting that water has very little effect at the higher fluences.

From a patient survey, in this author's practice, 70% would like a laser to be developed that could replace the dental drill. The ultimate question is whether a laser can be developed that can ablate at a speed similar to the high-speed air turbine dental handpiece (drill) that is used by dentists today, and whether a laser will be better tolerated by patients.

DENTAL CARIES SUSCEPTIBILITY

The effects of the infrared laser (9.0 to 11 μm) on dental hard tissues and on dental caries susceptibility has been investigated.[20–23] Two components of dental hard tissues, water and hydroxyapatite, have a moderate to high absorption in this area of the spectrum. Because of the moderate to high absorption in these substances infrared lasers have been shown to cause less thermal damage to hard tissues. For hydroxyapatite there are strong spectral absorption peaks at 9300 and 9600 nm, which are close to the main CO_2 emission of 10,600 nm. Because one of the major components of dental hard tissues is hydroxyapatite, it seems that there is a potential for these laser wavelengths to cut hard tissues efficiently. Combined with the high water absorption of hydroxyapatile in the 9.3- to 10.6-μm region, it seems that this area of the spectrum may have a role to play in hard tissue ablation. Featherstone and Nelson[24] and others use a low-powered CO_2 laser preferably tuned to the highly absorbed 9.3- and 9.6-μm wavelengths on extracted teeth leading to a reduction in the acid demineralization in sections of enamel. They suggest that the low-power laser has an effect on the carbonate ion in enamel by dramatically reducing its content in the hydroxyapatite crystal in enamel, thereby making this crystal less susceptible to demineralization by bacterial acids. These changes are caused by a thermal effect; however, the authors state that the actual mechanism of action is still not clear. Whether this same effect will be seen in vivo has yet to be determined.

LASER DENTAL DECAY DETECTION AND OPTICAL PROPERTIES OF TEETH

Zachariasen et al.[25] and Konig et al.[26] investigated the use of lasers to diagnose enamel decay. They found that when a laser is used to irradiate the enamel of teeth carious lesions will fluoresce. It is not understood why this occurs, but the authors suggest it may be due to the bacteria present in the lesion. Certain bacteria contain porphyrins in their cell walls that fluoresce when certain wavelengths of light are used. This characteristic may play a role in diagnosing caries before the lesions are detectable clinically. In another related study on hard-tissue laser effects Altschuler et al.[27] reviewed the optical properties of teeth. Their model suggests that the enamel prisms and dentinal tubules may affect laser light before the light is absorbed by the tissues. For instance, the dentinal tubules may act as guides directing the laser energy to the pulp of the tooth being treated. This directed and possibly concentrated laser energy may cause damage to the pulpal tissue instead of to the hard tissues at which the energy is being directed. The optical properties of teeth may cause unwanted damage to teeth and require more study for a better understanding of their possible influence.

LASER DENTAL MATERIALS PROCESSING

Another clinical application of lasers is in curing dental composite restorative materials. Research by Powell et al.[28] showed that composite materials exposed to argon laser light (488 nm) required shorter curing times than for conventional white light sources. The laser-cured materials also had a better bond strength to dentin at its interface with the composite. Kelsey et al.[29] investigated the physical properties of the composite materials cured with the argon laser and found them to be enhanced over conventional methods. Blankenau et al.[30] reported considerable difference in the physical properties as the time between curing and testing increased. They suggested that the autopolymerization of the composite was a factor in the differences seen. The FDA has cleared the use of the argon laser as a light source for the photopolymerization of dental composite materials. There is some controversy regarding whether the laser provides adequate benefit to compensate for its much higher cost.

Lasers have been used extensively in industry for cutting and welding of metals. New technology has been developed by Nobelpharma Industries (Nobelpharma AB, Gothenburg, Sweden) for the welding of dental implant supported bridges with a Nd:YAG laser. The method that is presently being used by dental laboratories for bridge assembly is either casting of a bridge in total or soldering components to fabricate the bridge. Both of these techniques can cause shrinkage of the metal and distortion of the bridge. Using the method developed by Nobelpharma, twin Nd:YAG laser beams weld the components on either side of the joint at the same time, thereby avoiding the differential shrinkage that normally occurs when welding is performed sequentially instead of simultaneously. The simultaneous welding of the titanium pieces enhances the precise adaptation of these implant bridges to the underlying implants. This method reduces distortion and therefore increases accuracy of fit.[31]

The laser system, developed by Nobelpharma Industries, is a flashlamp pumped Nd:YAG laser in which two laser beams are directed to the titanium bridge, which is then welded by the laser. Because of the tendency for the titanium to develop an oxide layer, the welding must occur under an atmosphere of argon gas. This atmosphere assures that the weld joint is oxide free and of maximum strength. With the lens system and mirror focal point used in this proprietary system a weld 600 to 800 μm deep is generated at the joint. The energy provided from the laser melts each piece of titanium on either side of the joint. As the metal cools the two pieces of titanium join together. This method is different from the soldering methods presently used because with the laser similar metals are welded, whereas in soldering impurities (flux) and dissimilar metals are soldered, which can lead to a weaker joint. This welding technique may be applied even to a complete arch bridge.

Preliminary investigational work suggests exciting areas of investigation for lasers in dentistry. Lasers have the potential for determining the vitality of a tooth based on the changes observed from laser irradiation on the buccal surface of a vital versus a nonvital tooth that can be detected by a laser. Nonionizing laser light has the potential for replacing the radiation now used to make dental radiographs. Lasers also may be used as a light source in conjunction with a microscope to evaluate the vasculature of the gingiva in vivo to diagnose active periodontal disease. The potential for laser applications in dentistry portends an exciting future.

REFERENCES

1. Stern RH, Sognnaes RF. Laser beam effect on dental hard tissues. *J Dent Res* 1964;43(suppl to no. 5):873 (abstract 307).
2. Stern RH, Sognnaes RF, Goodman F. Laser effect on in vitro enamel permeability and solubility. *J Am Dent Assoc* 1966;78:838–843.
3. Lobene RR, Bhussry BR, Fine S. Interaction of carbon dioxide laser radiation with enamel and dentin. *J Dent Res* 1968;47:311–317.
4. Goldman L, Hornby P, Meyer R, Goldman B. Impact of the laser on dental caries. *Nature* 1964;203:417.

5. Lobene RR, Fine SF. Interaction of laser radiation with oral hard tissues. *J Prosthet Dent* 1966;16:589–597.
6. Taylor R, Shklar G, Roeber F. The effects of laser radiation on teeth, dental pulp and oral mucosa of experimental animals. *Oral Surg* 1965;19:786–795.
7. Adrian JC, Bernier JL, Sprague WG. Laser and the dental pulp. *J Am Dent Assoc* 1971;83:113–117.
8. Abt E, Miserendino LJ, Carlson B. Histologic effects of Nd:YAG laser induced defects in bone. *Proceedings of International Society of Laser Dentistry;* 1992:71–72.
9. Hibst R, Keller U. Experimental studies of the application of the Er:YAG laser on dental hard substances: I. Measurement of the ablation rate. *Lasers Surg Med* 1989;9:338–344.
10. Hibst R, Keller U. Experimental studies of the application of the Er:YAG laser on dental hard substances: II. Light microscopic and SEM investigations. *Lasers Surg Med* 1989;9:345–351.
11. Fried D, Featherstone JDB, Glena RE, Seka W. The nature of light scattering in dental enamel and dentin at visible and near-IR wavelengths. *Appl Optics* 1995; 34(7):1278–1285.
12. Fried D, Featherstone JDB, Glena RE, Bordyn B, Seka W. The light scattering properties of dentin and enamel at 543, 632, and 1053 nm. In: Proceedings from lasers in *Orthopedic, Dental, and Veterinary Medicine,* vol 2. Bellingham, WA: SPIE; 1993:240–245.
13. Hibst R, Keller U. The mechanism of Er:YAG laser induced ablation of dental hard substances. In: *Proceedings from Lasers in Orthopedic, Dental, and Veterinary Medicine,* vol 2. Bellingham, WA: SPIE, 1993:156–162.
14. Wigdor HA, Abt E, Ashrafi S, Walsh JT. The effects of lasers on dental hard tissues. *J Am Dent Assoc* 1993;124:65–70.
15. Wigdor HA, Walsh JT, Cummings JP. New method for determination of ablation of hard tissues with the Er:YAG laser. *SPIE Proc* 1993;1880:142–148.
16. Wigdor HA, Walsh JT, Visuri S. Thermal effect of Er:YAG laser radiation on dental hard tissues. *SPIE Proc* 1993;2080:26–32.
17. Wigdor HA, Visuri SR, Walsh JT. Effect of water on dental material ablation of the Er:YAG Laser. *SPIE Proc* 1994; 2128: 267–272.
18. Visuri SR, Walsh JT, Wigdor HA. Erbium laser ablation of hard tissue: modeling and control of the thermal load. *SPIE Proc* 1994; 2134A:130–133.
19. Zach L, Cohen G. Pulp response to externally applied heat. *Endodontics* 1965;19(4):515–530.
20. Nelson DGA, Featherstone JDB. Preparation, analysis, and characterization of carbonated apatites. *Calcif Tissue Int* 1982;34:S69–S81.
21. Nelson DGA, Shariati M, Glena R, Shields CP, Featherstone JDB. Effect of pulsed low energy infrared laser irradiation on artificial caries-like lesion formation. *Caries Res* 1986; 20:289–299.
22. Nelson DGA, Williamson BE. Low-temperature laser Raman spectroscopy of synthetic carbonated appatites and dental enamel. *Aust J Chem* 1982;3S:715–727.
23. Meurman JH, Voegel JC, Rauhamaa-Makinen R, Gasser P, Thomann JM, Hemmerle J, Luomanen M, Paunio I, Frank RM. Effects of carbon dioxide, Nd:YAG and carbon dioxide-Nd:YAG combination lasers at high energy densities on synthetic hydroxyapatite. *Caries Res* 1992;26:77–83.
24. Featherstone JDB, Nelson DGA. Laser effects on dental hard tissue. *Adv Dent Res* 1987;1:21–26.
25. Zakariasen K, Barron J, Paton B. Laser scanned fluorescence of non-lased/normal, lased/normal, non-lased/carious and laser/carious enamel. *SPIE Proc* 1992;1643:493–502.
26. Konig K, Hibst R, Meyer H, Flemming G, Schneckenburger H. Laser-induced autofluorescence of carious regions of human teeth and caries-involved bacteria. *SPIE Proc* 1993;2080:170–180.
27. Altschuler GB, Belikov AV, Erofeev AV, Vitiaz IV. Optical model of human tooth. Proceedings of the *International Society of Laser Dentistry Proceedings.* 1992:247–248.
28. Powell GL, Kelsey WP, Blankenau RJ, Barkmeier WW. The use of an argon laser for polymerization of composite resin. *Esthetic Dentistry* 1989;1(1):34–37.
29. Kelsey WP, Blankenau RJ, Powell GL, Barkmeier WW, Cavel WT, Whisenant BK. Enhancement of physical properties of resin materials by laser polymerization. *Lasers Surg Med* 1989;9:623–627.
30. Blankenau RJ, Powell GL, Kelsey WP, Barkmeier WW. Post polymerization strength values of argon laser cured resin. *Lasers Surg Med* 1991;11:471–474.
31. Jemt T, Linden B. Fixed implant-supported prostheses with welded titanium frameworks. *Int J Periodont Restor Dent* 1992;12:177–183.

11 Phototherapy with Lasers and Dyes

Dan J. Castro, Romaine E. Saxton, Jacques Soudant

For years surgery and/or radiation therapy have been the therapy of choice for the successful treatment of superficial malignancies. However, each of these modalities is either invasive or destructive with some morbidity and restriction of further therapeutic options if and when recurrent disease occurs.

Laser phototherapy with dyes (activated by specific wavelengths of light) may become an attractive adjunctive modality for treatment of superficial malignancies when fluorochromes with high tumor specificity and low systemic toxicity are developed. This technique is simple and minimally invasive, with a potentially high effective cure rate and low morbidity. Most of these treatments can be performed as outpatient procedures thereby reducing the cost of hospitalization. Because lasers are nonionizing beams,[1] superficial tumors can be treated repeatedly by endoscopically delivered laser fiberoptics. This is particularly attractive because surgery and/or radiation therapy may still be used if and when recurrent disease occurs.

In the last two decades, the field of photodynamic therapy (PDT) has regained popularity, specifically since the introduction of lasers by Maiman,[1] the recent clinical evaluation of hematoporphyrin derivatives,[2] the current experimental testing of rhodamine-123,[3–7] and merocyanine 540[8] as photosensitizers for the treatment of superficial malignancies.

Laser phototherapy can be further subdivided into two major areas: PDT and photodiagnostic imaging (PDI). Both are used for eradication and imaging of cancers. Each of these potential applications will be reviewed.

HISTORY

This first use of light-sensitive substances (psoralens) in the treatment of disease can be traced back over 6000 years to the ancient Egyptians.[9] Crushed leaves from plants related to parsley were rubbed over an area of depigmented skin before exposure to the sun's rays to produce a severe form of sunburn only in the treated areas. After resolution of the sunburn the skin would return to its natural color. Reference to the use of a plant extract for the restoration of skin pigmentation was made in 1400 B.C.,[10] and phototoxic effects of psoralens were described in 1250 A.D.[11]

The pioneer of modern phototherapy in dermatology was Finsen[12] in 1901, whose extensive experiments on the treatment of skin tuberculosis with natural and artificial ultraviolet (UV) radiation stimulated the current interest in cutaneous photobiology. The first medical use of chemically enhanced phototherapy (other than for restoration of pigmentation) was reported by Jesionek and Tappeiner[13] in 1905. These pioneers in the study of photodynamic therapy treated five basal cell carcinomas by injecting eosin into the tumor and exposing it to light; three cures were reported. Haxthausen and Hausmann[14] in 1908 were the first to suggest that hematoporphyrin was a photodynamic photosensitizer. This finding was confirmed in 1913 by Meyer-Betz,[15] who injected himself intravenously with hematoporphyrin and became highly sensitive to light for 2 months, proving that these compounds can induce systemic photosensitization in man. Finally, in 1925 Goeckerman[16] successfully used the phototoxic effects of coal tar, together with UV radiation, to treat psoriasis.

PHOTODYNAMIC THERAPY

Definitions

Photodynamic therapy consists of the administration of a photosensitizing agent, i.e., a chemical at extremely low and nontoxic concentrations that is absorbed selectively by living tissues. This "sensitized" tissue is then exposed in the presence of oxygen to a light source of a specific wavelength, which results in the destruction of this tissue.

Mechanisms of Photooxygenation

Many chemicals, including natural cell constituents, can absorb light and by photochemical reactions damage the organism. This process, called "photodynamic action" requires oxygen and it damages biologic target molecules by photooxidation. Biochemical effects include enzyme deactivation (through destruction of specific amino acids, particularly methionine, histidine, and tryptophan), nucleic acid oxidation (primarily guanine), and membrane damage (by oxidation of unsaturated fatty acids and cholesterol). Photosensitized oxidation is initiated by the absorption of light by a sensitizer, which can be a dye or pigment, a ketone or quinone, or an aromatic molecule. The sensitizer (Sens), by capturing a photon, is elevated to a higher energy state where it may now act as an oxidizer.

There are two mechanisms of photosensitized oxidation, type I and type II, that are always in competition. Factors that govern the competition include oxygen concentration, the reactivities of the substrate and sensitizer excited state, substrate concentration, and singlet oxygen lifetime.

High sensitizer reactivity, high substrate reactivity and concentration, low oxygen concentration, and short singlet lifetimes favor the type I mechanism, while the opposite factors favor the type II.

Hematoporphyrin Derivatives

Hematoporphyrin derivatives (HPDs) were recently tested as a photosensitizer for specific laser treatment of superficial malignancies. This was based on observations that demonstrated that HPD was retained longer by malignant tissue than by many surrounding normal tissues and was detectable by tumor fluorescence.[17,18] This suggested that its activation would selectively damage only the abnormal tissue to which it had been bound.

The chemical composition of HPD has been shown to be a mixture of several porphyrins, but until recently, the active component responsible for its action was unknown.[19] The structure of the active element dihematoporphyrin ether (DHE) was elucidated by Dougherty et al.[18] in 1979. The absorption spectrum of HPD in human serum shows five major absorption peaks, at 402, 507, 540, 573, and 624 nm, all of which are in the visible spectrum of light. The least tissue penetration and the highest HPD absorption are at 402 nm; the greatest tissue penetration and least absorption are at 624 nm.

Attempts to demonstrate clear differences in affinity of porphyrins for normal or malignant cells in culture have given ambiguous results. Chang and Dougherty[20] examined two cell lines derived from normal tissue and two from malignant tissue under identical tissue culture conditions and they found no differences in porphyrin affinity or photodynamic killing for four cell lines of different oncogenic potential. However, these results may have been compromised by the presence of HPD impurities, rather than being attributable to the HPD component responsible for the in vivo effects. In fact, the result of studies by Henderson et al.[21] indicate that the uptake kinetics of the active component of HPD (DHE) are quite different from the HPD mixture. While numerous early reports indicated that most normal tissues do retain HPD, recent studies by Gomer and Dougherty[22] demonstrated that kidney, liver, and spleen of mice retain more HPD than does a transplanted mammary tumor.

The current interest in photodynamic therapy stems from studies begun in 1972 by Dougherty and colleagues at Roswell Park Memorial Institute in Buffalo. In 1978[17] and 1979[18] this group reported clinical studies showing that skin metastases could be eradicated with the proper combination of HPD and red light (630 nm), a wavelength selected for optimal activation of HPD, which also allowed maximum penetration through tissue (1–2 cm) as is necessary for this method to be useful for cancer therapy. The most important point common to both the diagnostic and therapeutic photoradiation systems employed with HPD is the requirement for sufficient amounts of light to reach tumor target sites. In addition, detection of tumor fluorescence is simplified when the exciting light is both coherent and of a different wavelength from the fluorescence emission of the tumor. Lasers are one type of light that can satisfy these conditions.

Current clinical applications of HPD for PDT have focused on accessible superficial malignancies, including cancer of the lung,[23,24] bladder,[25] vagina and cervix, gastrointestinal tract,[26] primary and metastatic skin cancers,[17] and tumors of the head and neck (laryngeal base of tongue, palatal, and floor of mouth tumors).[27–29] In a series of tumors treated with HPD and laser light, PDT has shown therapeutic effects.

The depth of tissue degeneration due to this therapy was influenced by the energy dose delivered to the treated tumor. At the same energy level, greater therapeutic effects were obtained when the light exposure was performed 96 to 168 hours after HPD administration than after 24 to 72 hours. However, therapeutic effectiveness varies according to each lesion, even in the same patient. Thus the inconsistent response implies that laser-tissue interactions and dosimetry remain as areas requiring further study.

The initial enthusiasm generated by the early successful results observed in patients treated with HPD and laser light was diminished substantially by its side effects and other treatment limitations.[30] Patients must be protected with adequate clothing or sunscreens against any sunlight and cannot even venture outside or sit near a window during this period. Pain is another common side effect, particularly involving the calvarium, with patients frequently experiencing severe headaches after light activation.[30] In addition, HPD has been shown to exhibit nonspecific uptake by inflammatory cells and traumatized tissues, which decreases its potential as a "tumor specific fluorescent dye." Also the low power (milliwatt range) of the dye lasers used for treatment have limited effectiveness for tumor therapy because of limited depth of tissue penetrance. These side effects and limitations of HPD will probably remain significant limiting factors for its future clinical applications. A variety of other photochemically active dyes, such as acridine orange, mercurochrome, nitro-red, methylene blue, psoralens, rose bengal, and sodium fluorescein have been investigated as potential photosensitizing agents with some advantages. They have not provided an advantage over the use of HPD.

Current Status of Laser Dyes

A large number of photosensitizers have been tested in laboratories around the world with promising results. Merocyanine-540 is currently used in phase I clinical trials for purging tumor cells from autologous bone marrow grafts in patients with leukemia, lymphoma, or metastatic neuroblastoma.[8] Rhodamine-123 (Rh-123) (Figs. 11–1 and 11–2) has recently been approved for phase I clinical trials in patients with recurrent head and neck carcinomas in our own studies at UCLA.

Recent work done by Riesz and Krishna[31] demonstrated the potential of sulfonated phthalocyanines as candidates for photodynamic therapy. Photocytotoxicity of phthalocyanines in mammalian cells has been demonstrated for various cell lines, and evidence for singlet-oxygen induced cell killings has been reported. Although the selective retention of phthalocyanine in tumor models appears to be similar to that of hematoporphyrin derivatives, a longer wavelength

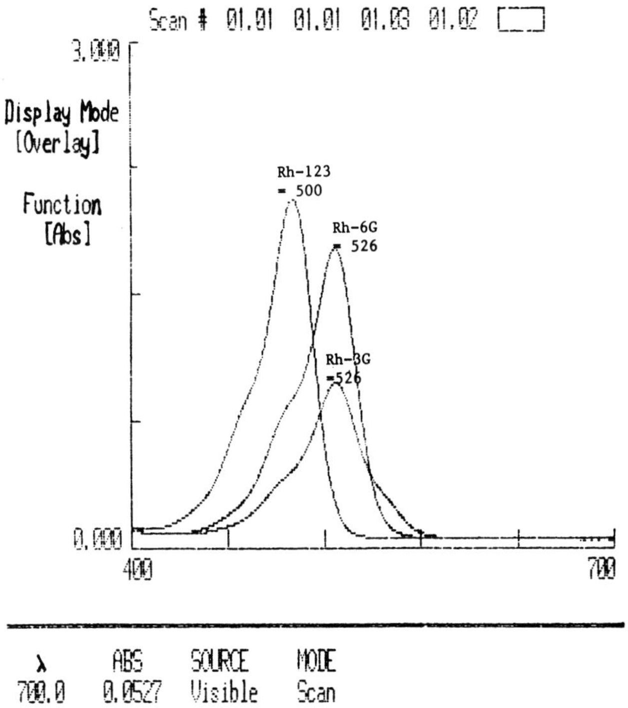

Figure 11–1. Absorption spectrum of rhodamine dyes (Rh-123, Rh-6G, Rh-3G).

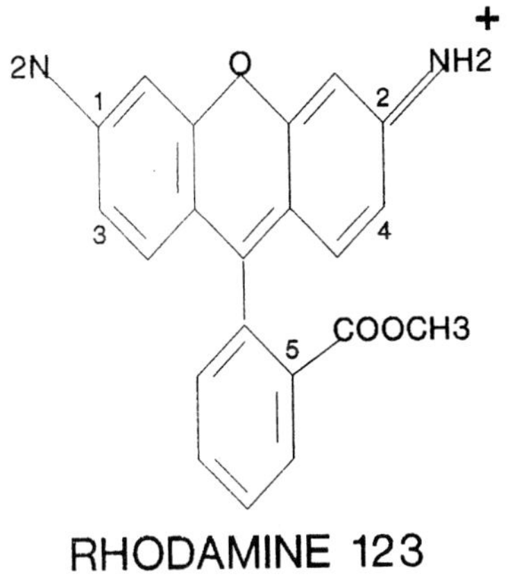

#	SUBSTITUTIONS RH3G	RH6G
1	N(CH3)2	NHC2H5
2	NH2+	NHC2H5·
3	CH3	CH3
4	CH3	CH3
5	COOC2H5	COOC2H

Figure 11–2. Molecular structure of rhodamine dyes.

(600 nm) with greater penetrating power in tissues than for hematoporphyrin has been used.

Two groups of photosensitizers were synthesized recently by Morgan et al.[32] These photochemicals include the purpurins and their metallo derivatives. Unlike HPD, they are homogeneous pure dyes of known structure. In addition, the purpurins have major absorption peaks between 630 and 715 nm, which are wavelengths capable of deep tissue penetration. From histologic studies in transplanted urothelial tumors, it is clear that purpurins and metallopurpurins are capable of causing extensive tumor necrosis when combined with visible light.

Detty[33] at the Eastman Kodak Laboratories recently demonstrated the potential usefulness of a new group of photosensitizers, the chalcogenapyrilium dyes, which are water soluble cationic compounds with various absorption maxima between 750 and 875 nm. The chalcogenapyrilium dyes represent a family of related compounds whose properties as a chromophore can be designed by proper choice of organic structural substitutions, which permit control of their wavelength absorption maxima, redox properties, fluorescence yields, and hydrolytic stability. These dyes should be compatible with commercially available gallium arsenide lasers. However, recent preliminary studies[34] show both relatively poor uptake and significant toxicity of the chalcogenapyriliums in cell cultures.

The kryptocyanine dye EDKC has been tested by Ara and Ohuoha[35] and exhibits preferential uptake by cancer cells of various origins, with an absorption maximum at 700 nm in saline. Kodak Q-Switch II dye (1051 nm) has recently been evaluated[36] in vitro in our laboratory as a near-infrared laser dye with promising results. Several oxazine dyes[37] and Nile blue A also have been tested as fluorescent cationic dyes. Pheophorbide, a chlorophyll derivative with a peak absorption at 670 nm, has been examined recently by Segelman.[38]

Future Directions: Photosensitizers and Light Sources

The field of photodynamic therapy with dyes and lasers for the treatment of cancer may become clinically useful only after performing extensive drug screening similar to antibiotic culture and sensitivity testing for infectious diseases. It is evident that there is not one "magic" antibiotic for all infectious processes. By analogy, there may not be one "magic" dye for all malignancies, but most likely many dyes will be suitable, each with a specific affinity for a specific cancer, perhaps based on the cell line of origin. For example, Rh-123 appears to have promising effects as a photosensitizer for argon laser treatment of squamous cell carcinoma (Fig. 11–3), melanoma, adenocarcinoma, leukemia, and lymphoma cell lines,[39] but has poor response in mesothelioma and sarcoma cell lines.[39] Merocyanine-540, on the other hand, is extremely efficient in leukemias, lymphomas, and neuroblastomas, but shows poor uptake and effects in lung and ovarian carcinomas.[37]

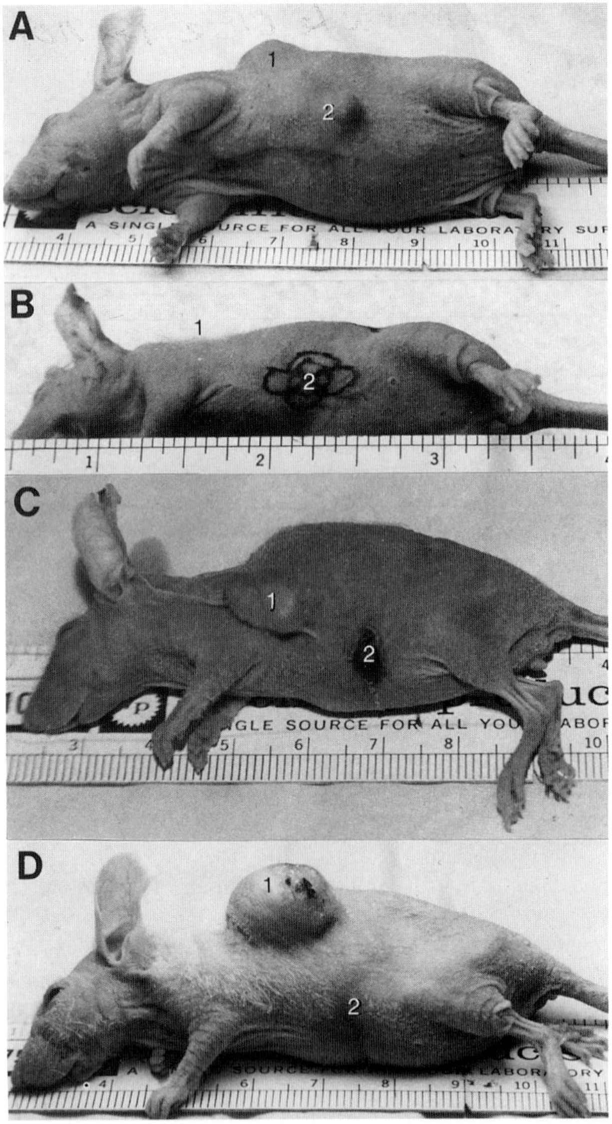

Figure 11–3. Argon laser phototherapy of experimental P_3 squamous carcinoma tumors in nu/nu mice after sensitization with Rh-123. Pretreatment (A2), immediately post–laser therapy (B2), 1 week (C2), and 10 weeks (D2) post–laser therapy. Complete cure is noted in the experimental tumors (Rh-123 + laser, D2) while continued growth is noted for control tumors (D1).

With the collaboration of clinicians, chemists, biologists, and photochemists, photochemical dyes may be "designed" in the laboratory, and then tested clinically. Dyes with higher affinity for specific neoplasms, with rapid metabolism, short half-life, and lower systemic toxicity can then be developed. Dyes with synergistic and/or antagonistic effects on various neoplasms may be found, and optimal fluorochromes for photodynamic therapy and/or photodiagnostic imaging with lasers can then be classified. The chalcogenapyrilium dyes are a good example of a "dye design" system, because their absorption wavelength maxima fluorescence versus singlet yields, redox properties, and aqueous stability can be now modified by changing different chalcogen atoms and substitutions in the dye chromophore.

A rapid technological advance in the design of diode lasers could also open a productive new approach for investigation and clinical applications of PDT for several reasons. First, diode lasers are the most efficient and stable lasers available. Second, this technology is becoming less expensive at the same time that the diode lasers are being miniaturized and increasing in power output.

Some new diode lasers have a power output of nearly 25 W from a device smaller than a Carousel slide tray. New tunable dye lasers with emissions from the visible to the near-infrared spectrum are continuously being developed. These diode lasers will certainly revolutionize the field of laser technology, and might even result in the development of powerful pocket-size portable lasers that might even be disposable because of their low cost.

New light delivery systems for photodynamic therapy are developing at a staggering pace. Flexible fiberoptic cables of 200 μm and smaller diameter are currently available. New fiberoptic devices for efficient laser light dosimetry and delivery to tumor during PDT are under development to optimize the effectiveness of this technique.

Photodiagnostic Imaging with Lasers

The ability to localize and map tumors has obvious oncologic applications for the clinician for potential identification of occult tumors as well as more precise tumor removal. The field of photodiagnostic imaging with laser may be further subdivided into several potential applications including laser spectroscopy, laser dye fluorescence, and dye-conjugated monoclonal antibody imaging.

CONCLUSIONS

A new and exciting approach to cancer diagnosis and therapy may be developed using lasers and dyes. Analogous to antibiotic therapy, tumor cultures may be initiated in the laboratory and then tested for sensitivity to many photosensitizers and laser wavelengths. The optimal tumoricidal effects of laser-dye combinations for a specific tumor may be defined and then applied clinically. With the collaboration of photochemists, physicists, tumor biologists, engineers, and clinicians, many different photosensitizers and new laser wavelengths will be developed. This may result in more specific dye uptake by tumors and longer retention in the target tumor, lower systemic toxicity, and deeper tissue penetration. This could lead to the identification of new dyes with synergistic effects that enhance the tumoricidal effect of laser light. The rapid technological revolution of magnetic resonance imaging, laser fiberoptics, and magnetic resonance–compatible probes will allow tumor detection and real-time monitoring of interstitial laser phototherapy for treatment of large-volume tumors using dyes and lasers in a wide range of the electromagnetic spectrum.

A new era is dawning in the diagnostic potential of laser

dye fluorescence, and laser-induced fluorescence spectroscopy is showing promising results for detection of occult carcinomas. Monoclonal antibodies can now be produced with specific antitumor binding capacity, be linked to photosensitizers, and then be injected into patients with cancer. Soon it may be possible for the clinician to examine and diagnose early recurrences by low-power illumination of dye-stained tumor nodules followed by treatment with high-power laser emission via interstitial fiberoptics.

Exploration is just beginning in a most promising new area that will require further collaborative research between the clinician and basic scientist to determine the usefulness of this exciting adjuctive modality for the treatment of cancer and other diseases.

Acknowledgments This study was supported by the Division of Head and Neck Surgery, and the Jonsson Comprehensive Cancer Center CICR Award, UCLA School of Medicine, NIH grant #USHHS DC 0031, and NIH grant #CA65053-O1R, the Elsa Pardee Foundation, the DuPont-Merck, E-ZEM, Inc., Laserscope, Resonance Technology, Ohmeda, Inc., Trimedyne, Valley Lab, Inc., In-Vivo Research Inc., GE Medical Systems, and the Association de Recherche sur le Cancer (A.R.C., BP 3-94801 Villejuif Cedex, France).

REFERENCES

1. Maiman TH. Stimulated optical radiation in ruby. *Nature* 1960;187:493–494.
2. Policard A. Etudes sur les aspects offerts pas des tumeur experimentales examinee a la lumiere de woods. *CR Soc Biol (Paris)* 1924;91:1423.
3. Castro DJ, Saxton RE, Fetterman HG, Castro DJ, Ward PH. Rhodamine-123 as a new photochemosensitizing agent with the argon laser: "Non-thermal" and thermal effects on human squamous carcinoma cells in-vitro. *Laryngoscope* 1987;97(5):554–561.
4. Castro DJ, Saxton RE, Fetterman HR, Ward PH. The effects of argon lasers on human melanoma cells sensitized with Rhodamine-123 in-vitro. *Am J Otolaryngol* 1988;9(1):18–29.
5. Castro DJ, Saxton RE, Fetterman HR, Ward PH. Phototherapy with the argon laser on human melanoma cells "sensitized" with Rhodamine-123: a new method for tumor growth inhibition. *Laryngoscope* 1988;98(4):369–376.
6. Castro DJ, Saxton RE, Fetterman HR, Castro DJ, Ward PH. Biostimulation of human carcinoma cells with the argon laser: a previously unreported potential iatrogenic effect of lasers. *Laryngoscope* 1987;98:109–116.
7. Castro DJ, Saxton RE, Fetterman HR, Castro DJ, Ward PH. Biostimulative effects of Nd:YAG Q-switch dye on normal fibroblast cultures: study of a new chemosensitizing agent for the Nd:YAG laser. *Laryngoscope* 1987;97(12):1454–1459.
8. Gaffney DK, Sieber F. Binding of merocyanine 540 by cells labeled with anthroyloxy fatty acids. *Photochem Photobiol* 1990;49 (suppl):315.
9. Forrest JB, Forrest HJ. Case report: malignant melanoma arising during therapy for vitiligo. *J Surg Oncol* 1980;13:337–340.
10. Whitney WD. Atharva-veda Samhita. (Translation and notes). *Harvard Oriental Series,* vol 7. Cambridge: Harvard University Press, 1905.
11. Ibn El-Bitar. *Mofradat Al Adwiya.* Cairo: Egyptian Government Press, 1877;1:4.
12. Finsen NR. Neue untersuchugen uber die einwirkung dess lichtes auf die haut. *Mitt Fisen Instit* 1900;1:8.
13. Jesionek A, Tappeiner HV. Zur behandlung de hautcarcinome mit fluoresierenden Stolle. *Dtsch Arch Klin Med* 1905;82:223–227.
14. Haxthausen H, Hausmann W. *Die lichterkrankugen der haut.* Vienna: Urban and Schwarzenberg, 1929.
15. Meyer-Betz F. Untersuchugen über die biologische (photodynamische). Wirkung des Hämatoporphyrins und anderer derivate des blut-und gallenfarbstoffs. *Dtsch Arch Klin Med* 1913;112:476–503.
16. Goeckerman WH. Treatment of psoriasis. *North West Med* 1925;24:229–231.
17. Dougherty TJ, Kaufman JE, Goldfarb A, et al. Photoradiation therapy for the treatment of malignant tumors. *Cancer Res* 1978;38:2628–2635.
18. Dougherty TJ, Lawrence G, Kaufman JH, et al. Photoradiation in the treatment of recurrent breast carcinoma. *J Natl Cancer Inst* 1979;62:231–237.
19. Hayata Y, Dougherty TJ. Lasers and hematoporphyrin derivative in cancer. In: Hayata Y, Dougherty TJ, eds. *Cancer.* Translation by Barron P. New York: Igaku-Shoin, Tokyo; 1982:1–114.
20. Chang CT, Dougherty TJ. Photoradiation therapy: kinetics of thermodynamics of porphyrin uptake and loss in normal and malignant cells in culture. *Radiat Res* 1978;74:498–499.
21. Henderson BW, Bellnier DA, Ziring B, Dougherty TJ. Aspects of the cellular uptake and retention of hematoporphyrin derivative and their correlation with the biological response to PRT in vitro. In: Kessel D, Dougherty TJ, eds. *Porphyrin Photosensitization.* New York: Plenum Press; 1983;129–138.
22. Gomer CJ, Dougherty TJ. Determination of [3H] and [19C] hematoporphyrin derivative distribution in malignant and normal tissue. *Cancer Res* 1979;39:146–151.
23. Balchum OJ, Doiron DR, Huth GC. Photoradiation therapy of endobronchial lung cancers employing the photodynamic action of hematoporphyrin derivative. *Laser Surg Med* 1984;4:13–30.
24. Hayata Y, Kato H, Konaka C, et al. Photoradiation therapy with hematoporphyrin derivative in early and stage I lung cancer. *Chest* 1984;86:169–177.
25. Benson RC, Kinsey JH, Cortese DA, et al. Treatment of transitional cell carcinoma of the bladder with hematoporphyrin derivative phototherapy. *J Urol* 1983;130:1090–1094.
26. Hayata Y, Kato H, Okitsu H, et al. Photodynamic therapy with hematoporphyrin derivative in cancer of the upper gastrointestinal tract. *Semin Surg Oncol* 1985;1:1–11.
27. Keller GS, Doiron DR, Fisher GU. Photodynamic therapy in otolaryngology—head and neck surgery. *Arch Otolaryngol* 1985;111:758–761.
28. Gluckman JL, Waner M, Shumrick K. Photodynamic therapy: a viable alternative to conventional therapy for early lesion of the upper aerodigestive tract. Presented at the Joint Meeting of the American Society for Head and Neck Surgery and the Society of Head and Neck Surgeons entitled, "Current Research and Clinical Concepts in Head and Neck Cancer," Dorado, Puerto Rico, May 5, 1985.
29. Kinsey JH, Cortese DA, Neel HB. Thermal considerations in murine tumor killing using hematoporphyrin derivative phototherapy. *Cancer Res* 1983;43:1562–1567.
30. Gregory RO, Goldman L. Application of photodynamic therapy in plastic surgery. *Laser Surg Med* 1986;6:62–66.
31. Riesz P, Krishna M. Phthalocyanines and their sulfonated derivatives as photosensitizers in photodynamic therapy.

New Directions in Photodynamic Therapy. *Proc SPIE* 1987;847:15–23.
32. Morgan AR, Kreimer-Birnbaum M, Selman SH. Purpurins improved photosensitizers for photodynamic therapy. New Directions in Photodynamic Therapy. *Proc SPIE* 1987;847:29–35.
33. Detty MR. Rational design of properties in chalcogenapyrlium dyes. New Directions in Photodynamic Therapy. *Proc SPIE* 1987;847:68–73.
34. Kessel D. Some observation of the photosensitization of neoplastic cells with a chalcogenacryrylium dye. *Photochem Photobiol* 1990;51(suppl):545.
35. Ara G, Ohuoha D, Oseroff A.R. Partial inhibition of glycolysis with 2-deoxy-D-glucose enhances EDKC medicated cellular photosensitization. New Directions in Photodynamic Therapy. *Proc SPIE* 1987;847:201–204.
36. Castro DJ, Saxton RE, Fetterman HR, et al. Bioinhibition of human fibroblast cultures sensitized to Q-switch II dye and treated with the Nd:YAG lasers. *Laryngoscope* 1989;99:421–428.
37. Osseroff A, Wan W, Wadwa KS, et al. Sensitive selection detection of carcinomas and melanomas using fluorescent cationic dyes. *Photochem Photobiol* 1990;51 (suppl):745.
38. Segelman AB. Highly purified pheophorbide as a photosensitizer in human bladder carcinoma. New Directions in Photodynamic Therapy. *Proc SPIE* 1987;847:205–208.
39. Sugita K, Giulliano AE, Sugita N, et al. Tumors of diverse histology are sensitive to rhodamine-123 laser phototherapy in vitro. *Am J Otolaryngol* 1990;11:1–7.

12 Laser Photothermal Therapy for Cancer Treatment

Dan J. Castro, Romaine E. Saxton, Jacques Soudant

The therapeutic value of heat was first recognized and reported in the time of the ancient Egyptians more than 2000 years ago. Breast tumors were treated using the glowing tip of a fire drill.[1] Classical Roman and Greek physicians also were aware of the homeostatic and destructive tissue capabilities of heat and used it widely in medical procedures.[2] Laser light has been used in a wide spectrum of applications both in medicine and surgery since its introduction in the early 1960s. Because most wavelengths are emitted via fiber optics, laser energy can be delivered to target sites endoscopically and/or interstitially using the principle of minimally invasive surgery, which reduces cost of treatment. In addition, because its energy is rapidly absorbed in tissues, its effects are predictable, reproducible, and controllable. Its nonionizing characteristic simplifies safety requirements. With the increasing cost of health care during the past 20 years, a great public interest in the relationship between cost and quality has developed. Laser technology has been permissive in the development of less invasive but highly effective surgical procedures that reduce both morbidity and cost. This is exemplified by laparoscopic surgery, which is replacing "open" laparatomy, resulting in reduced morbidity, accelerated functional recovery, and lowering of cost as ambulatory surgery has become a safe alternative to inpatient surgery. Image guided minimally invasive surgery is a new concept that uses ultrasound (UTZ) and/or fast magnetic resonance imaging (MRI) to guide various energy sources such as lasers, radio frequency, and ultrasonic and cryotherapy devices for therapy of deep tumors while monitoring tissue changes during energy deposition (Fig. 12–1). The use of lasers as a source of photothermal energy for treatment of cancer and other diseases, its physiologic effects, and background are reviewed in this chapter.

BACKGROUND

Localized hyperthermia may be delivered externally and/or interstitially using radio frequency, ultrasound, microwave, or laser energy. With all of these techniques the major problem is to precisely focus the energy on the target tissue to predictably induce the required cell death. The uneven heating achieved by local hyperthermia techniques presently available severely limits its utility, because the lowest temperature achieved in a tumor mass is the key predictor of treatment response.[3]

Other methods for inducing localized tissue necrosis such as topical or interstitial cryotherapy have been tested by Ravikumar et al.[4] and Zhou et al.[5] for the treatment of liver tumors. In several cases both tumor eradication and survival times for otherwise untreatable tumors have been increased.[4,5] Dritchilo et al.[6] used interstitial implantation of radioactive seeds in tumors to induce tumor necrosis, but the effect on survival was not clear. Livraghi et al.[7] and Shina et al.[8] injected 95% alcohol into the center of tumors using ultrasound guidance, which was associated with few complications and produced tumor necrosis. This method, however, is rather imprecise and treatment outcomes are unpredictable. Clearly these techniques are not ideal; cryotherapy requires a laparotomy for its application, which limits repeated treatment, and alcohol injection is subject to imprecision in administration and a requirement for repeat treatments. There is an obvious need to develop better techniques to induce tumor necrosis in a more predictable way, while using minimally invasive surgical access and improved "real" time monitoring systems.

Interstitial laser therapy of tumors is a promising new approach because it is minimally invasive and allows precise and controlled delivery of photothermal energy into tissues. However, it will become clinically useful only when noninvasive dosimetry systems deliver the energy in an accurate and reproducible way (Fig. 12–2). Invasive methods currently available use thermal probes, infrared thermography, and histologic assessment,[9,10] which are reliable but have limited clinical applications.

Since the mid-1970s, interstitial placement of laser fiberoptics has been applied successfully in large subcutaneous metastatic tumors.[11,12] In 1985 Svaasand et al.[13] developed preliminary optical dosimetry for interstitial phototherapy of malignant tumors. Bown[14] investigated the interstitial use of the neodymium:yttrium-aluminum-garnet (Nd:YAG) laser for hyperthermia. Matthewson et al.[15–17] used a single Nd:YAG laser fiber at low power (1–2 W), to produce areas of thermal necrosis in the normal rat liver (below the surface), and to eradicate induced rat colon tumors and implanted fibrosarcomas. Hashimoto et al.[18] applied 5 to 15 W of Nd:YAG laser power with a modified

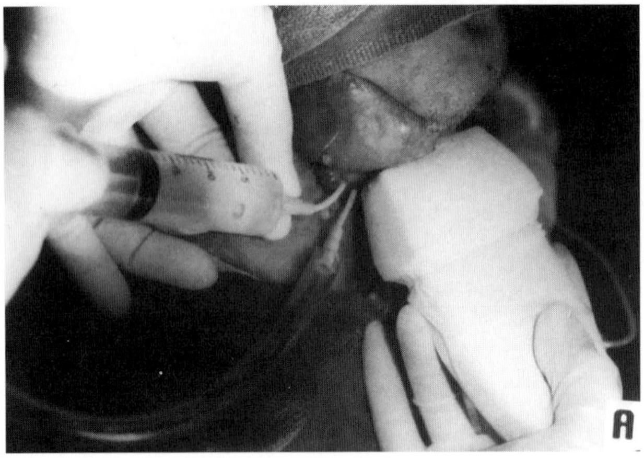

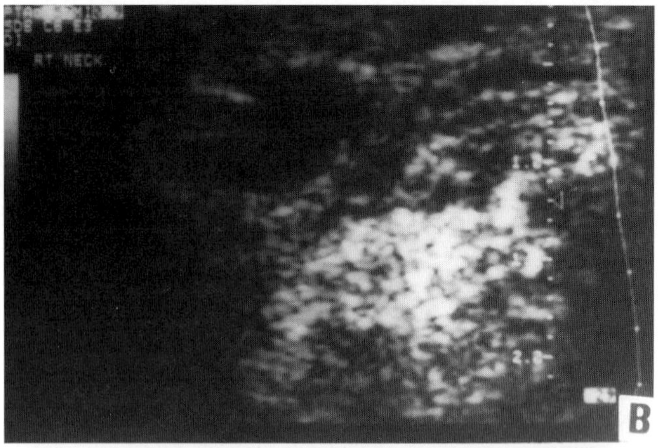

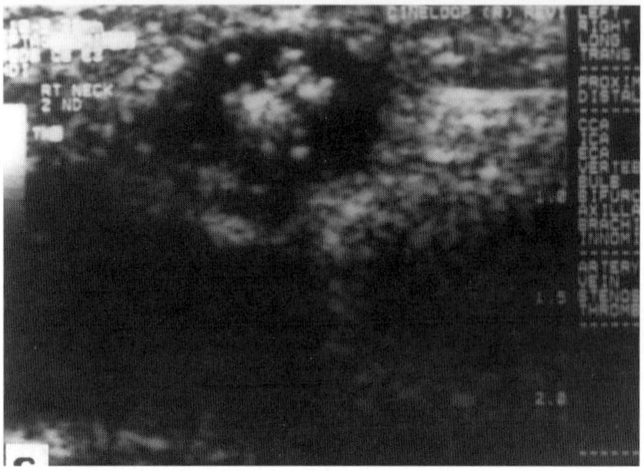

Figure 12–1. **(A)** Interstitial Nd:YAG laser treatment of a recurrent midline neck squamous cell carcinoma guided by ultrasound. **(B)** The 10-MHz transducer is placed on the skin while the laser needle is introduced transcutaneously in the tumor and its position confirmed by ultrasonography. **(C)** The Nd:YAG laser is then turned on while the ultrasound monitors the tissue effects, demonstrating a transient hyperechoic signal during energy deposition.

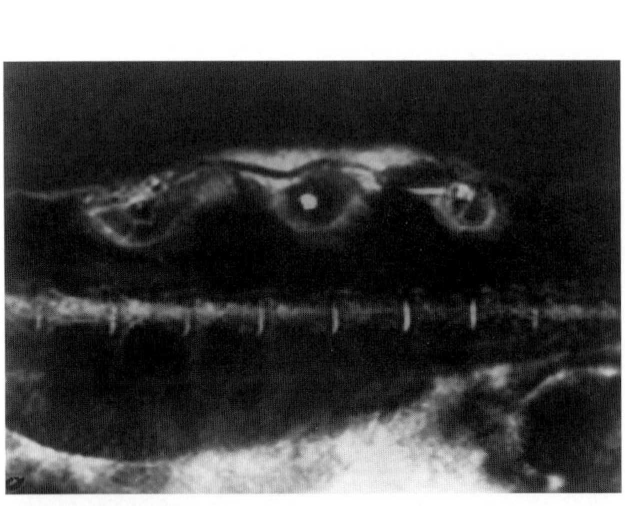

Figure 12–2. T2-weighted image of three in vivo laser lesions made at 2000 J in the normal muscle of a rabbit. Lesions were produced using 5 W × 400 sec, 10 W × 200 sec, and 20 W × 400 sec. Concentric layers of signal intensity change correspond to coagulated (dark) and interstitial edema (bright and diffused) zones. At the core of each lesion is the center filled with interstitial fluid, blood, or air.

diffuser fiber tip to treat liver tumors with evidence of reduction of tumor size. Godlewski et al.[19,20] used high-powered Nd:YAG of up to 100 W, of 1-second duration to produce areas of vaporization and necrosis of 16 to 22 mm in the porcine liver. However, the high power density at the distal end of the optical fiber resulted in frequent tip damage, burning, nonuniform distribution of laser energy, and poorly reproducible tissue effects. The recent introduction of synthetic sapphire probes,[21] which have high melting points (2020–2050°C), greater tensile strength, and a uniform pattern of laser beam delivery from the probe have allowed testing of Nd:YAG laser–induced hyperthermia in a dog model.[21,22] Daikuzono and Joffe[21] further developed a computer-controlled Nd:YAG system for interstital local hyperthermia.

To increase the area of necrosis that could be produced using a single laser as the energy source, Steger and Brown[22] employed fiber-optic coupling systems, which allow the insertion of multiple fibers. This concept, while attractive, has proved difficult to achieve in practice.

LASER TISSUE EFFECTS

The photobiologic effects of laser light on tissue can be separated into three categories: photochemical, photomechanical, and photothermal. Photochemical effects depend on the absorption of light to initiate chemical reactions such as the production of reactive chemical species in photodynamic therapy. It is associated with low fluence rates that do not produce a significant temperature increase in the treated tissue, but do interact with a natural or exogenous photosensitizer to produce the desired reaction. Photomechanical responses occur during application of extremely high fluence rates (greater than 10^8 W/cm^2), and short laser pulses (10^{-6} second or less), which produce shock waves and plasmas. Such effects occur, for example, when a laser is operated in the Q-switched mode.

Photothermal effects result from the transformation of absorbed light energy to heat. These photothermal effects can be further subdivided into three categories: (1) laser hyperthermia, (2) photoablation, and (3) photocarbonization or photoevaporation. In hyperthermia cells that are heated to temperatures ranging from 40° to 45°C can sustain reversible injury that becomes irreversible (death) after exposure from 25 minutes to several hours, depending on the type of tissue and experimental or therapeutic circumstances. Both systemic and local hyperthermia have been tested clinically with limited success, mainly because of the difficulties in delivering a uniform level of energy throughout the tumor mass. In addition this technique is slow, cumbersome, and difficult to apply.

In photoablation, the tissue is rapidly heated to a range of 60° to 100°C where visible whitening is seen, indicating thermal coagulation. Thermal coagulation of tissues is defined as thermally induced, irreversible alteration of proteins and other biologic molecules, organelles, membranes, cells, and extracellular components that are observable with the naked eye and/or microscope. Most of these alterations are due to thermal denaturation of structural proteins, although membrane rupture may result from alterations in lipids. By this definition, thermal tissue coagulation differs from low temperature injury in that the always lethal coagulative lesions are marked by structural changes seen immediately after heating. This process is easier and faster to deliver and control in tissues.

When tissue temperature is raised above 100°C, the process of photocarbonization and/or photoevaporation will occur with an explosive fragmentation of tissue loss. Subsurface heating generates bubbles that eventually explode in a series of events called the "popcorn effect." Water loss results in tissue desiccation, which radically changes the optical characteristics of tissues and their absorption efficiency of infrared lasers. In addition, water loss reduces the thermal conductivity and specific heat of tissues. Black char, yellow flames, and gray smoke are the prominent phenomena characterizing the clinical use of the process of photocarbonization.

BIOLOGIC EFFECTS OF HYPERTHERMIA

A number of biologic mechanisms have provided a rationale for considering hyperthermia as an antitumor agent. At a temperature range between 40° and 42.5°C, heat can increase cell killing in a synergistic way following exposure of a tumor to ionizing radiation or to chemotherapeutic drugs. This heat-induced radiosensitization is probably secondary to the inhibited repair of radiation induced DNA lesions. Bicher and Bruley,[23] Dethlefsen and Dewey,[24] Dietzel,[25] Hornback,[26] and Storm[27] demonstrated that the action of bleomycin, Adriamycin, and cis-platinum is enhanced by heat treatment (T = 40°–42.5°C). Hyperthermia acts as a cytotoxic agent at temperatures higher than 42.5°C because cells die after heating in a time-temperature– and cell cycle–dependent manner. The relationship between the temperature and time for which it is applied is not a simple linear product of these two variables.[28] Early observations of tissue hyperthermia were made in the late 1920s by Westermark[29] and Pincus and Fischer.[30] Moritz and Henriques[31] studied the effects of thermal burns induced in pig skin and humans after exposure to temperatures above 44°C, with heating times between 1 second and several hours. Pincus and Fischer[30] observed that above 44°C an increase in temperature of 1°C was equivalent to increasing the time of heating by a factor of two and vice versa.

One of the main subcellular targets for hyperthermia is cell membrane protein.[32] In addition, hyperthermia inhibits DNA replication and DNA and protein synthesis, and leads to changes in metabolic processes. During moderate increases in tissue temperature, an elevated rate of metabolism is seen, which is followed by an inhibition in energy production in most cells. This adenosine triphosphate (ATP) depletion plays an uncertain role during heat-induced cell killing, because the glycolytic pathway remains almost unaffected for a prolonged time. Tumor cells are preferentially killed in the S-phase during hyperthermia, specifically if their microenvironment is characterized by hypoxia, acidity, and energy deprivation. This enhanced effect of heat on tumor cells may also be attributed to blood flow, which may be poor and sluggish in tumors. In addition, because the perfusion rate is reduced with increasing size of a tumor,[33,34] it results in decreased heat dissipation and higher local temperatures for a given energy. The thermal distribution in tissues, the rate of temperature rise, and the steady state temperature are determined by multiple parameters including thermal conductivity, specific heat source, blood perfusion rate, tissue extinction coefficient, heat losses at exposed surfaces, and incident energy density. Factors such as optical wavelengths, heating conditions at the surface, and energy density can be controlled to shift the location of the maximum rise of tissue temperature at various depths. Cooling at the surface, for example, will shift the location of the maximum temperature rise from the surface to a deeper layer, previously inaccessible to the optical penetration of the wavelength used.

In most tumors, a significant reduction in blood flow will be observed if appropriate tissue temperature levels and heat exposure are chosen. However, despite the fact that blood flow inhibition may increase the cytocidal effects of hyperthermia, it may reduce its chemotherapy and/or radiosensitizing effects because heat diminishes the rate of drug delivery and makes the tumor more hypoxic. Therefore, appropriate timing and sequencing is required when using hyperthemia in conjunction with chemotherapeutic drugs and/or radiation therapy. The decreased blood flow to the tumor during hyperthemia also generates a cellular microenvironment that can sensitize cancer cells to heat. The intercellular space becomes hypoxic, acidic and deprived of nutrients, which further enhances the cytocidal effects of hyperthermia, thereby inhibiting the repair of the thermal damage and the development of thermotolerance.

IMAGING-GUIDED MINIMALLY INVASIVE THERAPY

The concept of imaging-controlled interstitial tumor therapy (ITT) employs MRI and/or UTZ systems to safely guide transcutaneous placement of an energy source in a tumor while avoiding surrounding obstacles, then serves as a monitor for tumor destruction in real or "near" real time.[32–41]

In recent years MRI has proven to be one of the most useful monitoring techniques for interstitial tumor therapy.[42–52] The availability of oblique and multiplanar imaging capabilities, a lack of ionizing radiation, high tissue contrast and resolution, the absence of beam-hardening artifacts from bone, and the recent development of ultrafast MR pulse sequences make MRI particularly useful during minimally invasive surgery (Fig. 12–3). However, several limitations of current MR systems must be resolved for its effective and safe use for interventional procedures. The high magnetic field (1.5 T) of the MR environment and the closed cylindrical shape of the magnet severely restrict both physical access to the patient as well as access to the monitoring and treatment devices in use. With the collaboration of a number of different manufacturers a variety of new MR-compatible devices were introduced in a standard superconducting 1.5 T Signa (GE Medical Systems, Milwaukee) MRI suite permitting the use of practical interventional procedures in this room (Fig. 12–4).

A series of 55 patients were treated over a 6-year period (1988–1994) at the UCLA School of Medicine, using the concept of imaging-guided minimally invasive therapy. Most patients were in the fifth and sixth decade of life and were treated for palliation in an attempt to control symptoms such as pain, dysphagia, dyspnea, and bleeding. Most treated tumors (90%) were squamous cell carcinomas, located in different anatomic sites within the head and neck. Most patients (83%) were treated in the operating room using UTZ as the guiding imaging modality (Fig. 12–1), while 17% were treated in an upgraded interventional MRI suite (Fig. 12–4). In 90% of the cases the neodymium:yttrium-aluminum-garnet (Nd:YAG) laser was used either externally or interstitially (600 μm bare fiber optic) to photoablate the tumors, while the CO_2 laser and ultrasonic energy were used in the remaining cases. Ninety percent of the patients were treated on an outpatient basis, with 80% showing improvement and/or resolution of symptoms after one to five sessions, with a mean of two treatments. In 50 to 80% of the patients, local tumor "control" or "cure" was observed (Fig. 12–5). This response was linearly related to the initial tumor volume, histology, and growth rate. Smaller, slow-growing, more differentiated tumors were

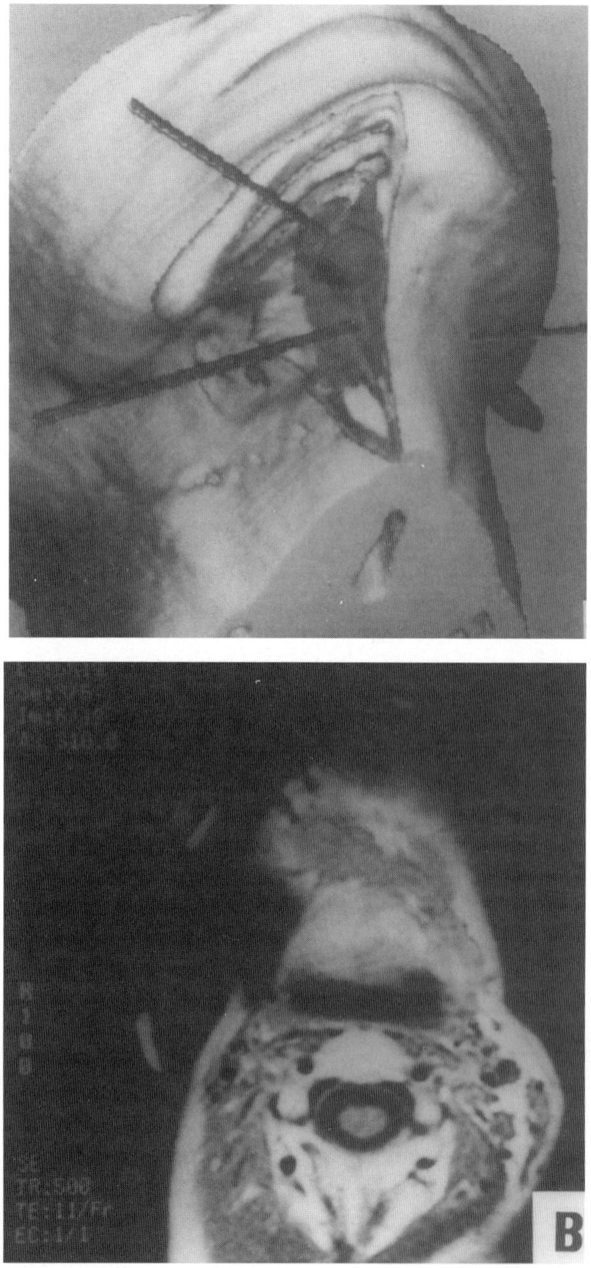

Figure 12–3. **(A)** Presurgical 3D-MRI of a patient with an unresectable recurrent submental carcinoma. Based on laser dosimetry study presurgical planning of the needle, introduction and position is made on the screen. **(B)** Presurgical MR images of the same patient showing the needles in the tumor during energy deposition.

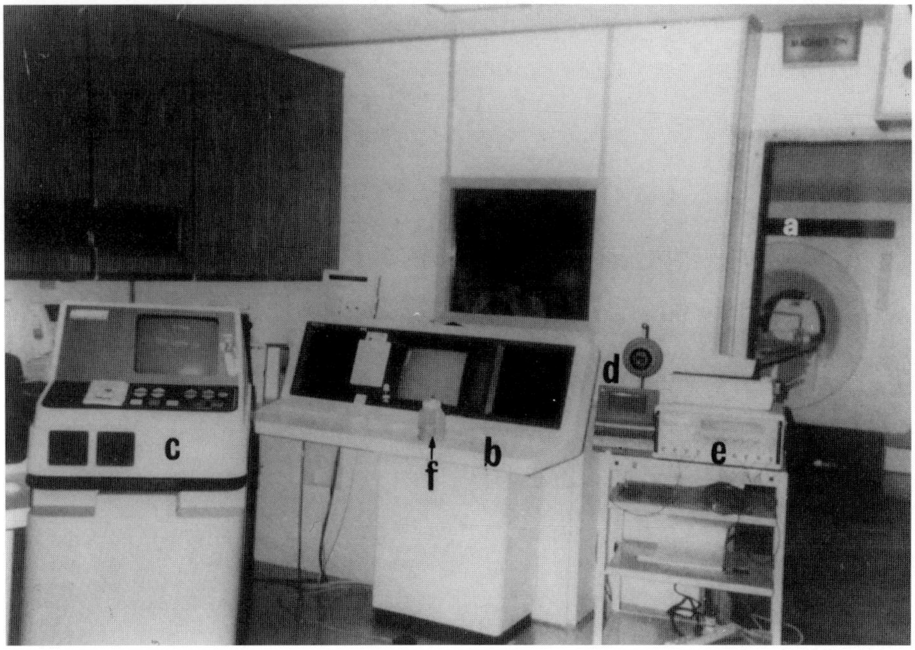

Figure 12–4. Setting of the MR suite showing the GE Signa MR magnet **(A),** the operator console **(B)**, the Laserscope KTP:YAG laser, which is kept outside the magnet **(C)**, the Coherent power meter and detector head **(D)**, the Luxtron fluoroptic thermometer **(E).**

palliated successfully and had a "better chance" for local cure than did rapidly dividing malignancies. Over 80% of the patients have shown significant functional and/or cosmetic improvement and were able to resume daily activities for periods of up to 4 years posttreatment with a mean of 18 months (range: 3 months to 5 years). Only one major complication was observed in a case early in this series. A perioperative bleed occurred during interstitial laser energy deposition that required embolization. Endotracheal intubation was required to protect the airway. This patient did well afterward and died of acute myocardial infarction 4 years after her initial palliative treatment. The only premature death occurred in the first patient 3 months postoperatively of unrelated cardiopulmonary disease. The mean survival for the study group was 18 months.

Procedures were carried out on inpatients using the operating room and on outpatients using an MRI unit specially equipped with a video monitoring system. After obtaining appropriate informed consent, the patients were placed on continuous cardiac and pulse oximetry monitoring and then heavily sedated or placed under general anesthesia by an anesthesiologst. The surgical field was prepared and draped in a sterile fashion, and the skin overlying the tumor mass was anesthetized with 1% lidocaine with 1:100,000 epinephrine. Based upon the tumor volume to be treated, a variable number of 16-gauge MRI-compatible needles (E-Z-EM, Inc.) were then passed percutaneously into the tumor mass. MRI (5 patients) or UTZ (25 patients) (Fig. 12–1) was used to confirm the position of the tip of the catheters within the tumor mass, with special attention given to their proximity to the great vessels and to tumor neovascularity.

A 600μm flexible Nd:YAG laser fiberoptic cable was then passed through the lumen of the needle and into the tumor mass. Nd:YAG laser energy (90% of cases) was applied interstially and/or externally while using T2 fast spin echo (FSE) MRI or UTZ as a monitoring technique. The CO_2 laser (7%) and ultrasonic (3%) energies were used externally in the remaining cases. As tissue photoablation occurred, the tumor mass was frequently irrigated with normal saline and suctioned (Fig. 12–1). During the procedure attempts were made to either excise the tumor with margins, debulk it, and/or induce photocoagulation necrosis and suction the debris. The initial tumor volume as calculated by 3D-MRI and/or with UTZ determined the number of treatment sessions with larger tumors requiring multiple treatments. At the end of each procedure a pressure dressing was applied and the patients were awakened from anesthesia.

CONCLUSION

The technique of interstitial therapy guided by MRI and/or UTZ is likely to become a minimally invasive method for initial treatment of benign tumors of the head and neck, breast, kidney, and prostate. Because it is performed under local anesthesia on an outpatient basis using a single needle stick, it will be much less expensive than open procedures. In addition, because laser light is nonionizing, treatment may be repeated many times without the morbidity of surgery and/or radiation therapy. Over three million "open" surgical procedures per year are performed to remove tu-

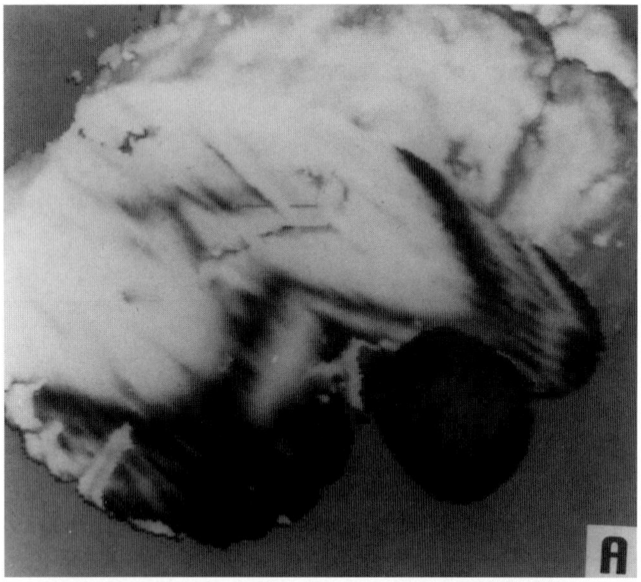

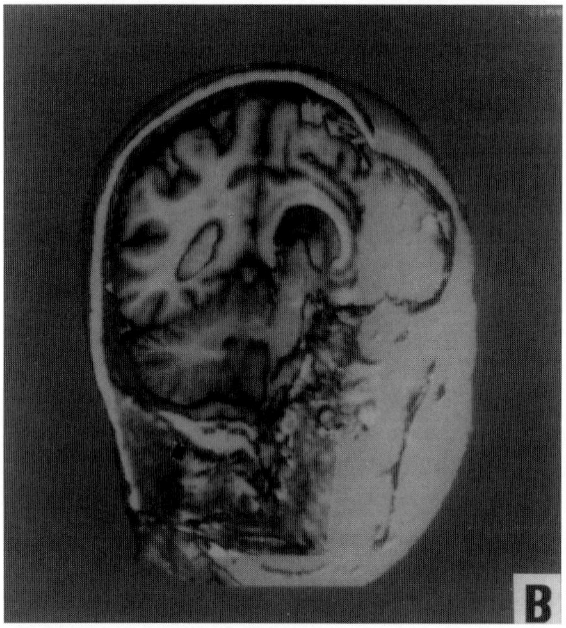

Figure 12–5. Pre- **(A)** and post- **(B)** 3D-MR images on a patient with a large base of skull carcinoma that was treated using the concept of imaging-guided surgery. The patient's tumor regressed completely and remained free of local recurrence 2 years post-treatment.

mors of the head and neck, breast, kidney, prostatic masses, and single-level disk diseases. If only 10% of these patients become candidates for this technique of interstitial therapy guided by imaging techniques, it could lead to substantial savings and benefit millions of patients. In the future, this technique may be extended to other diseases such as brain tumors, liver, chest, abdomen, all tumor metastases, and other pathologic conditions.

The techniques developed for Nd:YAG ITT may be adaptable to other forms of minimally invasive interstitial tumor therapy, employing lasers of other wavelengths, radio frequency, microwaves, cryotherapy, ethanol injection, or interstitial radioactive seed implantation. Such treatments have the potential to provide meaningful palliation for patients with advanced head and neck cancer on a cost-efficient, outpatient basis.

Acknowledgments This study was supported by the Division of Head and Neck Surgery, and the Jonsson Comprehensive Cancer Center CICR Award, UCLA School of Medicine, NIH grant #USHHS DC 0031, and NIH grant #CA65053-O1R, the Elsa Pardee Foundation, DuPont Merck, E-Z-EM, Inc., Laserscope, Resonance Technology, Ohmeda, Inc., Trimedyne, Valley Lab, Inc., In-Vivo Research Inc., GE Medical Systems, and the Association de Recherche sur le Cancer (A.R.C., BP 3-94801 Villejuif Cedex, France).

REFERENCES

1. Breasted JH. *The Edwin Smith Surgical Papyrus,* vol 1. Chicago: University of Chicago; 1930.
2. Milne JS. *Surgical Instruments in Greek and Roman Times.* Oxford: Clarendon Press; 1907.
3. Wagner von Jauregg J. Gutachten der Wiener Medizinischen Fakultaet. *Jahrb Psychiat Neurol* 1917–18;38:1–48.
4. Ravikumar TS, Kane R, Cady B, et al. Hepatic cryosurgery with intraoperative ultrasound monitoring for metastatic colon carcinoma. *Arch Surg* 1987;122:403–409.
5. Zhou XD, Tang ZY, Yu YQ, Ma ZC. Clinical evaluation of cryosurgery in the treatment of primary liver cancer (report of 60 cases). *Cancer* 1988;61:1889–1892.
6. Dritchilo AE, Grant EG, Harter KW, et al. Interstitial radiation therapy for hepatic metastases: sonographic guidance for applicator placement. *Am J Roentgenol* 1986;164:275–278.
7. Livraghi T, Salmi A, Bolondi L, et al. Small hepatocellular carcinoma: percutaneous alcohol injection results in 23 patients. *Radiology* 1988;168:313–317.
8. Shiina S, Yasuda H, Muto H, et al. Percutaneous ethanol injection in the treatment of liver neoplasms. *Am J Roentgenol* 1987;149:949–952.
9. Cummins L, Nauenberg M. Thermal effects of laser radiation in biological tissue. *Biophys J* 1983;42:99–102.
10. Welch AJ. The thermal response of laser irradiated tissue. *IEEE J Quant Electron* 1984;20:1471–1484.
11. Dougherty TJ, Lawrence G, Kaufman JH, et al. Photoradiation in the treatment of recurrent breast carcinoma. *J Natl Cancer Inst* 1979;62:231–237.
12. Dougherty TJ, Kaufman JE, Goldfarb A, et al. Photoradiation therapy for the treatment of malignant tumors. *Cancer Res.* 1985;38:2628–2635.
13. Svassand LO, Boerslid T, Oeveraasen M. Thermal and optical properties of living tissue: application of laser-induced hyperthermia. *Lasers Surg Med.* 1985;5:589–602.
14. Bown SG. Phototherapy to tumors. *World J Surg* 1983;7:700–709.
15. Matthewson K, Barr H, Tralau C, Bown SG. Low power interstitial Nd-YAG laser photocoagulation; studies in a transplantable fibrosarcoma. *Br J Surg* 1989;76(4):378–381.
16. Matthewson K, Barton T, Lewin MR, et al. Low power interstitial Nd-YAG laser photocoagulation in normal and neoplastic rat colon. *Gut* 1988;29:27–34.

17. Matthewson K, Coleridge-Smith P, O'Sullivan JP, et al. Biological effects of intrahepatic Nd-YAG laser photocoagulation in rats. *Gastroenterology* 1987;93:550–557.
18. Hashimoto D, Takami M, Idezuki Y. In depth radiation therapy by YAG laser for malignant tumors in the liver under ultrasonic imaging. *Gastroenterology* 1985;88:1663(abstract).
19. Godlewski G, Rouy S, Pignodel C, et al. Deep localized Nd-YAG laser photocoagulation in liver using a new water cooled and echo guided handpiece. *Laser Surg Med* 1988;8:501–509.
20. Godlewski G, Sambuc P, Eledjam JJ, et al. A new device for inducing deep localized vaporization in liver with the Nd:YAG laser. *Lasers Med. Sci* 1988;3(2):111–117.
21. Daikuzono N, Joffe SN. Artificial sapphire probe for contact photocoagulation and tissue vaporization with the Nd:YAG laser. *Med Instrum* 1985;19:173–178.
22. Steger AC, Brown GS. Use of multiple fiber optic systems in the medical application of lasers. *Proc SPIE—The International Society for Optical Engineering* (*SPIE Proceedings Series* vol 1067), Optical Fibers in Medicine IV (Katzir A, ed.), 1989:256–259.
23. Bicher HI, Bruley DF. *Hyperthermia.* New York: Plenum; 1982.
24. Dethlefsen LA, Dewey WC. *Cancer Therapy by Hyperthermia, Drugs, and Radiation.* National Cancer Institute Monograph 61, 1982.
25. Dietzel F. *Tumor und Temperatur.* Munich: Urban und Schwarzenberg; 1975.
26. Hornback NB. *Hyperthermia and Cancer: Human Clinical Trial Experience,* vols 1 and 2. Boca Raton: CRC; 1984.
27. Storm RK. *Hyperthermia in Cancer Therapy.* Boston: Hall; 1983.
28. Field SB, Morris CC. The relationship between heating time and temperature: its relevance to clinical hyperthermia. *Radiother Oncol* 1983;1(2):179–186.
29. Westermark N. The effects of heat upon rat tumors. *Scand Arch Physiol* 1927;51:257–322.
30. Pincus G, Fischer A. The growth and death of tissue cultures exposed to supranormal temperatures. *J Exp Med* 1931;54:323–332.
31. Moritz AR, Henriques FC. Studies of thermal injury. (II). The relative importance of time and surface temperature in the causation of cutaneous burns. *Am J Pathol* 1947;23:695–720.
32. Henriques FC. Studies of thermal injury. (V). The predictability and the significance of thermally induced rate processes leading to irreversible epidermal injury. *Arch Pathol* 1947;43:489–502.
33. Vaupel P, Gabbert H. Evidence for and against a tumor type-specific vascularity. *Strahlenther Onkol* 1986;162:633–638.
34. Vaupel P, Mueller-Klieser W. Heat susceptibility of tumor blood flow. Proceedings of the 31st Annual Meeting of the Radiation Research Society, San Antonio, 1983:68–69.
35. Field SB, Morris CC. Application of the relationship between heating time and temperature for use as a measure of thermal dose: In: Overgaard J, ed. *Hyperthermic Oncology, 1984.* London: Taylor and Francis; 1984;183–186.
36. Gatenby RA, Hammond ND, Brown DQ. Tumor therapy with hematoporphyrin derivative and lasers via a percutaneous fiberoptic technique: preclinical experiments. *Radiology* 1987;63:163–167.
37. Gatenby RA, Hartz WH, Engstrom PF, et al. CT-guided laser therapy in resistant human tumors: phase I clinical trials. *Radiology* 1987;63:172–175.
38. Godlewski G, Bourgeois JM, Sambuc P, et al. Ultrasonic and histopathological correlations of deep focal hepatic lesions induced by stereotactic Nd:YAG laser applications. *Ultrasound Med Biol* 1988;14:287–291.
39. Dachman AH, McBehee JA, Beam TE, Burris JA. US-guided percutaneous laser ablation of liver in a chronic pig model. *Radiology* 1989;173:425 (abstract).
40. Steger AC, Lees WR, Walmsley K, Bown SG. Interstitial laser hyperthermia: a new approach to local destruction of tumors. *Br Med J* 1989;299:362–365.
41. Masters A, Steger AC, Lees WR, Walmsley KM, Bown SG. Interstitial laser hyperthermia: a new approach for treating liver metastases. *Br J Cancer* 1992;66(3):518–522.
42. Anzai Y, Lufkin RB, Saxton R, Castro DJ, et al. Nd:YAG interstitial laser phototherapy guided by magnetic resonance image in an ex vivo model: dosimetry of laser-MR-tissue interaction. *Laryngoscope* 1991;101(7):755–760.
43. Castro DJ, Saxton RE, Layfield LJ, et al. Interstitial laser phototherapy assisted by magnetic resonance imaging: a new technique for monitoring laser tissue interaction. *Laryngoscope* 1990;100(5):541–547.
44. Robinson JD, Lufkin RB, Castro DJ, Layfield LJ. Magnetic resonance imaging of laser phototherapy: initial experience. *Eur Radiol* 1992;2:24–28.
45. Lufkin RB, Robinson JD, Castro DJ, Jabour BA, Duckwiler G, Layfield LJ, Hanafee HN. Interventional magnetic resonance imaging in the head and neck. *Topics MRI* 1990;2(4):76–80.
46. Castro DJ, Lufkin RB, Saxton RE, Nyerges A, Soudant J, Layfield LJ, Jabour BA, Ward PH, Kangarloo H. Metastatic head and neck malignancy treated using MRI guided interstitial laser phototherapy: an initial case report. *Laryngoscope* 1992;102(1):26–32.
47. Anzai Y, Lufkin RB, Castro DJ. Magnetic resonance-guided interventional procedures in the head and neck imaging. Zinreich JS, guest ed. *Radiology, Lippincott's Reviews* 1992;1(2):227–231.
48. Castro DJ, Saxton RE, Lufkin RB. Interstitial photoablative laser therapy guided by magnetic resonance imaging for the treatment of deep tumors. *Semin Surg Oncol* 1992;8:233–241.
49. Castro DJ, Farahani K, Soudant J, Zwarun A, Lufkin RB. Near "real" time magnetic resonance images as a monitoring system for interstitial laser therapy: experimental protocols. *Proc SPIE (Medical Laser and Systems)* (Harris DM, ed.) 1992;1650:20–32.
50. Ennevor SJ, Castro DJ, Schiller VL, Lufkin EB, Grant E. Real time transcutaneous vascular clipping guided by ultrasound: a minimally invasive technique for vascular control during interstitial tumor therapy. *Proc SPIE (Physiological Monitoring and Early Detection Diagnostic Methods)* (Mang TS, ed.) 1992;1641:113–121.
51. Anzai Y, Lufkin RB, Castro DJ. Superior contrast drives interventional MRI. *MR J* Summer: 1992;34–42.
52. Castro DJ, Lufkin RB. Minimally invasive laser tumor therapy guided by imaging modalities. *Optics Photonics News* 1992;3(10):21–25.

13 Laser-Assisted Temporomandibular Joint Surgery

Steven J. Butler

Advances in arthroscopic instrumentation and technique for small joint surgery have recently found application in surgery for the temporomandibular joint (TMJ). Coupled with the advent of high-resolution magnetic resonance imaging (MRI) the accuracy of diagnosis of TMJ disorders has been greatly enhanced. Arthroscopy of the TMJ has consequently progressed from an instrument of diagnosis to one of treatment. As its usefulness for the treatment of internal derangements, particularly nonreducing disk displacement (closed lock), has become generally accepted, the search for improved instrumentation has resulted in the development of various laser systems for TMJ surgery. As the safety and early success of arthroscopy of the TMJ became established,[1,2] continued technical developments resulted in the refinement of surgical technique. These included predictable and reproducible joint entry and distension, triangulation, and the introduction of arthroscopic hand instruments and mechanized shavers.[3,4] As a consequence of predictable successful outcomes with diminished morbidity in surgery of the upper TMJ space, arthroscopic surgery has become an alternative to open arthrotomy for the treatment of internal joint derangement involving the meniscus (disk). Fortunately, the demand created by the refinement of surgical skills by the profession has resulted in the rapid response by industry to produce arthroscopes and high-resolution video systems that are specifically designed for use in the TMJ. Consequently, new instruments have been developed that permit joint entry through cannulas less that 3 mm in diameter. Instruments for incising, sculpting, and cauterization of joint tissues have been similarly refined. However, they remained inefficient. The objective of incising of attachments of the lateral pterygoid muscle to the anterior band or resecting the meniscus would be achieved with electrocautery but only at the expense of excessive heat damage and carbonization (charring) of the target tissue and synovium. The surgical alternative of using a mechanical shaver was unsatisfactory because of its inefficiency and unpredictable results occurring as a consequence of limited access and maneuverability within the restricted confines of a small joint space.

The development of miniaturized laser delivery systems using optical fibers and "user friendly" control systems for small joint arthroscopic systems in orthopedics resulted in their adaptation for use in the TMJ.[5–8] Their ability to bloodlessly remove tissue in a predictable, reproducible way with minimal unwanted heat damage in a fluid medium compatible with good vision, excellent access, and controllable tissue removal has made this an exciting area for surgical development. Lasers, particularly the holmium:yttrium-aluminum-garnet (Ho:YAG) laser emitting at 2192 nm, are in use currently to remove degenerated fibrocartilage, synovium, or bone. They also are capable of making releasing incisions while cauterizing bleeding blood vessels or photoablating the neovascularization of synovitis.

THE Ho:YAG LASER

The Ho:YAG laser is a solid-state laser emitting at 2192 nm, which closely corresponds with a major spectral absorption peak for water in the infrared region of the electromagnetic spectrum. This laser operates in a pulsed mode at a pulse width of 350 μs, which is well below the thermal relaxation time for most tissues with high water content. Therefore, one would not expect to encounter significant heat effects. In fact, Koslin[7] demonstrated intraarticular temperature elevations of an average of 10°F (range = 1.2–22.6°F) measured with an intraarticular thermocouple during Ho:YAG arthroscopic surgery.

The Ho:YAG laser configured for arthroscopic surgery consists of a free-beam laser with a sterile fiber-optic delivery system and the appropriately adapted arthroscope and video system. Because the Ho:YAG emission is highly absorbed by water with an average depth of absorption of 0.3 mm, it removes tissue precisely. Because the target tissue itself has a high water content and the laser operates within a fluid medium, there is very little unwanted thermal damage lateral to the vaporization crater. Nevertheless, even with minimal unwanted heat effects the actual thermal injury may vary from 0.1 to 1.0 mm depending on tissue type and the exposure parameters of the individual laser. Tarro[8] measured tissue necrosis with Ho:YAG and found it to be 0.4 to 0.6 mm, whereas electrocautery produced necrosis of

0.7 to 1.8 mm. In addition to the thermal effects the short pulse width of 350 μs associated with high fluence rates may also induce photomechanical and photoacoustic effects that also contribute to tissue ablation.

Commercially available low output Ho:YAG lasers are quite adaptable for TMJ arthroscopic surgery. Several fiber delivery methods are available. The specific styles and specifications vary among manufacturers. Some surgeons prefer a side firing tip to access the lateral aspects of the joint while others prefer to bend the fiber slightly or use alternate port placements to reach this area. It is rare to require an output power in excess of 10 W or a post-repetition rate (PRR) exceeding 10 Hz to resect fibrocartilage or recontour bone. Lower settings are suggested for making releasing incisions. Table 13–1 summarizes suitable energy levels for different procedures.

Table 13–1. Suitable energy levels for the Ho:YAG pulsed TMJ unit

45 WATT MODEL	60 WATT MODEL (0.5–7.0 J; 5–55 Hz; 350 μs)
2.1 μm	2.1 μm
0.5–2.8 J	0.5–2.8 J
250 μs	250 μs
45 W	60 W
2.5 mW at 650 ns up to 11 kW	2.5 mW at 650 ns

Average power—actual use in TMJ arthroscopic surgery:
Aiming Beam—0.6–1.0 J/pulse at 8–12 Hz; Avg P = 6–12 W.
Peak Power—[up to 5 J/pulse: Surgilase Ho:YAG].

CASE 1

A 26-year-old woman with a 5-year history of popping in the right TMJ developed a spontaneously reducing intermittent closed lock immediately after childbirth. Three months later she developed limitation on opening of 32 mm, and a diagnosis of nonreducing TMJ disk displacement (closed lock) was made. Her remote past history included bruxism and use of a soft interocclusal night guard. She complained of severe pain in her right joint when attempting to force her mouth open and described a dull tight feeling in the joint "all the time." The patient drew a diagram that outlined her pain only in the preauricular area on the right side. There was no pain on the left side. Her examinations showed a maximum interincisal opening of 32 mm with significant deviation to the right when her opening reached 28 mm. There were no joint sounds or crepitus. She had an angle class I molar occlusion but the incisors were retroclined and crowded. The masticatory muscles on the right were slightly more tender than those on the left but essentially all of her pain was focused in and around the right TMJ itself. Joint imaging showed an anterior dislocation of the right meniscus. The left joint was normal. After discussing nonsurgical and surgical treatment alternatives she chose the surgical option.

An arthroscopic release and repositioning procedure was carried out under a general anesthetic using conventional arthroscopic techniques as described by McCain.[2] The meniscus was found to be anteriorly and medially dislocated (Fig. 13–1), and reduction with a blunt probe produced an audible "snap." The Ho:YAG laser was used for anterior release and posterior band cauterization. The laser was set at 8 W output power, pulsed mode at 5 Hz. This resulted in a bloodless releasing incision (Fig. 13–2). The laser was defocused at the same settings and was used to cauterize and shrink the posterior tissues. A resorbable suture, O-PDS Ethicon, was passed percutaneously through the posterior band of the disk. The entire procedure lasted 32 minutes and the total laser usage was less than 5 minutes. Postoperatively, recovery was uneventful and physical therapy was given in six sessions. A predicted right posterior open bite was present after surgery and this occlusal change was maintained during the postoperative phase using a prefabricated hard acrylic occlusal splint. Within 3 weeks of her surgery she had regained a maximum opening of 42 mm with no detectable opening click and 8 mm of lateral excursive movements. She reported little or no discomfort with mastication or opening but did notice occasional abnormal noises in the joint, which were not problematic for her. The patient ultimately chose comprehensive orthodontic treatment to correct her occlusion. She remains pain free and functional since then.

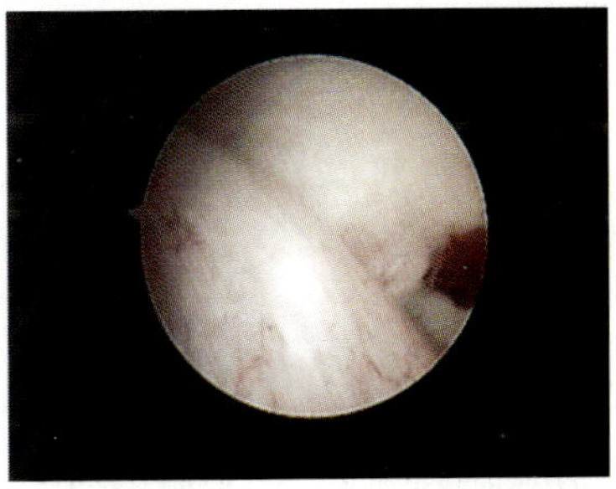

Figure 13–1. Anterior and medial dislocation of TMJ mensicus. Retrodiscal tissues are shown stretched over posterior portion of condylar head.

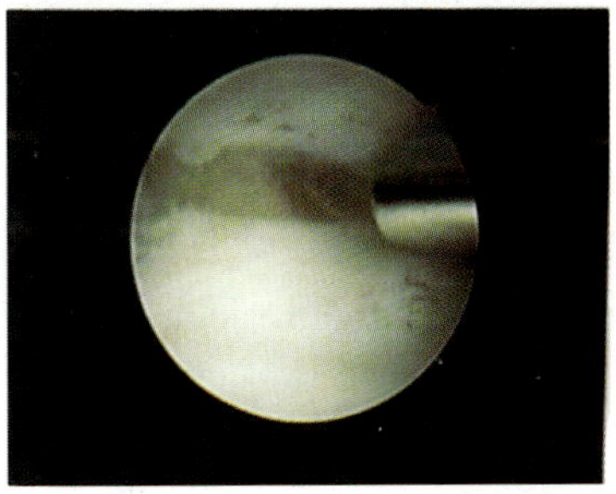

Figure 13–2. Bloodless releasing incision created through synovium and superior aspect of lateral pterygoid muscle using the Holmium:YAG laser.

CASE 2

A 46-year-old woman presented with pain in and around her right temporomandibular joint. She had complained of noise in the joint and intermittent episodes of locking that had been treated over several years with various types of splints with some improvement in her symptoms. She denied a history of recent trauma but noticed increasing crepitus and pain over the past 6 months. She described her current pain as a periodic "jolt" in her right ear and temple area that would be followed by a headache and tightness in her jaw. Two weeks prior to her presentation she noted the onset of inability to open her mouth fully and stated that her level of pain had greatly increased. Physical examination showed a maximal interincisal opening of 18 mm with essentially no translation to the left. She had mandibular retrognathia with a deep bite. Palpation of the right preauricular area demonstrated crepitus and tenderness while the left side was normal. There were no areas of defined muscle tenderness. Tomograms of the temporomandibular joints showed a small flattened mandibular condyle on the right. MRI confirmed a grade IV dislocation of the right meniscus with possible fragmentation. The left side was normal.

Arthroscopic surgery was chosen as the treatment of choice with a diagnostic suspicion of a perforated meniscus. The right TMJ was entered without difficulty using standard triangulation techniques.[2,4] A large disruption in the meniscus was seen (Fig. 13–3). The anterior recess contained adhesions and areas of ecchymosis and a prominent bony protuberance on the anteromedial portion of the condylar head. Consequently, the decision was made to remove the meniscus using the Ho:YAG laser. The laser fiber was placed in the anterior portal and serial sections of meniscus were removed and the joint mechanics evaluated (Fig. 13–4). Some difficulty was encountered in accessing the most lateral aspect of the anterior joint space, and a monopolar coagulation probe was used to isolate several large pieces of disk. Varied energy levels and pulse settings were used ranging from 5 to 8 pulses per second at an average power of 8 to 10 W. Bleeding was minimal, even with resection of the anteromedial portion of the meniscus. After completing the menisectomy (Fig. 13–5), the joint was injected with a 0.5% bupivacaine with dilute epinephrine solution after removal of the cannulas, and the patient recovered uneventfully. Aggressive physical therapy was initiated on the second postoperative day and no postoperative complications were observed. Her postoperative interincisal opening was 28 mm after 5 days and 34 mm after 7 weeks. She continued to have a mildly decreased left lateral excursive movement of the mandible but related that although she still had some mild discomfort in the joint her pain was 90% improved and she had no restrictions in her diet. Her occlusion demonstrated prematurities on the right side and orthodontic follow-up was recommended.

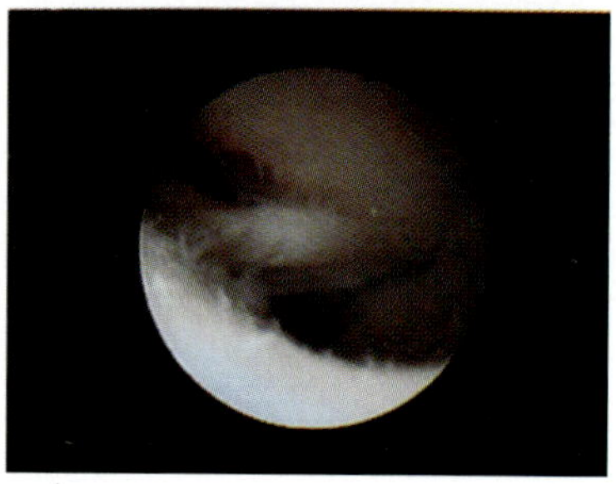

Figure 13–3. Large perforation of meniscus with visible deformed condylar head.

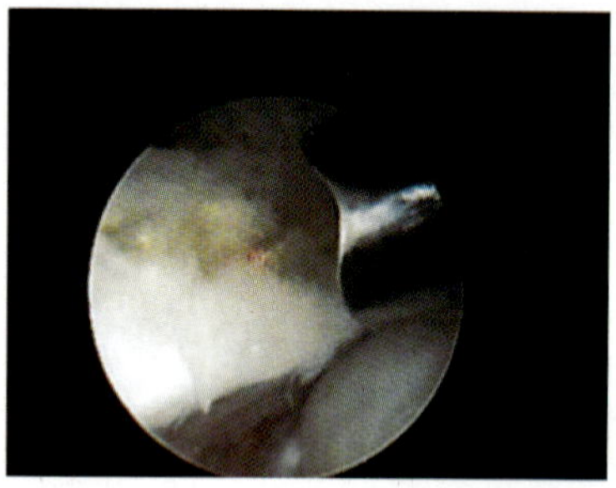

Figure 13–4. Resection of residual perforated meniscus using the Holmium:YAG laser.

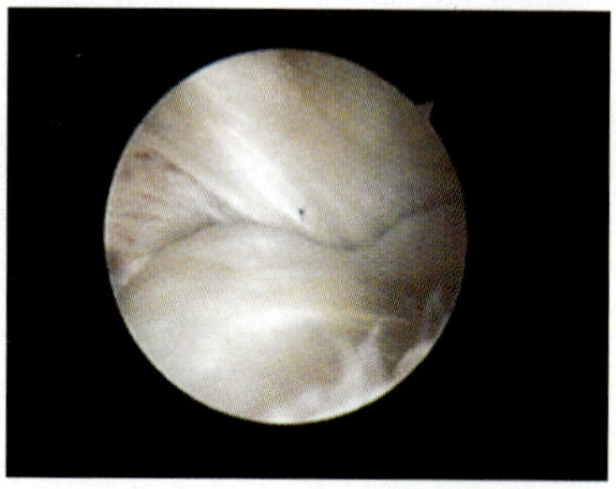

Figure 13–5. Completed laser-assisted menisectomy: View of intact cartilidge over deformed condylar head.

CONCLUSION

Arthroscopic surgery of the temporomandibular joint has become a valuable treatment modality that is rapidly replacing open joint procedures for internal derangement. While anterior releasing incision and posterior scarification can easily be accomplished by the trained arthroscopist using electrocautery, removal of the meniscus with conventional shavers, and rotary instruments is tedious and inaccurate. In contradistinction, use of the laser for arthroscopic surgery permits precise intraarticular tissue removal with excellent hemostasis without the resultant heat damage to tissue that electrocautery produces. In addition, because the fiber is smaller and more maneuverable than conventional rotary instruments, it minimizes scuffing of condylar surfaces. Because the depth of tissue penetration is usually only 0.4 to 0.6 mm, ablation is readily confined to the abnormal meniscus, thereby maximally preserving the normal areas of meniscus. Consequent to its excellent hemostatic properties, postoperative hemarthroses have been eliminated as a complication of intraarticular surgery. Lasers are safe and effective when standard precautions are taken. The Ho:YAG laser is amazingly versatile, permitting the performance of a wide range of procedures on various tissue types. Continued study of the intraarticular applications of lasers will result in the development of more sophisticated laser systems permitting the arthroscopist of the future even more choices when treating the diseased temporomandibular joint.

REFERENCES

1. McCain JP, De la Rua H. Principles: practices of operative arthroscopy of the human temporomandibular joint. *Oral Maxillofac Surg Clin North Am* 1989;1:135–151.
2. McCain JP. Puncture technique and portals of entry for diagnostic and operative arthroscopy of the temporomandibular joint. *Arthroscopy* 1991;2:221–232.
3. McCain JP. *An Illustrated Guide to TMJ Arthroscopy.* Andover, MD: Dyonics; 1987.
4. Sanders B. *TMJ Internal Derangement and Arthrosis: Surgical Atlas.* St. Louis: Mosby; 1985.
5. Hendler BH, Gateno J, Mooar P, et al. Holmium:YAG laser arthroscopy of the temporomandibular joint. *J Oral Maxillofac Surg* 1992;50:931–934.
6. Koslin MG, Martin JC. The use of the holmium laser for temporomandibular joint arthroscopic surgery. *J Oral Maxillofac Surg* 1993;51:122–123.
7. Koslin MG. *Arthroscopic Laser Debridement of Perforated Articular Disc Using the Versa Pulse Surgical Laser.* Palo Alto CA: Coherent, 1992.
8. Tarro AW. *Arthroscopy: A Diagnostic and Surgical Atlas.* Philadelphia: J.B. Lippincott; 1993.

14 Endoscopic Sinus Surgery: A Significant Adjunct to Maxillofacial Surgery

Jeffrey J. Moses, Claus R. Lange

With the use of Le Fort osteotomies for the correction of skeletofacial deformities there has developed within the discipline of oral and maxillofacial surgery (OMS) a renewed interest in the management of sinonasal pathology. As enhanced awareness of the importance of the patency of the osteomeatal unit (OMU) grew, it has become evident that some cases of postoperative sinusitis occurred consequent to midfacial orthognathic surgery. High-level septal deviations could lead to distortion of the middle turbinate on the convex side of the septum, which lateralizes the uncinate process and hiatus semilunaris of the infundibular outflow pathway, which subsequently also becomes tortuous. These anatomic alterations predispose to the development of postoperative sinusitis.

Occasional cases were noted with direct interruption of infundibular patency attributable to inadvertent mucous membrane synechial web and wall formation, or the creation of narrowed or blocked ostia in conjunction with altered airway flow patterns occurring after high-level Le Fort I osteotomy. If symptoms arise, direct diagnostic assessment of the maxillary sinus and endonasal structures is now possible with endoscopic techniques. This permits assessment of the mucosal and bony response to autogenous, allogeneic, and alloplastic materials placed adjacent to the sinus during surgery. Most importantly, these techniques also permit complete evaluation of the endonasal anatomy, especially as it relates to its permissive role in sinus aeration.

RATIONALE FOR ENDOSCOPIC SINONASAL SURGERY

The concept of reversibility of sinus disease based upon the restoration of normal drainage patterns and aeration led to the development of several surgical techniques. Two of these in common use are the Messerklinger and Wiegand techniques. Messerklinger (A, B) technique evaluates and alters structure from an anterior to posterior approach, concentrating on the maxillary, ethmoidal, and frontal sinuses. In contrast, Wiegand (C) developed his pansinus evaluation and treatment from posterior to anterior structures associated with more aggressive eradication of the same sinuses, including extension to the sphenoid sinus. For the majority of orthognathic surgery patients who have developed sinusitis postoperatively, the Messerklinger approach provides adequate treatment. With increasing familiarity and sophistication, the application of endoscopic evaluation of the middle meatus has given OMS a new diagnostic aid to predict patients at risk for the postoperative development of sinusitis. Those with preexisting sinus disease also may be considered for treatment prior to orthognathic surgery.

The essence of endoscopic surgery is to restore aeration and mucociliary flow patterns (Fig. 14–1). Ciliary function is both temperature and humidity sensitive. Below 18°C and 50% humidity, impairment occurs. If contact occurs between mucosal surfaces, as can happen when the infundibular mucosa swells, normal ciliary beats of 10 to 15 strikes per minute cease altogether. Since these beats are required to move the thicker mucinous blanket along the less viscous

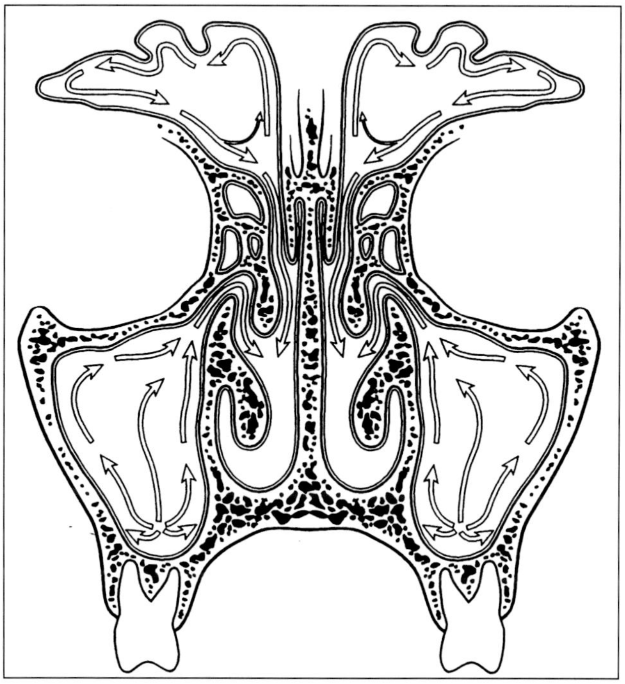

Figure 14–1. Coronal view of paranasal sinuses. Arrows indicate direction of normal ciliary directed mucous flow toward natural ostea.

A
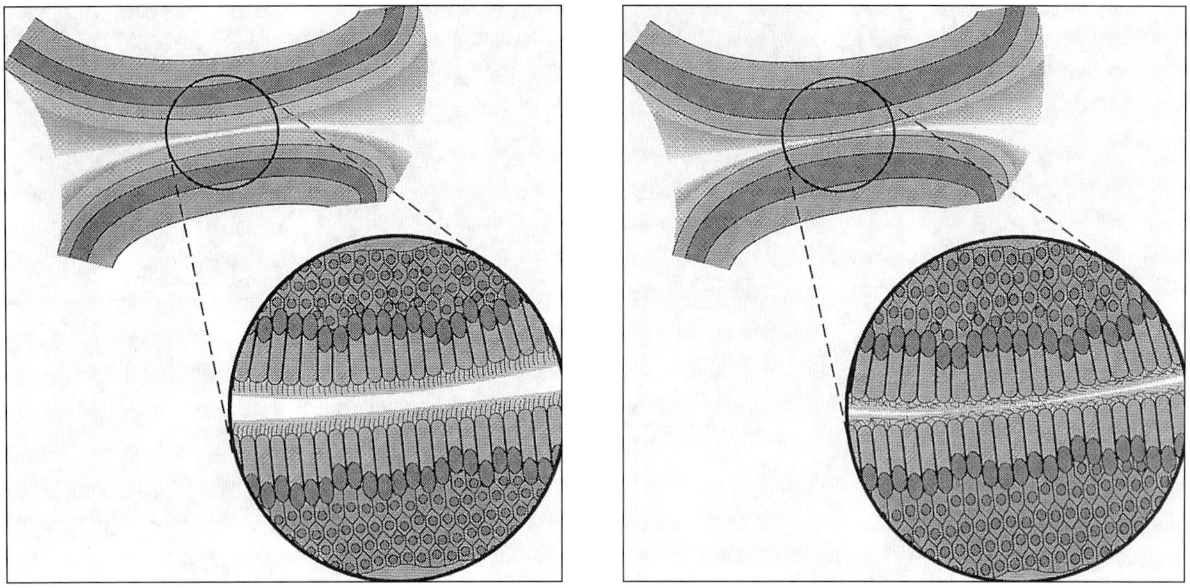
B

Figure 14–2. **(A)** Diagram of stylistic ostea lumen of greater than 2.5 mm diameter indicating healthy cilia and aeration. **(B)** Diagram of cross section of ostea lumen with less than 2.5 mm diameter indicating paralysis of ciliary motion and inadequate aeration potential due to mucous stagnation.

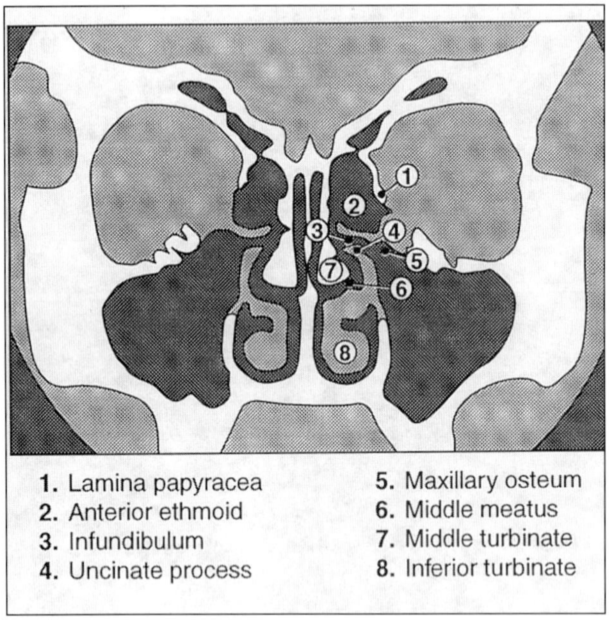

Figure 14–3. Cross-sectional coronal diagram of normal structure in the nose and osteo-meatal complex.

layer immediately adjacent to the cilia, stasis occurs, providing a culture medium for bacterial infections. Thus, the common rhinitis occurring after a viral upper respiratory tract infection induces mucosal edema and ciliary paralysis, leading to mucosal secondary bacterial infection within 24 to 48 hours. Infundibular mucosal swelling induced by alterations in airflow patterns, as may occasionally occur after Le Fort osteotomies in the lateral nasal wall, similarly impairs mucociliary function.

Structurally, the infundibulum receives drainage from the ethmoidal, frontal, and maxillary sinuses within the hiatus semilunaris which, along with the middle turbinate, occupies the middle meatus. Ostia diameters less than 2.5 mm are predisposed to infections primarily because of the phenomenon of cilia impairment secondary to mucosal approximation (Fig. 14–2A,B). Additionally, deviations of the superior and middle aspects of the septum, swollen or paradoxical turbinate positioning and anatomic variations of the uncinate process all can lead to obstruction of the OMU, resulting in chronic sinus disease.

The focus of endoscopic sinonasal surgery is on the mucociliary and lower concha system, and location and patency of the ostia and OMU (Fig. 14–3).

PREOPERATIVE EXAMINATION

Preoperative examination should include speculum and headlight-assisted inspection of the nasal cavity both before and after the application of the decongestant spray. Additional tests such as those of Mueller and Cottle (Smith and Nephew Richard, Inc., 7450 Brooks Rd., Memphis, TN 38776 USA) to assess the nasal valve, and lateral wall airway resistance should also be done before and after the decongestant treatment.

Any deviations of the septum, laterally or in a vertical to inferior S-shaped fashion, should be noted. Of particular importance is a visual check of the middle meatus for the presence of high septal deviations or spurs and contralateral compensatory turbinate hyperplasia. The convex side of the spur or deviation can cause a paradoxical form of the middle turbinate. This may lead to a delicate balance between OMU patency and obstruction. Le Fort I osteotomy may alter airflow patterns, which induce compensatory mucosal responses that block OMU patency.

In addition, septal deviations can lead to lateralization and toruosity of the infundibulum, with subsequent risk of mucosal approximation and narrowing of the maxillary ostia. Minor alterations in airflow cause approximation of the mucosa lining the ostia, thereby narrowing its lumen to less than 2.5 mm, which leads to a cessation of ciliary motion that blocks OMU function.

For patients with midfacial skeletal asymmetries or preexisting obstructive nasal respiration (ONR) as exemplified by those patients with apertognathia or "long face syndrome" who are mouth breathers, preoperative computed tomography (CT) of the sinuses documents disease or predisposition for postorthognathic surgery development of OMU dysfunction. Surgical management of sinonasal disease is tailored to eliminate abnormalities such as polyps, hypertrophic turbinates, and symptomatic OMU blockage. Should these symptoms first appear postoperatively, then CT scanning becomes necessary as a first diagnostic step in establishing a diagnosis and treatment plan.

INSTRUMENTATION

These procedures are usually accomplished under general anesthesia with oral endotracheal intubation. A Richard's 30° angled endoscope of 3.5- or 4.0-mm diameter is used, which is then attached to a Stryker solid-state video optical-enhancement and monitoring camera system. A simple setup of instrumentation is preferred by the author; this simplifies maintenance of equipment and minimizes the need for assistance. Most of the surgery can be performed with straight and 45° angled Weil-Blakesley forceps, along with a sharp Cottle elevator. If required, soft tissue resections are performed with a medium "thru-cutter" and medium reverse biting instruments. A curved ostium-seeking probe and suction-assisted sound are used to palpate the maxillary ostium. Additional instrumentation for endoantral triangulation procedures occasionally requires use of the Storz cannula trocar system, #10 French catheter tubing, and irrigation. Larger mucinous structures, such as engorged turbinates or intranasal polyps, can readily be removed with the Stryker "Hummer."

Occasionally, mucosal hemorrhage is encountered despite the injection of local anesthetic, 0.5% bupivacaine with epinephrine 1:100,000, and timed nasal cottonoid packing soaked with 4% cocaine. It is therefore helpful to have laser-assisted carbon dioxide (CO_2) or Holmium:yttrium-aluminum-garnet (Ho:YAG) photocoagulation available. If not available, insulated electrocautery should be accessible.

The Ho:YAG laser (New Star Lasers, 77802 Kemper Rd., Auburn, CA 95603 USA) with a quartz fiber handpiece can be utilized for endonasal soft tissue ablation, photocoagulation, and turbinoplasty when indicated. Settings of 10 W of power and high-speed plume evacuation are utilized. The CO_2 laser (Luxar Corporation, 79206 North Center Parkway, Bothell, WA 90877-8205; LXS-BD 120-090 Beam Deflector Sheath for LX220 Laser System) can also be used for these procedures, and convenient tips are available for directed beam localization.

On selected cases, septoplasty is performed first if there is deviation or high posterior septal spurs. This condition prevents access to the middle meatus or pushes the middle turbinate against the lateral nasal wall, inhibiting access to the hiatus semilunaris, uncinate process, and infundibulum. Otherwise, the septoplasty is performed following the functional endoscopic sinus surgery in order to reduce the incidence of hemorrhage, which obstructs vision.

TECHNIQUE OF FUNCTIONAL ENDOSCOPIC SINUS SURGERY (FESS)

Introducing the endoscope along the nasal floor just beyond the sill permits better access and control for instrumentation and aids in visibility. First, the uncinate process is identified and a vertical incision made with the sharp edge of the Cottle elevator. The uncinate process is grasped at the superior margin of this incision with the Weil-Blakesley forceps and pulled inferiorly to the level of the middle turbinate. These same forceps are then used to open the bulla ethmoidalis, with care being taken to orient the beaks of the forceps vertically to prevent inadvertent extension laterally through the lamina papyracea and thereby entering the orbit.

Decompression of the infundibulum by this maneuver frequently requires enlargement of the maxillary ostium, especially in patients who have had high-level Le Fort osteotomies with resultant abnormal bony architecture or synechial webbing. Use of a curved probe is essential to identify the maxillary ostium. After its identification, the ostium is enlarged with the reverse biting forceps working anteriorly until sufficient diameter (3.0 mm plus) is achieved. We have found that a curved laser-delivering probe or a beam-deflecting probe (CO_2 Luxar or modified Ho:YAG Coherent) is useful in reestablishing adequate patency of this ostium.

The indications for the judicious removal of portions of the middle turbinate are concha bullosa, turbinate hypertrophy, or paradoxical turbinate morphology, or even normal turbinates that have been pushed into obstructive positioning within the OMU by posterior septal deviations. In these cases, both the "thru-cut" Richards forceps and the laser-assisted endoscopic nasal turbinoplasty are indicated.

Following these procedures, a FESS silicone stent, bacitracin-coated Telfa strip, and nasal drip pads are applied to prevent the formation of lateral synechiae and to aid mucosal wound healing. If septoplasty was performed, its mucosa is reapproximated with 4-0 chromic mattress sutures to prevent septal hematoma.

Other areas of antral access are sometimes utilized, such as the Hosaka window (Fig. 14–4). During the course of down-fracturing of the maxilla in the Le Fort I operation, patients with chronic sinusitis and obstructive nasal respiration undergoing rigid fixation receive nasoantral notching procedures of the lateral nasal walls. These are placed at the junction of the anterior maxillary walls and the lateral nasal walls at the anterior aspect of the maxillary antrum. This is accomplished using an end-cutting bone rongeur, thereby allowing the drainage of the maxillary antrum during healing. Additionally, the author utilizes this window to place a small endoscope postoperatively through a Storz cannula placed transnasally to view the sinus mucosa (Fig. 14–5). The status of bone healing, fixation hardware, hydroxyapatite, and bone grafts can also be evaluated with this access.

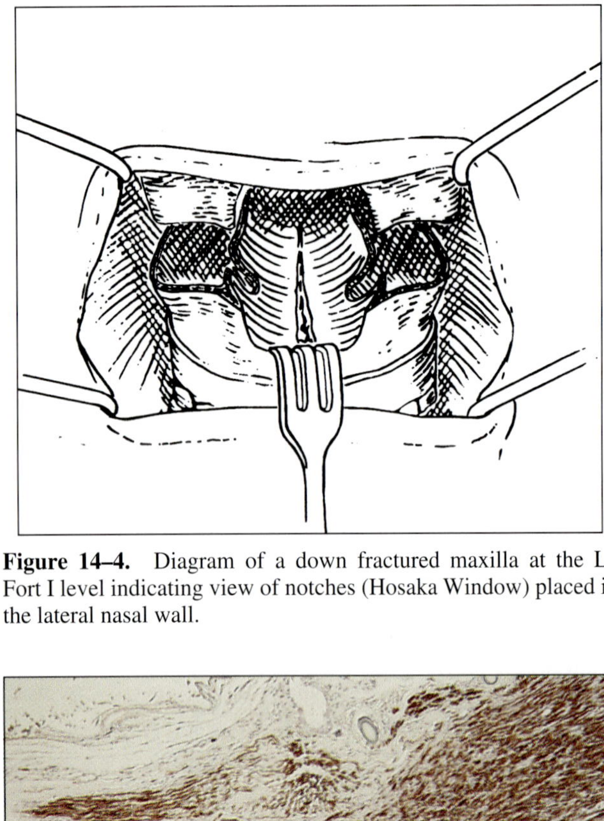

Figure 14–4. Diagram of a down fractured maxilla at the Le Fort I level indicating view of notches (Hosaka Window) placed in the lateral nasal wall.

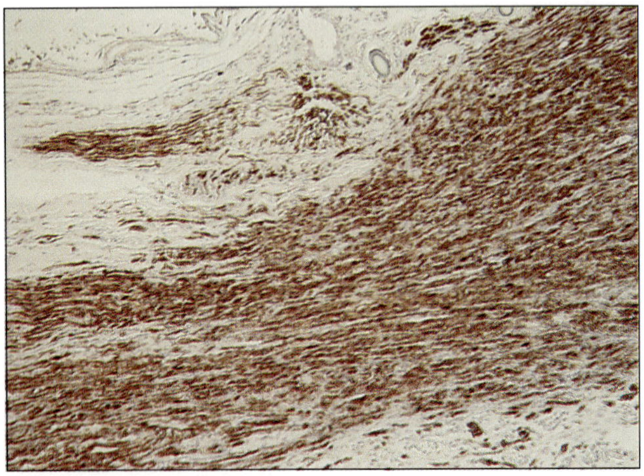

Figure 14–5. Placement of endoantral cannula and endoscope through a "Hosaka Window" approach.

In certain cases mucosal webs and/or shelf-life plicae, which may inhibit physiologic mucous flow, may also be present and require lysis.

The maxillary–antral trochar–cannula puncture can be utilized at the area of the canine fossa for surgical access, transantral polyp, tooth or foreign body removals, and endoscopically assisted laser debridement of reactive mucosa. Punctures are usually left open to heal by secondary intention once the instrumentation is removed.

COMPLICATIONS AND POSTOPERATIVE CONSIDERATIONS

Occasionally, nasal irrigation and even steroid nasal sprays are required in the postoperative period following pack and stent removal. Follow-up antibiotics are given routinely with all patients. Endonasal examinations are done with a headlight and speculum to detect early synechial formation since these can frequently be interrupted with antibiotic-coated cotton applicators or with minimally invasive manipulations. More mature adhesions may require surgical or laser-assisted lysis.

CASE ILLUSTRATIONS

Case 1

This is a 42-year-old man status post–segmental Le Fort I osteotomy combined with mandibular osteotomy, septoplasty, and partial turbinectomies. These procedures were accomplished for treatment of facial skeletal asymmetry, vertical maxillary hyperplasia and retrognathism, as well as obstructive nasal respirations due to septal deviation and hypertrophic turbinates. Significant findings at the time of the Le Fort I revealed a cyst of the left maxillary antrum, and severe septal spurs and deviations. Pathology reports were consistent with cholesterol granuloma initially read from tissue pathology specimens.

Within 2 to 3 weeks after surgery, the patient reported a large tissue obstruction of the right nasal passageway. Intranasal examination revealed a polypoid mass present and nasal topical steroids were employed to assist management. These were unsuccessful in reducing the size of the tissue and a CT scan was ordered. A large (2–3 cm) oblong soft tissue mass was discovered in the right lateral aspect of the nasal cavity (Fig. 14–6). Functional endoscopically assisted nasal surgery was performed with surgical removal of the polyposis, followed by Ho:YAG laser ablation of soft tissue tags remaining. Pathologic confirmation of polyps and the mucous-retention cyst phenomenon with mucous gland hyperplasia were obtained. Postoperative intranasal steroids were applied, and there have been no recurrences in the past 16 months.

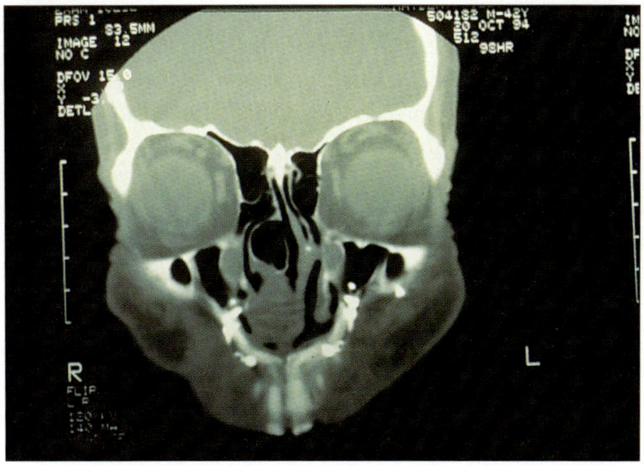

Figure 14–6. Coronal CT scan of patient (Case 1) having a large Concha Bullosa and nasal polyp in right nasal parragenay.

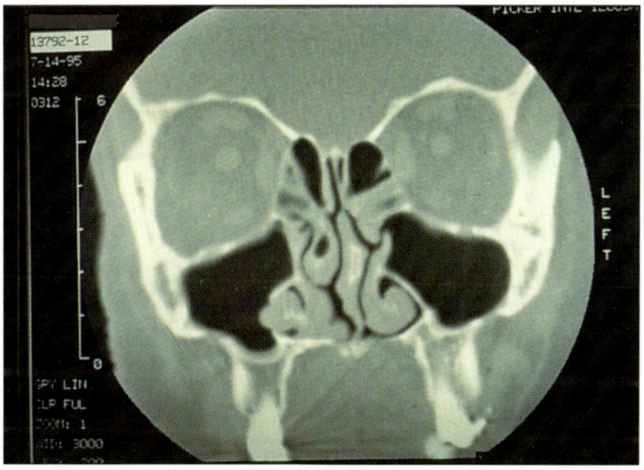

Figure 14–7. Coronal CT scan of patient (Case 2) showing Concha Bullosa, obstructed OMU, and evagination of inferior turbinates into the maxillary antrum.

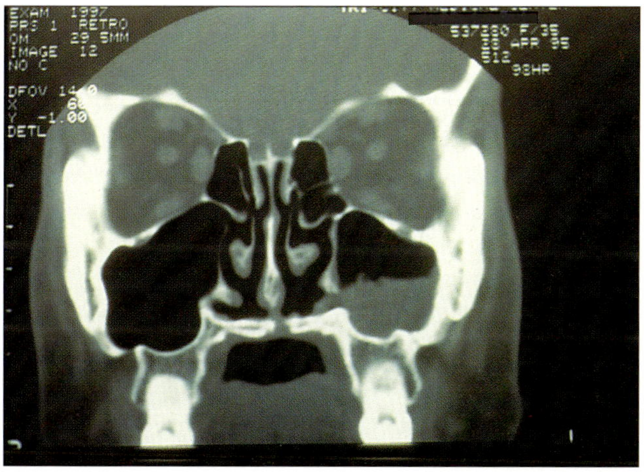

Figure 14–8. Coronal CT scan of patient (Case 3) with OMU blockage and synechial web obstruction of the maxillary ostea.

Case 2

This is a 54-year-old white woman who presented status post–multiple facial osteotomies for correction of posterior vertical maxillary hyperplasia with apertognathism and retrognathism. Segmental Le Fort I osteotomies, along with mandibular osteotomies, were accomplished without septoplasty or turbinectomies. The maxillary nasal sinuses had polyps present, which were sent for pathologic confirmation of inflammatory polyps with increased number of eosinophils of the nasal mucosa.

Several years later, the patient returned with a complaint of headaches and chronic sinusitis resistant to medical management. CT scan revealed that the left maxillary sinus had extensive inflammatory changes that extended throughout the ethmoidal air cells. Additionally, the patient had nocturnal snoring and clinical evidence of hypertrophy of the uvula and redundancy of the soft palate. Blockage of the OMU was noted on the left side (Fig. 14–7). A surgical plan for treatment involved FESS with opening of the maxillary ostium and OMU with anterior ethmoidectomy, Ho:YAG laser-assisted middle turbinoplasty, and CO_2 laser-assisted uvulopalatoplasty, which was accomplished.

Case 3

This is a 35-year-old white woman who was treated in 1987 with temporomandibular joint (TMJ) arthroscopic surgery for temporomandibular dysfunction (TMD) with internal joint derangement (IJD), and in 1989 with Le Fort I osteotomy with superior repositioning, sagittal split ramus osteotomy, turbinectomies, and septoplasty. Her treatment was related to management of her posterior vertical maxillary hyperplasia with resultant apertognathia, mandibular asymmetric prognathism and concurrent hypertrophic turbinates, and obstructive nasal respirations.

The patient returned in 1995 with a complaint of sinusitis and chronic nasal rhinorrhea. A combination of endoscopically assisted endonasal examinations and CT scan analysis revealed synechial web blockage of the maxillary ostium, resulting in physiologic flow restriction of maxillary sinus mucous (Fig. 14–8). This was present despite the patency of a large nasal antral window placed at the time of the original Le Fort I osteotomy (Hosaka window).

FESS treatment consisted of partial laser-assisted turbinoplasty, synechial lysis, and enlargement of the maxillary ostium on the left side.

DISCUSSION

Examination of the maxillary antral walls through the Hosaka window placed at the time of the Le Fort osteotomy in most cases revealed absence of diseased mucosa next to the rigid fixation hardware protruding into the sinus.

This was independent of the type of metal used for the hardware (Fig. 14–9).

Utilization of the 70° endoscope and careful rotation for better visualization revealed synechial webs and shelves in some patients at the Le Fort I osteotomy site in the maxillary antrum. This probably led to a "fall back" inhibition of normal physiologic mucous flow toward the natural ostium (Fig. 14–10). In our experience, several patients have required lysis of synechial webs at the level of the maxillary ostium in order to restore aeration of the maxillary sinus.

Other etiologic factors to consider include predisposing anatomic variants, such as concha bullosa and enlargements of the middle turbinate, creating the contact phenomenon that inhibits ciliary movement at the hiatus semilunaris and infundibulum. The presence of high septal spurs and asymmetric deviations lead to a predisposition of the narrowed airway passages and drainage spaces to become obstructed after orthognathic surgery. Whereas normal airway anatomy and mucosal health might have been able to tolerate these changes, the impaired mucosa and airway patencies of patients with obstructive nasal respiration, such as those with the classic apertognathia—long face syndrome—with concurrent mouth breathing patterns, may not be able to adapt rapidly enough after Le Fort osteotomy to avoid these airway problems.

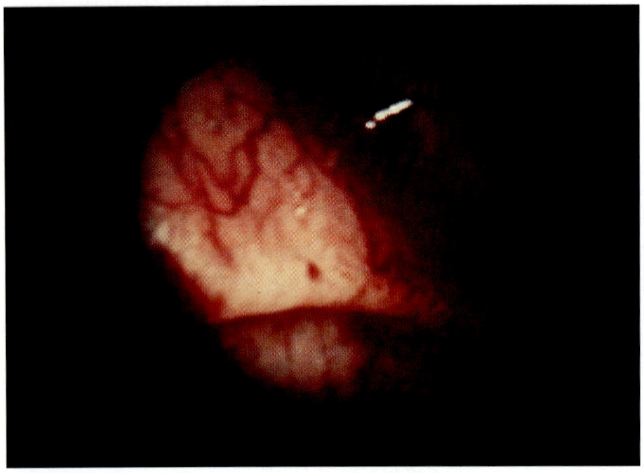

Figure 14–9. Endoscopic view of maxillary antral wall showing step and hardware entrance into the maxillary sinus.

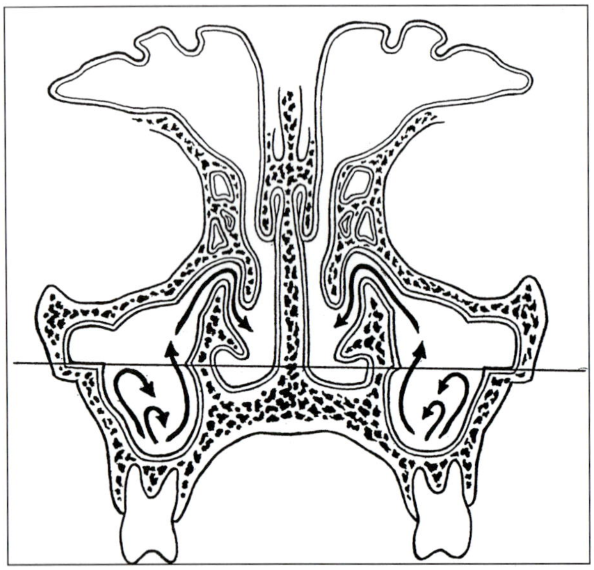

Figure 14–10. Cross-sectional coronal view diagram of steps formed within the maxillary antrum and resultant potential for redirected/inhibited ciliary mucous flow following Le Fort I osteotomy.

SUMMARY

Certain patterns of facial skeletal asymmetries with high-level septal deviations and others with obstructive nasal respiration/mouth breathing, and skeletal growth disturbances such as long face syndrome or apertognathia may be predisposed to the development of clinically significant sinonasal disease postoperatively. These may in part be due to the OMU blockage or with synechial shelves and webs blocking normal maxillary antral mucosal flow.

The use of nasoantral windows placed in the anterolateral nasal wall at the time of Le Fort I down-fracture (Hosaka window) does not appear to enhance drainage of the maxillary antrum because the physiologic flow pattern of the mucous bypasses this region.

With the advent of office-based endoscopic instrumentation, the oral and maxillofacial surgeon is better equipped to immediately evaluate and treat postoperative untoward sequelae such as synechial webs, polyps, and OMU blockage, as well as to view the healing of the lateral nasal wall within the maxillary sinus. Regions exposed to sinus lift implants and interpositional hydroxyapatite or bone grafts can be visualized and evaluated. Evaluation of patients by both endoscopically assisted intranasal examination and axial and coronal CT scan analysis is recommended. FESS with the minimally invasive Messerklinger approach, combined with intranasal use of laser-assisted turbinoplasty and soft tissue lysis, has been successful in the management of the majority of these cases.

REFERENCES

1. Heetderks DL. Observations on the reactions of normal nasal mucous membrane. *Am J Med Sci.* 1927; 174:231.
2. Hilding AC. The role of respiratory mucosa in health and disease. *Man Med.* 1967; 50:915–919.
3. Holliday RA, Shiptner BA. Avoiding complications of endoscopic sinus surgery: analysis of coronal, axial, and sagittal computed tomographic images. *Operative Tech Otolaryngol Head Neck Surg.* 1995; (3):149–157.

4. Lang J. *Clinical Anatomy of the Nose, Nasal Cavity, and Paranasal Sinuses.* New York: Thieme; 1989.
5. Levine HL, May M. *Endoscopic Sinus Surgery.* New York: Thieme; 1993.
6. Lucas AM, Douglas LC. Principles underlying ciliary activity in the respiratory tract. II. A comparison of nasal clearance in man, monkey and other mammals. *Arch Otolaryngol.* 1934; 20:518–541.
7. Messerklinger W. Uber die Drainage der menschlichen Nasennebenhohlen unter normalen und pathologischen Bedingungen, II. Mitteilung: Die Stirnhohle und ihr Ausfuhrungssystem. *Monatsschr Ohrenheilhd.* 1967; 101:313–326.
8. Messerklinger W. Endoskopische Diagnose und Chirurgie der rezidivierenden Sinusitis. In: Krajina Z, ed. *Advances in Nose and Sinus Surgery.* Zagreb, Yugoslavia: Zagreb University; 1985.
9. Rice DH. Management of the middle turbinate in endoscopic surgery. *Operative Tech Otolaryngol Head Neck Surg.* 1995; 6(3):144–149.
10. Rice DH, Schaefer SD. *Endoscopic Paranasal Sinus Surgery.* New York: Raven Press, 1988.
11. Rosenberger HC. The clinical availability of the ostium maxillae: a clinical and cadaver study. *Ann Otol Rhinol Laryngol.* 1938; 47:177–182.
12. Simon E. Anatomy of the opening of the maxillary sinus. *Arch Otolaryngol.* 1993; 29:640–649.
13. Stammberger H. Endoscopic surgery for a cystic and chronic recurring sinusitis. *Ann Otol Rhinol Laryngol Suppl.* 1985; 119:1–11.
14. Stammberger H. Endoscopic endonasal surgery—concepts in treatment of recurring rhinosinusitis. Part I. Anatomic and pathophysiologic considerations. *Otolaryngol Head Neck Surg.* 1986; 94:143–155.
15. Stammberger H. Endoscopic endonasal surgery—concepts in treatment of recurring rhinosinusitis. Part II. Surgical technique. *Otolaryngol Head Neck Surg.* 1986; 94:147–156.
16. Stammberger MS. *Essentials of Functional Endoscopic Sinus Surgery.* St. Louis: Mosby Year Book; 1993.
17. Stankiewich JA. *Advanced Endoscopic Sinus Surgery.* St. Louis: Mosby Year Book; 1995.
18. Wiegand ME, Steiner W, Jaumann MP. Endonasal sinus surgery with endoscopical control: from radical operation to rehabilitation of the mucosa. *Endoscopy.* 1978; 10:255–260.

15 Laser Biostimulation: Photobioactivation, A Modulation of Biologic Processes by Low-Intensity Laser Radiation

Joseph S. Rosenshein

BACKGROUND

Therapeutic Use of Light in Medicine

HELIOTHERAPY

Light therapy can be traced back to healing practices of the ancient Egyptians and Greeks who praised Ra or Helios as the god of light, sun, and healing. Greek and Roman physicians, Celsus and Galen for example, recommended sunbathing as therapy for a variety of conditions including epilepsy, arthritis, and asthma. Exposure to sunlight was considered to be preventive medicine and its effects on bone growth were recognized by the 6th century B.C. The worship of the sun was practiced throughout the Roman Empire until it was suppressed by early Christianity. As a consequence of the Industrial Revolution, there was a large transfer of rural populations to cities with poorly illuminated housing, poor diets, long hours in dark workplaces, and few opportunities for adequate exposure to sunlight. These conditions resulted in outbreaks of scurvy, rickets, edema, rheumatic arthritis, and depression, for which sunbathing was often prescribed as a cure. A number of scientific investigations into the biologic effects of sunlight eventually resulted in the discovery of its bactericidal effects and its role both in the prevention and treatment of rickets by the end of the 19th century.

ULTRAVIOLET (UV) THERAPY

At the turn of the 20th century, attempts to artificially duplicate the sun's radiation using artificial light resulted in the development of convenient sources of UV radiation that were effective in treating the open wounds found in tuberculosis and rickets. By the 1930s, UV light therapy was claimed to be successful in treating hundreds of conditions including nephritis, rheumatoid arthritis, hemophilia, and herpes zoster. The conditions for which UV therapy was, at that time, the only effective treatment are today successfully treated by medications, dietary supplements, etc. The use of UV therapy has undergone alternating periods of enthusiastic endorsement and denouncement. Despite the current concerns regarding the poor findings from controlled clinical research and the potential for harmful effects from UV exposure, actinotherapy is still recommended, although not universally accepted, for stimulation of wound healing in ulcers, boils, and carbuncles, and for treatment of acne vulgaris and neonatal jaundice when used cautiously and prudently.[1,2]

LASERS IN MEDICINE

The development of light sources for medical purposes took a giant leap forward with the building of the first laser by Theodore Maiman in 1960. Since that time, medical applications of the intense, coherent, monochromatic radiation available from a variety of pulsed and continuous wave (CW) solid-state, dye, and gas lasers have multiplied. Shortly after the introduction of this new source of light, ophthalmologists became the first users of medical lasers by applying the ruby laser to photocoagulation of the retina to weld detached retinas back into place. With the availability of other lasers, applications of the intense electromagnetic radiation at different wavelengths became possible. The following are some examples of medical laser applications:

The CO_2 laser, an infrared (IR) emitter at 10,600-nm wavelength, is used in both CW and pulsed modes as a surgical laser because of its excellent hemostasis and shallow penetration depth in neurosurgery, dermatology, plastic surgery, gynecology, ophthalmology, oncology, oral and maxillofacial surgery, otolaryngology, and general surgery.

The neodymium:yttrium-aluminum-garnet (Nd:YAG) laser produces IR radiation at a 1060-nm wavelength. It is used in ophthalmology to remove opacities that sometimes develop in the posterior capsule after removal of a cataract and insertion of an intraocular lens and for transcleral destruction of portions of the ciliary body in intractable cases of glaucoma.

Solid-state lasers produce wavelengths in the visible and infrared regions of the spectrum. Arrays of these lasers can produce pulses with peak powers of 100 W or CW radiation with an average power of tens of watts. Many of the most common of these solid-state near-IR lasers are constructed from gallium arsenide (GaAs) or gallium aluminum arsenide (GaAlAs), which produces radiation of 820- to 904-nm wavelengths. These lasers promise to deliver even greater power densities with greater reliability and lower cost as they come into common use in the near future.

Helium-neon (HeNe) gas lasers are perhaps the most commonly known visible light producing lasers because of their relatively low cost and availability. These lasers emit light primarily at 632.8-nm wavelength and commonly are used as aiming beams for IR lasers.

Argon ion gas lasers produce visible light wavelengths of blue and blue-green. These lasers are employed in ophthalmology to treat proliferative retinopathy and glaucoma because their light is highly absorbed by vascularized tissue. Similarly, they are useful for the treatment of vascular malformations and port-wine stains. Another recent application of argon lasers is in photodynamic therapy (PDT) of cancer.

Tunable dye lasers and more recently tunable Ti:sapphire lasers provide a wide range of visible and IR wavelengths for use in ophthalmology and dermatology.

Most recently argon fluoride excimer lasers producing extreme UV radiation of 193 nm have been developed for use in photoablative refractive keratectomy for correction of myopia and astigmatism.

Almost all the lasers used in surgical applications employ the photothermal effects of light absorption, which involve protein denaturation, coagulation, and vaporization with the increased temperatures associated with energy absorption. The extreme ultraviolet radiation of high-energy photons from the excimer laser disrupt molecular and atomic bonds, resulting in ablation relatively free of thermal effects.

LOW-INTENSITY LASER THERAPY

The use of low-intensity laser radiation (LILR) for therapy was pioneered by Endre Mester in Budapest in the late 1960s,[3,4] and independently by Dr. Friedrich Plog[5] in Canada. The use of low-intensity laser light for therapy is distinct from the use of lasers in surgery in that the therapeutic effects apparently arise either directly or indirectly from the electromagnetic interaction of the light with tissue and not from thermal effects. Early researchers used very low power lasers of less than 1 milliwatt (mW) but present research is being conducted at powers between 1 and 75 mW. The typical low-intensity laser currently used in biostimulation research or in a clinical setting has a power of at least 15 mW and may be as high as several hundred milliwatts. Treatment times are typically short ($\leq$ 30 sec), resulting in delivery of energies of only a few joules per square centimeter to the treated site.[6]

Although laser therapy or laser biostimulation is frequently used in Europe and Asia as a therapy for a variety of diseases, it has not been generally accepted in the United States due to the difficulty in gaining Food and Drug Administration (FDA) approval for new medical devices as safe and effective. There is no clear evidence that laser biostimulation is superior to existing therapy options. Until such evidence is presented, it seems unlikely that the FDA will grant approval for use of this therapy in the United States.

Clinical Areas of Application

Low-intensity laser biostimulation has been applied to some of the following areas:

1. Physiotherapy
   a. Wound healing
   b. Soft tissue injuries
   c. Pain relief
   d. Arthritis
2. Dentistry
   a. Reduction of edema and hyperemia
   b. Wound healing
   c. Pain relief
   d. Treatment of herpes labialis and herpetic gingivostomatitis
   e. Activation of bone growth
3. Veterinary practice
   a. Pain relief
   b. Wound healing
   c. Treatment of respiratory tract infections
   d. Reversal of neuropraxia
   e. Improvement of foot growth in horses
4. Laser acupuncture

CONTROVERSY

Since Mester's initial work, there has been considerable controversy regarding the effectiveness and even the existence of low-intensity laser biostimulation.[7,8] The early reports of LILR-induced photobiostimulation were published in Russian and Eastern European journals that were inaccessible to most researchers in America. Even when translated, the initial work suffered from incomplete description of experimental parameters, protocols that were not blinded or controlled, and flawed methodologies. In particular, the specifications of LILR research were inconsistently presented, making comparisons and replication of results difficult if not impossible. As the field has matured, the rigor of reporting has improved, leading to more credible and reliable results. Modern research in this field should specifically report:

In vitro vs. In vivo studies—How do the cellular studies compare to applications in animals or humans?

Laser light sources—What are the characteristics of the light source, including intensity, beam profiles, polarization, and stability? Was the light pulsed or continuous? If pulsed, what were the pulse characteristics?

Wavelengths—What are the wavelengths and bandwidths of the light used in the research?
Dosimetry—How was the energy delivered? Over what area? What were the peak and average powers per unit area? How long was the exposure?
Techniques—What were the treatment schedules? Describe the controls and limited blinding by researchers.[8,9]

LASER PARAMETERS

The specific characteristics of LILR research need to be considered when evaluating the effects produced.

A. Inherent Laser Parameters

1. Wavelength
2. Polarization
3. Beam mode and profile
   a. TEM_{00}—gaussian
   b. Multimode
   c. Homogeneous
4. Beam temporal type
   a. CW
   b. Pulsed

B. Adjustable Parameters

1. Power density
2. Energy density
3. Pulse width
4. Pulse repetition rate
5. Duration of exposure
6. Exposure schedule

These parameters are essential to understanding the mechanism underlying the effects of photobiostimulation because too low an exposure will have no effect and too high an exposure can produce deterioration or even destruction of the cells and tissues. This lack of complete description of the LILR parameters used in research may account for the confusion and contradiction present in this field.

Parameters Used in Studies

WOUND HEALING

The early work of Mester on wound healing of chronic ulcers involved the effect of LILR photobiostimulation on ulcers that had been unresponsive to other treatment modalities. After treating 1120 ulcers and other nonhealing wounds with 4 J/cm^2 of HeNe laser light and later with an argon laser twice per week on the entire wound surface, 78% healed and another 14% were improved, while only 8% remained unhealed. The average healing time was 12 to 16 weeks. Other uncontrolled trials of the effect of LILR on healing of decubitus ulcers[10] and of leg ulcers from various causes[11] showed significant beneficial results. Other investigators[12] have found no benefit of LILR on venous leg ulcers. The extent of the investigation of the effect of LILR on wound healing is shown in Table 15–1. An overview of these results indicates that LILR may demonstrate effects of photobiostimulation on wound healing, particularly in its early phases. These effects may depend on the species of animal used. Loose-skinned animals such as rabbits, rats, and mice seem to show a prominent response to LILR, possibly due to enhanced collagen accumulation in the wounded area.[14] There are, however, negative results reported for pigs that are more similar to humans.[15]

EXAMPLES OF LASER-MEDIATED ANALGESIA

Examples of laser-mediated analgesia shown in Table 15–2 are not exhaustive but indicative of scope of work done in this area of clinical pain management and therapy.

Rheumatoid arthritis (RA) is the subject of considerable research interest because of its prevalence in the general population. A number of well-designed and controlled studies find pain lessened, swelling diminished, medication use reduced and morning stiffness improved following multiweek courses of both visible and IR LILR. However, benefits may be limited. Alterations of sedimentation rates, leukocyte counts, platelet aggregation, and C reactive protein concentrations, which may be associated with LILR effects on the immune system, are frequently reported but occur sporadically. The relationship of these factors to clinical effectiveness is still unclear. A multicenter, multiyear study involving HeNe LILR photobiostimulation of hands with RA was presented to an FDA advisory committee in 1988. The study was not approved due to concerns about design limitations, patient selection, and benefit. Another well-controlled multicenter study in 1990 and 1991 evaluated the effect of LILR therapy on RA of the hands with control patients treated conventionally. The study was stopped before completion due to concerns that improvements, if any, were too limited to justify continuation.[6,8]

CURRENT RESEARCH

Cellular Effects

Research on the effects of LILR has been most extensive and systematically carried out in the area of cell processes.[8] However, because of the diversity of experimental protocols and the nonstandard methods of reporting the conditions of exposure and results, the interpretation of the published information presents difficulties.[1] Photoactivation apparently occurs at two levels in biologic systems: the cellular level, which is the localized primary response, and then over a larger contiguous area, which is more of a systemic secondary response.[2] By radioactive labeling of cellular components, Mester and his sons,[16] over a 20-year period, have examined the influence of LILR on the following:

Table 15–1. In vivo animal experiments

AUTHOR	ANIMAL	WOUND	EVALUATED	LASER WAVELENGTH	POWER DENSITY (mW/cm^2)	ENERGY DENSITY (J/cm^2)	EXPOSURE SCHEDULE	EFFECT
Mester (1971) [35]	Mouse	Burn	Diameter	Ruby 694 nm	N/A	0.5, 1, 4, 5, 10	2 × weekly	1 J/cm^2 increased healing
Mester (1973) [36]	Rat	Open skin	Complete wound and collagen synthesis	Ruby 694 nm	N/A	1 4 6	Day 5 Postop Postop	4 J/cm^2 increased healing and collagen synthesis
Mester (1975) [37]	Rat	Muscle injury	Regeneration of muscle	Ruby 694 nm	N/A	1	Every 3rd day × 4	Immediate: increased regeneration but adverse with repeated treatment
Haina (1981) [38]	Rat	Open skin	Granulation tissue formation	HeNe 633 nm	50	0.5, 1.5, 4, 10, 20	Once daily	Increase up to 4 J/cm^2, then decrease
Kana (1981) [39]	Rat	Open skin	Rate of wound closure and collagen synthesis	HeNe 633 nm	45	4, 10, 20	Once daily	None but 4 J/cm^2 increased 3–12 days
Surinchak (1983) [40]	Rabbits	Open skin	Wound area, effect of eschar removal, tensile strength	HeNe 633 nm	Variable	1.1 2.2 4.5	Every 3rd day 2× daily 2× daily	None
Jongsma (1983) [41]	Rats	Open skin	Wound area	Argon 488 and 514 nm	50 200	1 4	After 4 days then 2× weekly	None
Mashiko (1983) [42]	Guinea pig	Open skin	Wound area	830 nm	17	2	Every 2 days	Increased rate of healing
Hunter (1984) [43]	Pig	Open skin	Wound area	HeNe 633 nm	64	0.96	N/A	None
McCaughan (1985) [44]	Guinea pig	Open skin	Wound area	Argon 488 and 514 nm	20	2	Every 2–3 days	None
Mester (1985) [45]	Mice	Open skin	Wound area, cellular content of granulation tissue	Ruby 694 nm	N/A	1.1	2× weekly	Increased rate of closure
Abergel (1987) [46]	Mice	Open skin	Wound area, collagen content, tensile strength	HeNe 633 nm	4.05	1.22	Every other day	Increased collagen and tensile strength
Abergel (1987) [46]	Pig	Open skin	Procollagen levels	HeNe 633 nm	1.56	0.6	3× weekly	Increased levels
Lyons (1987) [47]	Mice	Open skin	Wound area, tensile strength, collagen content	HeNe 633 nm	4.05	1.22	Every other day	Increased collagen and tensile strength
Rochkind (1989) [48]	Rats	Open skin, burns, peripheral and CNS	Wound area, action potential, neuron degeneration	HeNe 633 nm	N/A	7.6 10 10	Daily for 20–21days	Increased rate of healing, action potential increased and degeneration reduced
Braverman (1989) [49]	Rabbits	Open skin	Wound area, tensile strength, epidermal thickness, collagen area	HeNe 633 nm and infrared	N/A	1.65 HeNe 8.25 IR	N/A	None, except increased tensile strength
Enwemeka (1990) [50]	Rabbits	Tendons	Size, tensile strength, energy absorption, strain	HeNe 633 nm	N/A	1, 2, 3, 4, 5mJ/cm^2	Daily	Size decreased, no other difference, but fibroblasts and collagen aligned
Zarkovic (1991) [51]	Mice	Open skin	Wound area, serum lipoprotein content	GaAs 830 nm	50-W pulses	N/A	210 seconds daily, 7 days	Increased rate of healing, decrease in LDLs
Rossetti (1991) [52]	Rat	Brain	Superoxide dismutase	HeNe 633 nm	5	1.08	N/A	Increased SOD

Table 15–2. Examples of laser-mediated analgesia

REFERENCE	LASER	TREATMENT	DIAGNOSIS	N	D	P	EFF	MEASURE	COMMENTS
Atsumi et al. (1987) [53]	830	60 mW CW and pulsed	RA pain	163	Y	Y	82%*	Report	*40% placebo
Basford et al. (1987) [54]	633	0.9 mW, 90 s, CW ×3 pw, 3/52, T	OA thumb pain	81	Y	Y	ns	Numeric*	*+ROM, strength, etc.
Bieglio et al. (1987) [55]	633	N + IR	Radicular pain	?	?	?	+ve*	Report	*inflamm phase; ?neural/vasc mechanisms
Bliddal et al. (1987) [56]	633	10 mW, 5 min, ×3 pw, 3/52, T	RA pain	17	Y	Y	ns	VAS*	*+EMG etc; ?systemic effects
Burgudjieva et al. (1985) [57]	633	T	Postop pain (gynecologic)	179	-	-	+ve	Report	[FLA]
Choi et al. (1986) [58]	904	<1 mW, 60 s, ×2 pw, Acu	Painful elbow	1	N	N	67%	Report*	*+glucocorticoid excretion
Dubenko et al. (1976) [59]	?	?	Tri neuralgia	106	-	-	+ve	Report	[FLA]
Emmanouilidis and Diamantopoulos (1986) [60]	820	15 mW, 90s, CW, ×5 pw, 2/52, T	Sports injuries	62	Y	Y	90%*	Scott/VAS**	Cumulative effect *25%; placebo, **+thermography
England et al. (1989) [61]	904	3 mW, 5 min, 4000 Hz, T, ×3 pw, 2/52	Tendinitis	30	Y	Y	+ve*	VAS**	*$p < .001$; **+goniometry
Galperti et al (1987) [62]	633	<60s, <7.2J/cm^2	PA pain	60	-	-	+ve	Quest	
Gartner et al. (1987) [63]	IR	10–20 min, ×5 pw, 4/52, T	AS, PA, LBP, etc.	546			87%	Report*	*+functional; cumulative effect
Glykofridis and Diamantopoulos (1987) [64]	633; 660–950	<25 mW, var time, CW, ×5 pw, T	Locomotor pain	200	N	N*	+ve	Numeric	*Comparative study; ?analysis
Gussetti et al. (1986) [65]	904/633	5–20 min, ×5 pw, T	PA shoulder	30	-	-	80%	Report*	*+X-ray invest
Jensen et al. (1987) [66]	904	0.3 mW, 30 min, 250 Hz, ×5 pw, T	PA knee	29	Y	Y	nil	Report*	crossover study; *+drug intake
Kamikawa and Kyoto (1985) [67]	IR	× 14 Rx, T	Various	60		Y	79%*	Numeric	*46% "effective"/ 34% fair
Kats et al. (1985) [68]	633	?	Oral pain*	88	?	?	+ve	Report	[FLA], *sialadenitis
Kreczi and Klinger (1986) [69]	633	2 mW, 30 s, 100 Hz, 1 Rx, Acu	Radicular pain	21	N	Y	+ve*	Adapt VAS	*$p<.001$, max post 1 h; effects <9.6 h
Lonauer (1986) [70]	633/IR*	10 min, 15/365, T	OA pain hand	40	N	Y	+ve**	?	*combination preferable; **+ grip strength, etc.
Lukashevich (1985) [71]	633	T	PHN	150			+ve*	Report	[FLA] *versus alternatives
Martino (1987) [72]	CO_2	5 mW, CW?, <20 min, ×5 pw, 3/52, N + T	Mastalgia	50			32%	Keele/Lasa/ Map	[Ab]
Mayordomo et al. (1986) [73]	CO_2	<25 W, scan, CW, 5–10 min, ×2 pday	Locomotor pain	82	?	N	;lt80%	Numeric*	*+thermography
Mester and Mester (1987) [74]	Clust	50 mW	Wound pain	?	?	?	+ve		[Ab]
Morselli et al. (1985a) [75]	CO_2	<25 W scan, CW, 5–10 min, ×3 pw	OA pain	200	N	N	>70%*	?	[Ab], *62% acute effect; effects extend>1 h
Morselli et al. (1985b) [76]	CO_2	<25W, scan, CW?; 10–15 min, ×2 pday	Sports injuries	>100	-	-	+ve	Report	[Ab]
Roumeliotis et al. (1985) [77]	820	15 mW, CW, <25 min, ×5pw, 2/52, T	Sports injuries	31	N	Y	+ve	VAS*	[Ab] *+thermography
Shiroto et al. (1986) [78]	830	<30 s/pt, <7 min, TP+ Acu	Various pain	1600	N	N	85%	Report	[Ab]
Siebert et al. (1987) [79]	633; 904	<30 mW, 1200 Hz, 15 min, 10/365, T	Tendinopathies	64	Y	Y	ns	Numeric*	*+thermography; ?placebo: 10-cm distance
Simunovic (1987) [80]	633	?	Oral pain	?	-	-	+ve	Report	[Ab]
Ternovoy (1984) [81]	633	T + TP	Locomotor pain	400	-	-	+ve	Report*	[FLA]

Table 15–2. Examples of laser-mediated analgesia (continued)

REFERENCE	LASER	TREATMENT	DIAGNOSIS	N	D	P	EFF	MEASURE	COMMENTS
Vidovich et al. (1987) [82]	CO_2	1 mW	RA pain	272	-	-	75%	VAS*	[Ab] *+drug intake, etc.
Walker (1983) [83]	633	1 mW, <30s, 20 Hz, ×3 pw, 10/52, N + T	Chronic pains	36	Y	Y	73%	VAS*	Chronic effect, * +5-HIAA
Walker et al. (1986) [84]	633	1 mW, ×3 pw, 10/52	RA pain	64	S	Y	+ve*	VAS**	*p <.001, **+drug intake
Willner et al, (1985) [85]	904	60 s, 1000 Hz,	OA pain hands	67	?	Y	62%	MPQ*	[Ab], *+drug intake
Zhou Yo Cheng (1987) [86]	CO_2	30 mW, Acu	Minor surgery	40	-	-	95%	Report*	[Ab], *+drug intake

D, double-blind; P, placebo-controlled; Eff, efficacy; Measure, pain measurement method used; RA, rheumatoid arthritis; [Ab], abstract; pw, per week, e.g., 3/52 = 3 weeks; T, topically applied to lesion; ns, nonsignificant findings; ROM, range of movement; N, applied to nerves/nerve roots; VAS, visual analogue scale; EMG, electromyography; [FLA], foreign language abstract; Acu, applied to acupuncture points; Tri, trigeminal; PA, periarthritic pain; AS, ankylosing spondylitis; LBP, low back pain; Rx, treatment; OA, osteoarthritis; PHN, postherpetic neuralgia; Scan laser used in conjunction with scanning

1. Protein synthesis—The effect of ruby laser LILR on RNA and DNA protein synthesis in human fibroblast cultures was studied. There was a significant incorporation of thymidine related to the number of fibroblasts in the S-stage of the cell cycle. The S-stage is the stage of DNA synthesis prior to cell division. The incorporation of uridine and valine was only increased by a small amount. This implies an increase in the number of cells in the process of reproduction.
2. Collagen synthesis—A series of experiments involving ulcers and nonhealing wounds, using LILR from HeNe and argon ion lasers of about 4 J/cm^2, showed a significant increase in collagen fibers, which increased with subsequent exposures to LILR. It was thought that the rates of incorporation of glycine and proline indicated that the primary effect of LILR was in the synthesis of collagen during the collagenous phase of wound healing. There was also an appearance of vesicles having electron-dense nuclei in both intracytoplasmic and intercellular material. These vesicles were thought to release bioactive substances that promoted healing in nonirradiated areas of the wound.
3. DNA synthesis—Human lymphocyte cultures stimulated with phytohemagglutinin (PHA) and treated with 1 J/cm^2 of LILR had a 20% increase in transformation of lymphocytes to large-size, blast-type cells compared with cultures that were only stimulated with PHA but not treated with LILR. This was associated with an increase in the rate of synthesis of DNA of the lymphocytes. There was no effect of LILR on lymphocytes that had not been stimulated with PHA.
4. Cell replication and proliferation—Healing of artificially created skin defects in white mice was significantly accelerated when treated by ruby laser LILR. In the treated wounds, there was a higher number of dividing cells and the wounds closed more quickly. LILR of 1 J/cm^2 from a HeNe laser produced a significant accumulation of the E and F types of prostaglandin in the first 4 days after wounding.

Many other researchers examining the effects of LILR on cell function have reported changes in cell proliferation, motility, phagocytosis, immune response, and respiration. Basford[6,8] has observed increases in RNA synthesis, cell granule release, cell motility, membrane potential, cell binding affinities, neurotransmitter release, oxyhemoglobin dissociation, phagocytosis, adenosine triphosphate (ATP) synthesis, intercellular matrix, and prostaglandin synthesis.

Recently, investigators have shown that an enhancement of cultured human keratinocyte migration subsequent to LILR exposure could be attributed to an increase in keratinocyte motility, but not to proliferation.[17] The effect of LILR on collagen and protein synthesis and cell proliferation has been found by some researchers to produce both increases and decreases in those processes.

Irradiation of normal human mucosal fibroblasts with infrared diode lasers has been shown to have a biostimulative effect on DNA synthesis[18] similar to that observed in HeLa cells.[19]

These effects generally are significant and are too widespread to be easily dismissed. Although the effects of LILR on cell function have been repeatedly demonstrated, to this date there has been no elaboration of the precise mechanisms by which these effects are produced. There has been speculation that the respiratory chain components of the mitochondria—the cytochromes and the prophyrins—might be the primary photoabsorbers in the visible and near-IR wavelengths.[20,21] It has been suggested that LILR may activate the enzymes in the electron-transport chain directly, alter cellular signaling, or increase production of ATP, followed by the augmentation of DNA synthesis and cell proliferation. The action spectrum of LILR for wavelengths from 300 to 900 nm measured by the synthesis rate of nucleic acids in HeLa cell cultures has been determined. The action spectra reveal maxima in the synthesis of DNA and RNA at 400, 630, 680, 760, and 820 nm.[22] However, the direct activation of enzymes as the basis for increased DNA synthesis and consequent therapeutic effects has not yet been verified.

One of the most obvious candidates for absorption of the longer wavelengths is a hemoprotein, probably one or more components of the mitochondrial oxidative phosphorylation system and its constituent cytochromes.[23] The formation of ATP following exposure to HeNe LILR at an energy density of 5 J/cm^2 points to the oxidative phosphorylation system in the inner mitochondrial membranes.[24] Cytochromes A-A3 and copper complex, or cytochrome oxidase, form a functional component of the terminal electron transport system that absorbs light energy in the reduced but not in the oxidized state.[25] Cytochrome oxidase has an absorption peak at 830 nm and also at 605 nm.[26] Cytochromes of the mitochondrial oxidative phosphorylation system might produce a series of chromophores that absorb light over the wide range of wavelengths in which LILR photobiostimulation is observed to occur. Because of the low absorptivities, relatively high power may be required to initiate photon conversion into high-energy phosphate (ATP). Because ascorbic acid crosses the cell membrane against a concentration gradient through a process that can be blocked by uncoupling oxidative phosphorylation, inhibiting electron transport, or anaerobiosis, the change in intracellular ascorbate concentration can selectively alter collagen synthesis.[27]

Thus, one hypothesis proposed for the basis of the photobiostimulative effects of LILR has been the direct stimulation of ATP production. However, this hypothesis seems to be ruled out by the contradicting observation that biostimulation by HeNe laser radiation of HeLa cells increases the stress from trypsinization and plating 5 minutes after exposure; a significant degradation occurred in the exposed cells compared with the nonirradiated control cells. If the trypsinization was delayed until 30 to 240 minutes after exposure to LILR, the number of irradiated cells increased within the first week and later decreased to below the level of the control cells. Thus, the initial and short-term effect of LILR cannot be a result of direct stimulation of the ATP production.[18]

It has been shown that free radicals are present after exposure of biologic materials to LILR.[28,29] The photochemical or photodynamic production of free radicals and oxidants has been proposed as the cause of the effects on cellular function produced by LILR.[30,31]

There have been suggestions that the effects of LILR may be due to the absorption of light in chromophores producing photophysical vibrational and local thermal effects.[32] The changes in the stereotaxic configuration of biologic molecules produced by excitation of vibrational states by the LILR as well as by localized heating could alter the kinetics of biochemical reactions at specific sites during those phases of cellular processes that are particularly vulnerable to alteration. Timing of exposure to the cellular phases would be critical and difficult to control unless careful synchronization of the cultures were maintained. The variability of the effects of LILR in some of the studies cited may be explained by this sensitivity to timing of exposure. These factors only serve to further obscure an already confused area of research. Only careful research in the future can elucidate the mechanisms responsible for the effects of LILR on biologic materials.

FURTHER RESEARCH

Effects of Repetition Rates

In pulsed laser application, the pulse rate may be an important experimental parameter to examine. The lifetime of some excited molecular states may be longer than the period of the pulse, allowing for less efficient absorption of energy. Also, there may be a relaxation time for the biochemical processes resulting from photon absorption, which may be longer than the pulse period that would reduce the efficiency of energy transport into the cellular process.

Timing of Exposure to Cellular Processes

As mentioned in the previous section, the timing of exposure to LILR may be critical in determining the effectiveness of the exposure to alter cellular processes. For example, during DNA synthesis the bonds of the DNA molecule are altered, producing a change in the molecular absorption spectra. This change in absorption spectra would depend on the stage of replication in the cellular cycle. Thus, maintaining a synchronized cell culture may enhance the effects observed in LILR photobiostimulation.

Effects of Exposure to Simultaneous Multiple Wavelengths

Only a few reports of multiple wavelength exposure to LILR biostimulation can be found in the literature.[33,34] The combined effects of multiple wavelength LILR (MWLILR) may result in enhanced photobiostimulation because of synergistic action. The absorption of a photon of one wavelength by a chromophore can excite that molecule into a long-lived state. The molecule in the excited state may have enhanced absorption of a photon with a wavelength that would not be absorbed by the molecule were it in its unexcited state. The combined absorption of two sequential photons can result in greater energy transfer to the cell containing the biomolecule than would be expected from the absorptivity of each photon individually. Because laser light is highly monochromatic, MWLILR exposes biologic materials to much higher photon densities at specific wavelengths than would be encountered in light from ordinary, incoherent sources. The problem is quite complex because the action spectra of multiple wavelengths in cellular processes are not easily measured. However, such information would enable the mechanisms of photobiostimulation to be more precisely elucidated and perhaps be used more effectively.

REFERENCES

1. Baxter GD, Diamantopoulos C, O'Kane S, Shields TD, eds. *Therapeutic Lasers—Theory and Practice.* Edinburgh: Churchill-Livingstone; 1994.
2. Ohshiro T, Calderhead RG, eds. *Low Level Laser Therapy: A Practical Introduction.* Chichester: John Wiley and Sons; 1988.
3. Mester E, Ludany G, Vajda J, Razgha A, Karika J, Tota J. Laser beam actions on bacteriophagocytosis of leukocytes. *Acta Biol Med Germ* 1968;21:317–321.
4. Mester E, Ludany G, Sellyei M, et al. The stimulating effects of low power laser rays on biological systems. *Laser Rev (Lond)* 1968;1:3.
5. Plog FMW. Biophysical application of the laser beam. In: Koebner HK, ed. *Lasers in Medicine.* New York: Wiley; 1980.
6. Basford JR. Laser therapy: scientific basis and clinical role. *Orthopedics* 1993;16(5):541.
7. Nemeth AJ. Lasers and wound healing (review). *Dermatol Clin* 1993;11(4):783–789.
8. Basford JR. Low-energy laser therapy: controversies and new research findings. *Lasers Surg Med* 1989;9:1–5.
9. Basford JR. Low energy laser treatment of pain and wounds: hype, hope or hokum? *Mayo Clinic Proc* 1986;61:671–675.
10. Lievens P. Infrared laser therapy and bedsores. *Lasers Surg Med Suppl* 1992;4:12.
11. Telfer J, Filomencko N, Salansky N. Low energy laser therapy for leg ulcers. *Lasers Surg Med Suppl* 1993;5:56.
12. Santoianni P, Monfrecola G, Martelotta D, Ayala F. Inadequate effect of helium-neon laser on venous leg ulcers. *Photodermatology* 1984;1:245–249.
13. Baxter GD, et al. *Therapeutic Lasers.* 1994.
14. Abergel RP, Lyons RF, Castel JC, et al. Biostimulation of wound healing by lasers: experimental approaches in animal models and in fibroblast cultures. *J Dermatol Surg Oncol* 1987;13:127–133.
15. Hunter J, Leonard K, Wilson R, et al. Effects of low-energy laser on wound healing in a porcine model. *Lasers Surg Med* 1984;3:285–290.
16. Mester E, Mester AF, Mester A. The biomedical effects of laser application. *Lasers Surg Med* 1985;5:31.
17. Hass Af, Isseroff RR, Wheeland RG, et al. Low-energy helium-neon laser irradiation increases the motility of cultured human keratinocytes. *J Invest Dermatol* 1990;94:822–826.
18. Loevschall H, Arenholt-Bindslev D. Effect of low level diode laser irradiation of human oral mucosa fibroblasts in vitro. *Lasers Surg Med* 1994;14:347–354.
19. Karu TI, Kaloenda GS, Letokhov VS, Lobko VV. Biostimulation of HeLa cells by low-intensity visible light. *Il Nuovo Cimento* 1984;3D(2):309–317.
20. Lubart R, Wollman Y, Friedmann H, Rochkind S, Laulicht I. Effects of visible and near infrared lasers on cell cultures. *J Photochem Photobio B* 1992;12:305–310.
21. Karu TI. *Photobiology of Low-Power Laser Therapy.* Chur, Switzerland: Harwood; 1989.
22. Karu TI. Photobiology of low-power laser effects. *Health Phys* 1989;56:691–704.
23. Tiphlova O, Karu T. Role of primary photo-acceptors in low-power laser effects: action of the He-Ne laser radiation on bacteriophage T4–*Escherichia coli* interaction. *Lasers Surg Med* 1989;9:67–69.
24. Passarella S, Casamassima E, Molinare S, Pastore D, Quagliariella E, Catalano IM, Cingolani A. Increase of proton electrochemical potential and ATP synthesis in rat liver mitochondria irradiated in vitro by helium-neon laser. *FEBS Lett* 1984;175:95–99.
25. Yong FC, King TE. The interactions of copper and A3 in cytochrome oxidase. *Biochem Biophys Res Commun* 1970; 38:940–946.
26. Wharton DC, Tzagoloff A. Studies on the electron transfer system. LVII. The near infrared absorption band of cytochrome oxidase. *J Biol Chem* 1964;239:2036–2040.
27. Labbe RF, Skogerboe KJ, Davis HA, Rettmer RL. Laser photobioactivation mechanism: in vitro studies using ascorbic acid uptake and hydroxyproline formation as biochemical markers of irradiation response. *Lasers Surg Med* 1990;10:201–207.
28. Gameleya NF. Laser biostimulation. In: Wolbarsht ML, ed. *Laser Biomedical Research in the USSR.* New York: Plenum Press; 1977:114–145.
29. Derr VE, Klein E, Fine S. Free radical occurrence in some laser-irradiated biologic materials. *Fed Proc* 1965;24(suppl 14):99–103.
30. Ambartzumian RV, Arutunian AA, Voskanian KH, Melkonian AD. Cytotoxic effect of laser radiation. In: Galletti G, Bolognani L, Ussia G, eds. *Laser Applications in Surgery and Medicine.* Bologna: Monduzzi; 1992:247–251.
31. Jori G. The molecular biology of photodynamic action. In: Prateri R, Sacchi CA, eds. *Lasers in Photomedicine and Photobiology.* New York: Springer-Verlag; 1980:58–66.
32. Friedmann H, Lubart R, Laulicht I, Rochkind S. A possible explanation of laser-induced stimulation and damage of cell cultures. *J Photochem Photobiol B* 1991;11:87–95.
33. Becker J. Biostimulation of wound healing in rats with combined soft- and middle-power laser. *Biomed Tech (Berlin)* 1990;35:98–101.
34. Rezvani M, Nissan M, Hopewell HW, van den Aardweg GJMJ, Robbins MEC, Whitehouse EM. Prevention of x-ray induced later dermal necrosis in the pig by treatment with multi-wavelength light. *Lasers Surg Med* 1992;12:288–293.
35. Mester E., Spiry B., Szende B., Tota JG. Effect of laser rays on wound healing. American Journal of Surgery 1971; 122(4):532–5.
36. Mester E., Jaszsage-Nagy E. The effect of laser radiation on wound healing and collagen synthesis. Studia Biophysica 1973;35:227–230.
37. Mester E., Korenyi-Both A., Spiry T., et al. The effect of laser irradiation on the regeneration of muscle fibers. Zeitschrift fur Experimentelle Chirurgie 1975;8:258–262.
38. Haina D., Brunner R., Landthaler M., et al. Animal experiments in light induced wound healing. Laser in Basic Biomedical Research 1982;22:1.
39. Kana JS., Jutschenreiter G., Haina D., et al. Effect of low power density laser radiation on healing of open skin wounds in rats. Archives of Surgery 1981;116:293–296.
40. Surinchak JS., Alago ML., Bellamy RF., et al. Effects of low-level energy lasers on the healing of full-thickness skin defects. Lasers in Surgery and Medicine 1983;2:267–274.
41. Jongsma FMH., van de Bogaard AEJM., van Gemert MJC., et al. Is closure of open skin wounds in rats accelerated by argon laser exposure? Lasers in Surgery and Medicine 1983;3:75–80.
42. Mashiko S., Shimamoto M., Inaba H., et al. Effect of near infra-red light irradiation on wound healing using high power light emitting diodes. Journal of the Japanese Society of Laser Medicine 1983;4:187–192.
43. Hunter JG., Leonard LG., Snider GR., et al. Effects of low-

energy laser on wound healing in a porcine model. Lasers in Surgery and Medicine 1984;3:328.
44. McCaughan JS., Bethel BKH., Johnston T., et al. Effect of low-dose argon irradiation on rate of wound closure. Lasers in Surgery and Medicine 1985;5:607–614.
45. Mester E., Mester AF., Mester A. The biomedical effects of laser application. Lasers in Surgery and Medicine 1985;5:31–39. (See Reference 16.)
46. Abergel RP, Lyons RF., Caster JC. Biostimulation of wound healing by lasers: experimental approaches in animal models and fibroblast cultures. Journal of Dermatological Surgery Oncology 1987;13:127–133. (See Reference 14.).
47. Lyons RF., Abergel RP., White RA., et al. Biostimulation of wound healing in vivo by a helium neon laser. Annals of Plastic Surgery 1987;18:47–50.
48. Rochkind S., Rousso M., Nissan M., et al. Systemic effects of low power laser irradiation on the peripheral and central nervous system, cutaneous wounds and burns. Lasers in Surgery and Medicine 1989;9:174–182.
49. Braverman B., McCarthy RJ., Ivankovich AD., et al. Effect of helium neon and infra-red laser irradiation on wound healing in rabbits. Lasers in Surgery and Medicine 1989;9: 50–58.
50. Enwemeka CS., Rodriquez O., Gall NG., et al. Correlative ultrastructural and biomechanical changes induced in regenerating tendons exposed to laser photostimulation. Lasers in Surgery and Medicine 1990;(Suppl. 2):12.
51. Zarkovic N., Saltzer B., Hrzenjak M, et al. The effect of gallium arsenide laser irradiation and partial hepatectomy on murine skin wound healing and lipoprotein composition. Period Biology 1991;93:359–361.
52. Rossetti V., Lombard A., Urciuoli R., Cassone MC., Rolfo PM. Rat brain metabolism enzyme activity variations following HE-Ne laser irradiation. Molecular & Chemical Neuropathology 1991;15(2):185–191.
53. Atsumi K., Fujimasa I., Abe Y., et al. Biostimulation effect of low-power energy of diode laser for pain relief. Lasers in Surgery and Medicine 1987;7:77.
54. Basford JR., Sheffield CG., Mair SD., et al. Low energy helium-neon laser treatment of thumb osteoarthritis. Archives of Physical Medicine and Rehabilitation 1987;68:794–797.
55. Bieglio C., Bisschop G. de. Physical treatment for radicular pain with low-power laser stimulation. Lasers in Surgery and Medicine 1986;6:173.
56. Bliddal H., Hellesen C., Ditlevsen P., et al. Soft laser therapy of rheumatoid arthritis. Scandinavian Journal of Rheumatology 1987;16:225–228.
57. Burgudjieva T., Katranushkova N., Blazeva P. Laser therapy of complicated wounds after obstetric and gynecologic operations. Akusherstvo I Ginekologiia 1985;6:60–69.
58. Choi JJ., Srikantha K., Wu W-H. A comparison of electroacupuncture, transcutaneous electrical nerve stimulation and laser photobiostimulation on pain relief and glucocorticoid excretion. International Journal of Acupuncture and Electrotherapeutics Research 1986;11:45–51.
59. Dubenko EG., Shuk AA., Safronov GB., et al. Experience with lasers of low intensity radiation in the clinic of nervous diseases. Vrachebnoe Delo 1976:114–119.
60. Emmanoulidis O., Diamantopoulos C., CW IR low-power laser application significantly accelerates chronic pain relief rehabilitation of professional athletes. Lasers in Surgery and Medicine 1986;6:173.
61. England S., Farrell AJ., Coppock JS., et al. Low-power laser therapy of shoulder tendonitis. Scandinavian Journal of Rheumatology 1989;18:427–431.
62. Galperti KG., Fava G., Martino G., et al. Breast cancer: pain therapy in post surgery. Lasers in Surgery and Medicine 1987;7:79.
63. Gartner CH., Becker M., Dusoir T. Pain control in spondylarthritis with infrared laser. Lasers in Surgery and Medicine 1987;7:79.
64. Glykofridis S., Diamantopoluos C. Comparison between laser acupuncture and physiotherapy. Acupuncture in Medicine 1987;4:6–9.
65. Gussetti P., Moroso P., Palazzo C., et al. Calcific shoulder joint periarthritis. Disappearance of calcifications after laser therapy. Radiologia Medica 1986;72:934–936.
66. Jensen H., Harregy M., Kjer J. Is infra-red laser effective in painful arthrosis of the knee? Ugeskr Laeger 1987;149: 3104–3106.
67. Kamikawa K., Kyoto J. Double blind experiences with midlasers in Japan. International Congress Laser Medicine Surgery. Monduzzi Editore, Bologna, 1985.
68. Kats AG., Belostotskava I., Malomud AP., et al. Remote results of the complex treatment of chronic sialoadenitis with the use of helium-neon laser. Vestnik Khirurgii Imeni II Grekova 1985;135:P39–P42.
69. Kreczi T., Klinger D. A comparison of laser acupuncture versus placebo in radicular and pseudoradicular pain syndromes as recorded by subjective responses of pain. International Journal of Acupuncture and Electrotherapeutics Research 1986;11:207–216.
70. Lonauer G. Controlled double blind study on the efficacy of He-Ne laser beams versus Ne-Ne plus infra-red laser beams in the therapy of activated osteoarthritis of finger joints. Lasers in Surgery and Medicine 1986;6:172.
71. Lukashevich IG. Use of helium-neon laser in facial pains. Stomatologiia 1985;64:29–31.
72. Martino G., Fava G., Galperti G., et al. CO_2 laser therapy for women with mastalgia. Lasers in Surgery and Medicine 1987;7:78.
73. Mayordomo MM., Failde JMG., Cabrero MV., et al. Laser in painful processes of locomotor system: our experience. International Congress on Laser in Medicine and Surgery. Monduzzi Editore, Bologna, 1985.
74. Mester AF., Mester AR. Biotherapy 3 and Argon ion, He-Ne, ruby lasers, comparative study of their biostimulative effects. Abstracts, Fifth Annual Congress, 28-30 January 1987. British Medical Laser Association, 1987.
75. Morselli M., Soragni O., Anselmi C., et al. Very low energy-density treatments by CO_2 laser in sports medicine. Lasers in Surgery and Medicine 1985;5:150.
76. Morselli M., Soragni O., Lupia BP. Effects of very low energy-density treatment of joint pain by CO_2 laser. Lasers in Surgery and Medicine 1985;5:149.
77. Roumeliotis D., Emmanouilidis O., Diamantopoulos C. CW 820 nm 15 mW, 4J/cm^2, laser diode application in sports injuries. A double blind study. Abstracts, Fifth Annual Congress, 28–30 January 1987, British Medical Laser Association, 1987.
78. Shiroto C., Ono K., Ohshiro T. Laser stimulation therapy using a diode laser: 1600 patients. Lasers in Surgery and Medicine 1986;6:172–173.
79. Siebert W., Siechert N., Siebert B., et al. What is the efficacy of "soft" and "mid" lasers in therapy of tendinopathies? Archives of Orthopaedic and Traumatic Surgery 1987; 106:358–363.
80. Simunovic Z. Application of He-Ne laser therapy in major and minor oral surgery. Lasers in Surgery and Medicine 1987;7:125.
81. Ternovoy KS. Analgesic laser therapy of patients with post-

traumatic and involutional lesions of the weightbearing locomotor apparatus. Ortopediia Travmatologiia I Protezirovani 1984;7:1–7.

82. Vidovich D., Olson DR. Neodymium YAG laser stimulation as a treatment modality in acute and chronic pain syndromes and in rheumatoid arthritis. Lasers in Surgery and Medicine 1987;7:79.
83. Walker JB. Relief from chronic pain by low-power laser irradiation. Neuroscience Letters 1983;43:339–344.
84. Walker JB., Akhanjee LK., Cooney MM. Laser therapy for pain of rheumatoid arthritis. Lasers in Surgery and Medicine 1986;6:171.
85. Willner R., Abeles M., Myerson G., et al. Low-power infrared laser biostimulation of chronic osteoarthritis in hand. Lasers in Surgery and Medicine 1985;5:1149–1150.
86. Zhou Yo Cheng. Facial cosmetic surgery under laser acupuncture anesthesia. Lasers in Surgery and Medicine 1987;7:94.

16 Tissue Fusion

Paul Kuo

Laser technology has blossomed in recent years, along with the emergence of new, active media and wavelengths. In addition, laser delivery systems are being miniaturized and have become more flexible and convenient to use. With these impressive advances, potential has increased for further clinical application of lasers in surgery and medicine. Two such areas are laser tissue fusion and photoactivation. Photoactivation refers to the use of laser wavelengths to initiate solidification of protein tissue adhesives and tissue substrates, which facilitates laser tissue-welding.

Clinical use of lasers in surgery and dentistry has not yet been universally accepted for a number of reasons. These included the large size and cost of equipment, lack of portability, and the unfamiliarity of a newer system that requires training and practice as compared with conventional surgical instruments such as scalpel or electrocautery. The myriad wavelengths and systems available, each with its own specific properties and hence clinical application, adds to the confusion in this field. For widespread laser use in surgery and medicine, the system should be compact, reliable, inexpensive, and easy to use. To achieve these ideals, miniaturized models of CO_2 laser with flexible waveguide delivery systems and neodymium:yttrium-aluminum-garnet (Nd:YAG) lasers without need for water cooling have been developed. But the system that has the best prospect for wide acceptance in surgery and dentistry is that of the diode lasers. These are desktop and handheld units that are small, portable, and relatively inexpensive. Dye-enhanced photoablation and photoactivation will facilitate the use of these lower-power lasers. At the same time, research is being conducted to increase the power output of diode lasers with the expectation that they may become the dominant laser system in surgery, especially for aerospace and military applications (see Chapter 17).

Laser tissue fusion is being investigated as an alternative to surgical closure with sutures. Although sutures and staple have worked well in general, laser tissue fusion technology is particularly suited to endoscopic and laparoscopic surgery.[1] Laser tissue fusion has the advantage of smaller instrumentation, greater speed, ease of use, and decreased inflammatory response with little or no foreign body reaction. It also allows welded tissue the ability to grow, as compared with conventional sutures that inhibit growth.[2] Furthermore, it offers a complete, circumferential seal of the wound for a watertight closure and decreases leakage, especially when glue reinforcement is added. Experiments comparing bursting pressures of sutured versus laser-glue–reinforced anastomoses in a rabbit aortotomy model showed greater early strength in the latter, using indocyanine green dye–fibrinogen glue exposed to 808-nm diode laser.[3]

DEVELOPING FRONTS

As with laser photoablation, laser tissue fusion requires training, and its success and reliability are dependent on operator skill and judgment. Dew and coworkers[4] used computer-controlled Nd:YAG laser welding in 169 laser skin closures in pigs. They reported good healing without dehiscence with good cosmetic results. The Nd:YAG provided similar penetration depth regardless of tissue wetness or pigmentation. More importantly, the automated welding with computer controlled laser dosimetry (power density, exposure duration, duty cycle) tends to provide a more uniform result, although it does not entirely obviate operator judgment in the final outcome.

Tissue glue or "solder" refers to fibrinogen or other protein compounds that are used to absorb laser energy during welding. This further provides selective localization of the laser energy, thus sparing the underlying host or native tissue from collateral thermal damage regardless of water content or pigmentation. In addition to forming stronger bonds, the presence of tissue glue requires less energy for welding and allows the use of simpler laser systems. Moreover, the margin for error is greater as unsuccessful or imperfect "welds" may be adjusted by secondary treatments without ill effects to the host tissue.

To achieve dye-enhanced photoactivation, the laser/dye pairs are chosen so that their wavelengths/absorption peaks are closely maintained. This allows efficient target-specific delivery of laser energy and enhancement of laser tissue fusion. One such laser/dye combination uses fibrinogen extracts with indocyanine green and an 808-nm solid-state diode laser.[7] The 808-nm wavelength corresponds to an optical window[8] for vascular and other tissues. In addition, adding indocyanine green dye permits selective tissue effects at the area of dye application while sparing adjacent native tissue, because the latter does not absorb within the

808-nm window. Clearly, this minimizes damage to the native host tissue. The physical and optical properties of tissue glue are determined by the protein and carrier ground substance as well as by the dye. Theoretically, by manipulating the proportions of these substances, properties of the tissue glue can be altered to suit specific uses and requirements. However, obtaining fibrinogen for clinical use is problematic, because homologous sources present a risk of acquired infection.

MECHANISM

The exact mechanism of tissue fusion is not clear. It is generally accepted that fusion is a result of photothermal action. There is also speculation as to whether photochemical bonds are formed or changed during the fusion process. Studies of the effect of laser welding on structural protein (collagen) are not conclusive. This is in part due to the use of different wavelengths and welding parameters. Nevertheless, there are some suggestions of formation or degradation of covalent bonds. Overall, a high enough energy or temperature is needed to cause protein denaturation in target tissues so that an amorphous coagulum is formed that infiltrates the native tissue. In this sense, the fibrin glue or solder constitutes a biodegradable scaffold on which tissue edges heal.[9]

IN VIVO STUDIES

In vivo studies performed on blood vessels have provided some insight into the process of laser annealing or coaptation. Assessment of these studies has been made difficult by the use of different laser wavelengths and parameters in different studies. In general, laser-bonded vessels are found to be smoother and less rigid than sutured controls. Theoretically this results in less turbulent flow downstream and hence less trauma to the intima. Moreover, fibrinogen glue is reabsorbed without a foreign body reaction, in contradistinction to the case when sutures are used. Studies of stress-strain analyses reveal similar strength in laser-repaired vessels.[9] The advantage of laser welding is especially evident in small vessels anastomoses where suturing is difficult. They are simpler to weld, particularly when the use of tissue glue obviates the need for precise tissue edge approximation while also preventing excessive heating of host tissues. Reapplication and retrial of fusion can also be carried out without damage to native tissue, and welded vessel tissue has been observed to grow freely as compared with restricted growth of suture-repaired tissue.[9]

Similar observations of decreased foreign body reaction and ease of operation was noted for skin closure. Increased collagen formation was found, with greater strength of laser-fusion skin repair without any long-term wound compromise in strength or cosmesis.[10]

The first successful nerve regeneration of transected rat sciatic nerve after epineurial repair using CO_2 laser was reported by Dew et al.[11] in 1982. The electrophysiology, axoplasmic transport, and light electron microscopic studies of the laser-repaired nerves demonstrated comparability to conventional suture repairs.

Regeneration of transected nerves is predicated upon successful axonal growth into endoneurial tubes left patent by wallerian degeneration of distal segments. Coaptation of transected nerve with sutures inherently does not provide a watertight seal. Axons sprout outside the fascicular and epineurial confines, forming a neuroma with incomplete reinnervation. Investigators have attempted to block such aberrant axonal growth by using different materials such as collagen sleeves, vein, silicon, glass, and fibrin glue. Laser tissue fusion provides a circumferential seal with less constriction at the repair site because of the lack of foreign body reaction. Campion and coworkers[12] used an argon laser to repair transected peroneal nerve of rabbits (power density 100 W/cm^2, pulse duration 200 ms, spot size 0.5 mm via microscope with micromanipulator). They noted enhanced, parallel alignment of nerve fibers at the laser neurorrhaphy site without inflammatory reaction or carbonaceous debris. Changes in collagen substructure were also evident, with actual interdigitation of the layered fibrils occurring, thus allowing for a more complete epineurial seal than was possible by suture repair. Moreover, laser-assisted nerve coaptation could be performed in difficult to reach places and could be done more rapidly.

Bailes and coworkers[13] studied laser-assisted anastomoses in primate peroneal nerves using autogenous sural interpositional fascicular grafts. They used a single stay suture, which was later removed, to aid in the repair and found no difference between the laser experimental group as compared with the suture control group with respect to continuity of nerve, conduction velocity, axon fiber density, and distal/proximal myelinated fiber density. Notably, there was less axonal escape into extrafascicular space in the laser-assisted group, whose sites of repair were not discernible grossly or microscopically at harvest. Other workers have noted weaker tensile strength at coaptation sites in nerve treated with laser tissue fusion.[14,15] Again, a wide range of wavelengths and energy were used in these studies on peripheral nerve or interpositional grafts to decrease tension at coaptation sites and support the laser fusion. Potentially, these adaptations would compromise nerve regeneration. Attempts to circumvent problems with sutures and additional anastomosis sites from interpositional grafts by using other methods such as subcutaneous (SQ) welding with a SQ tissue sleeve[16] to boost strength of the anastomoses have only had limited success. Further work in this area is clearly needed, because the full potential for physically coapting severed nerve ends with sutures has seemingly been reached (Figs. 16–1 to 16–4).

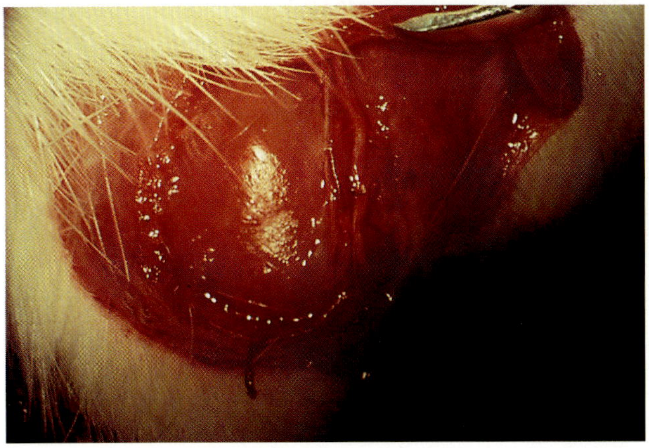

Figure 16–1. Rat sciatic nerve. Nerve transected and then fused with 810-nm dye laser, CW at 680 mW for 20 seconds, 660-μm spot size. (10×.) (Courtesy of Lewis Clayman, D.M.D., M.D.)

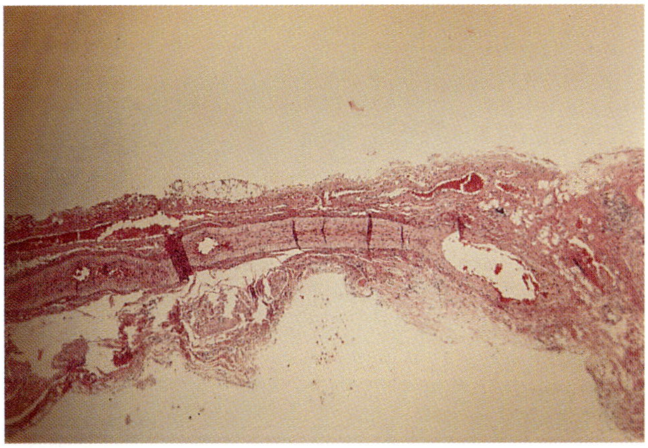

Figure 16–2. Sciatic nerve at 6 weeks. Dense staining vertical band indicates persistent scar. (50×.) (Courtesy of Lewis Clayman, D.M.D., M.D.)

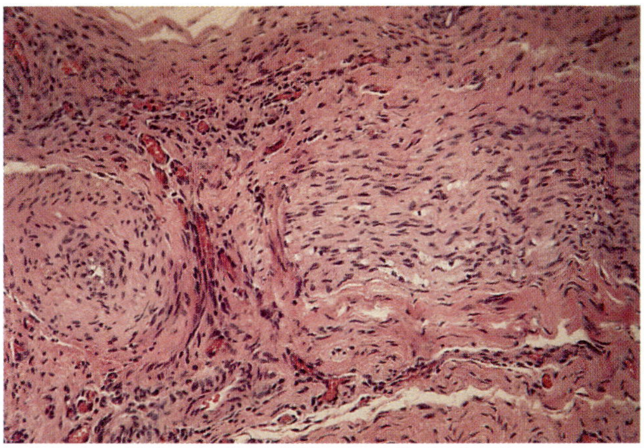

Figure 16–3. Same rat. Residual histologic signs of thermal damage and incomplete nerve healing still present. (250×.) (Courtesy of Lewis Clayman, D.M.D., M.D.)

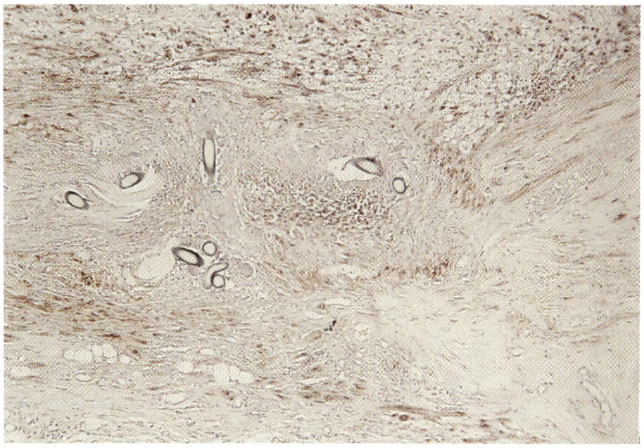

Figure 16–4. Rat sciatic nerve. CW CO_2 laser, 600-μm spot size, P = 0.4 W. PW = 0.2 sec. Six weeks: nerve continuous. (S100 stain.) Partial neuroma at site of stay suture. (25×.) (Courtesy of Lewis Clayman, D.M.D., M.D.)

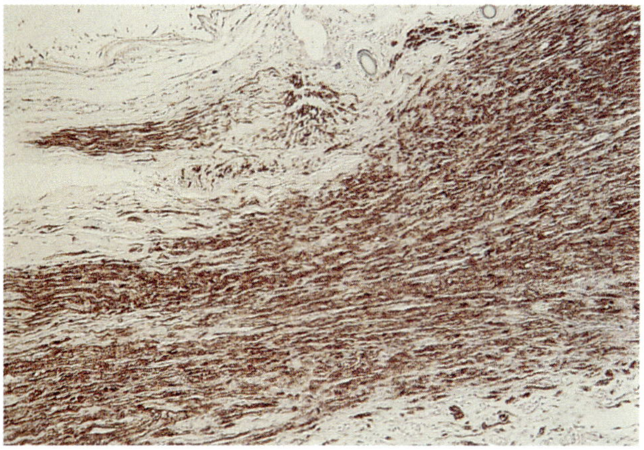

Figure 16–5. Six weeks. Healing complete. Minor disturbance of axonal architecture. (S100 stain.) (25×.) (Courtesy of Lewis Clayman, D.M.D., M.D.)

REFERENCES

1. Bass LS, Ozc MC, Auteri JS, et al. Laparoscopic applications of laser-activated tissue glues. *Proc SPIE* 1991; 1421: 164–168.
2. Frazier OH, Painvin GA, Morris JR, et al. Laser-assisted microvascular anastomoses: angiographic and anatomopathologic studies on growing microvascular anastomoses: preliminary report. *Surgery* 1985;97:585–590.
3. Oz MC, Johnson JP, Parangi S, et al. Tissue soldering using indocyanine green dye enhanced fibrinogen with the near infrared diode laser. *J Vasc Surg* 1980;11:718–725.
4. Dew DK, Hsu TM, Hsu LS, et al. Laser assisted skin closure at 1.32 microns: The use of a software driven medical laser system. *Proc SPIE* 1991;1422:111–115.
5. Grubbs PE, Wang S, Marini C, et al. Enhancement of CO_2 laser microvascular anastomoses by fibrin glues. *J Surg Res* 1988;45:112–119.
6. Poppas DP, Schlossburg SM, Richmond IL, et al. Laser welding in urethral surgery: improved results with a protein solder. *J Urol* 1988;139:415–417.

7. Oz MC, Chuch RS, Johnson JP, et al. Indocyanine green dye enhanced vascular welding with the near infrared diode laser. *Vasc Surg* 1990;24:564–670.
8. Anderson RP, Parrish JA. Selective photothermolysis: precise microsurgery by selective absorption of pulsed radiation. *Science* 1983;220:524–527.
9. Oz MC, Steven K, Libutti MD, et al. Comparison of laser-assisted fibrinogen-bonded and sutured canine arteriovenous anastomoses. *Surgery* 1992;112:76–83.
10. Wider TM, Steven K, Libutti MD, et al. Skin closure with dye-enhanced laser welding and fibrinogen. *Plast Reconstr Surg* 1991;88:1018–1025.
11. Dew DK, Verdeja JC, Shebert RT, et al. CO_2 laser is successful in repair of transected rat sciatic nerve [abstract]. *Neurology* 1982;32(2):A132.
12. Campion ER, Bynum DK, Steven KP. Repair of peripheral nerves with the argon laser. *J Bone Joint Surg* 1990;72-A:715–723.
13. Bailes JE, Jeffrey W, Cozzens MD, et al. Laser-assisted nerve repair in primates. *J Neurosug* 1989;71:266–272.
14. Maragh H, Hawn RS, Gould JD, et al. Is laser nerve repair comparable to microsuture coaptation? *J Reconstr Microsurg* 1988;71:266–272.
15. Benke TA, Clark JW, Wisoff PJ, et al. Comparative study of suture and laser-assisted anastomoses in rat sciatic nerves. *Laser Surg Med* 1989;9:602–615.
16. Korff M, Bent SW, Havig MT, et al. An investigation of the potential for laser nerve welding. *Otolaryngol Head Neck Surg* 1992;106:345–350.

17 Laser Application in Microgravity, Aerospace, and Military Operations

Paul C. Kuo, Michael D. Colvard

Research in space medicine suggests that traumatic injuries in space are reduced, but not eliminated, due to microgravity.[1,2] The need for surgical repair is clear. Conventional surgical techniques are possible in microgravity, but it is difficult to control, contain, and collect fluids, and there is a tendency for arterial blood to scatter.[3–6]

The first use of a CO_2 laser to perform facial and abdominal surgery on rats while aboard an aircraft during high-altitude pressurized flight was recorded in 1992.[7] The experiment demonstrated that aircraft safety and operations are not compromised by the use of a medical laser in flight. Environmental contamination by tissues and fluids was minimal with the use of laser photoablation and photocoagulation for control and stabilization of bleeding wounds. Furthermore, the reduced flotsam and the reusable nature of the portable laser allowed for a reduction in the quantity of surgical materials required without compromising proper surgical and wound care in experimental rats. The investigators observed that surgical precision could be enhanced by the use of a contact laser to counter to some extent the unpredictable nature of air turbulence. In this light, the miniaturization of laser technology with smaller diode lasers of various wavelengths will provide the flight surgeon with portable, reliable, re-usable lasers for expedient stabilization of wounds in aviation and possibly in the zero-gravity, weightless space environments.

Similar miniaturized and compact laser units can be used in trauma care and in field military operations by (combat) medics for wound stabilization and emergency procedures. Early hemostasis and wound sealing reduces bacterial exposure as well as blood and fluid loss and improves wound healing. Recently, a small, totally rechargeable, N:–Cad battery powered diode laser that emits 7 W of energy at 810–900 nm capable of cutting, coagulating and closing wounds in the search and rescue enviroment has been developed.[8] To be effective, these miniaturized units should be configured with pre-set, controlled parameters for predictable wound tissue response. In addition, they must be extremely lightweight, small, and rugged to withstand weather extremes, vibration, and shock. They must have self-contained power sources and be compatible with an external power supply. Biological dressing and dye-enhanced superstrength tissue glue or solder capable of photoactivation, when developed, will further enhance the potential for rapid wound closure using these laser systems. As previously discussed, the use of tissue solder allows for a greater margin of safety to native tissues as well as more uniform, reproducible results, particularly in unskilled hands with less surgical expertise. Currently, diode lasers are the most promising in terms of size and cost. Appropriate clinical features are being developed as mentioned above, and the introduction of diode laser systems with further improved features and delivery parameters should be forthcoming.

REFERENCES

1. Gardener RM, Ostler DV, Nelson BD, et al. The role of smart medical systems in the space station. *Int J Monit Comp* 1989;6:91.
2. Nelson BD, Gardener RM, Ostler V, et al. Medical impact analysis for the space station. *Aviat Space Environ Med* 1990;61:170.
3. Markham SM, Rock JA. Deploying and testing an expandable surgical chamber in microgravity. *Aviat Space Environ Med* 1989;60:76.
4. Rock JA. An expandable surgical chamber for use in conditions of weightlessness. *Aviat Space Environ Med* 1984;55:403.
5. Yaroshenko, GL, Terentyn VG, Mokov MD. Characteristics of surgical intervention under conditions of weightlessness. *Voen-Med ZH* 1967;10:69.
6. Space Life Sciences: A status report. Offices of Space Science and Applications. *NASA* 1990;Feb:5.
7. Colvard MC, Kuo PC, Caleel R, et al. Laser surgery procedures in the operational KC-135 aviation environment. *Aviat Space Environ Med* 1992;63:619.
8. Keipert AG, Garber DD, Colvard MD. *Field Medical Laser System (FMLS) for the Special Operations Command.* Kirkland AFB, New Mexico. Phillips Laboratory Laser and Imaging Directorate, Airforce Material Command, 1994.

Appendix

CO_2 λ = 10.6 μm/10,600 nm Power: CW—up to 100 W, RSP—up to 25W

- Pulse width 350–1200 μs
- Peak power 500–1200 W/pulse
- Pulsed: 10–600 mJ/pulse (up to 400 mJ with Surgilase 150; 200 mJ/pulse with Ultrapulse system)
- Minimum spot size: 0.15–0.30 mm (0.3 mm with 125 mm focal length handpiece)
- 0.6–0.8 mm for microscope units with microslad attachment
- Delivery systems
  - Waveguide
  - Articulated arm (with coaxial HeNe aiming beam)
  - Incision: spot size 0.3 mm: PD ≈ 10^4 W/cm^2 (10,000 to >50,000 W/cm^2)
  - Ablation: spot size 2.0–2.5 mm PD ≈ 400–750 W/cm^2
- Estimation of PD ≅ 100 W/d^2 (d = diameter of spot in mm)

Representative Articulated Arm System (Sharplan)

- CW: 0.1–100 W
- RSP 0.5–2.0 W
- Peak P = 430 W @ 450 mJ/pulse
- Energy/pulse = 150 mJ/200 mJ
- Pulse width = 770 μs
- Aiming beam: 5 mW HeNe
- Duty cycle: up to 15%

CO_2 Scanning Lasers

- Automated scanner: 175–300 mJ/pulse
- Preset output for wrinkle removal

The majority of the cases presented in Chapters 4 and 7 were performed with an RSP CO_2 laser with the following characteristics:

Contact Nd:YAG

- Silica tips: varied
- Typical power
  - Up to 10 W to mark periphery of tumor
  - To incise: 5–25 W depending on tissue

Nd:YAG: free beam: λ = 1064 nm

- Aiming beam: HeNe: 5 mW
- Power: 100 mW to 100W
- Pulse capability: 0.1 to 1.0 sec and CW fiber
- delivery system

SLT Contact Nd:YAG

- λ = 1064 nm

Absorption characteristics

	ABSORPTION COEFFICIENT		PENETRATION IN MEDIUM	
	water (*cm^{-1}*)	*blood* (*cm^{-1}*)	*water* (*cm^{-1}*)	*blood* (*cm^{-1}*)
CO_2	778	800	0.001	0.001
Nd:YAG	0.40	4	2.5	0.25
Argon	0.0001	330	10,000	0.003

From Fuller TA. Chapter 1: Fundamentals of Laser Surgery (pp. 1–17). In: *Surgical Lasers: A Clinical Guide.* New York, NY: Macmillan, 1987.

Erbium:YAG

- λ = 2.94 nm

Argon/argon:dye

- λ = 488, 514, 585
  - Up to 5.0 W
- Spot size: 50 μm to 6 mm

CO_2 Sharplan Laser Pulse Characteristics*

Actual (pulses per second	46	42	92	86	165	157
Avg. power (watts)	20	25	20	25	20	25
Pulse width (millisec)	4.24	6.40	1.62	2.40	0.85	1.15
Pulse period (millisec)	21.74	23.90	10.82	11.60	6.05	6.35
Duty cycle (%)	19.50	93.50	133.60	120.90	142.30	138.10
Avg. pulse power (watts)	102.60	93.50	133.60	120.90	142.30	138.10
Pulse energy (millijoules)	435	597	216	290	121	159

*Note: Pulse characteristics measured from pulse generating circuitry, *not* from actual output. Data courtesy J. Rosenshein, Ph.D.

P = up to 5.0 W
Dye lasers
Candela SPTL vascular lesions laser
Pulsed dye laser, flashlamp excited
10 J/cm^2
2-mm spot size
Alexandrite
Pulsed dye/alexandrite
4 J/cm^2, 8 J/cm^2
3-mm, 5-mm spot size
Gold vapor laser
2.0 W
$\lambda = 627.8$ nm
For PDT
Copper vapor

Matching Laser to Chromophere

LASER		CHROMOPHORE	
NAME	WAVELENGTH(S)	NAME	PEAK ABSORPTION
ArF	193 nm	Peptide bonds	220 nm
XeCl	308 nm	Bilirubin, Beta-carotene	≈310 nm
Ar	488 and 514 nm	Hemoglobin, Melanin, Bilirubin, Beta-carotene	400 – 500 nm
KTP (Nd:YAG freq. doubling)	532 nm	Hemoglobin, Melanin	550–600 nm
Cu vapor	511 & 578 nm	Hemoglobin, Cytochrome a-a3, Red & orange tattoos	550–600 nm, ≈600 nm 510–532 nm
Au vapor	627.3 nm	HpD	350–630 nm
Kr	647 nm	Melanin	400–700 nm
Dye	500–800 nm	Hemoglobin, Tattoos, Melanin, Cytochrome PDT	550–600 nm 350–630 nm
Ruby	694.3 nm	Green/Blue/Black Tattoo ink	694, 755, 1064 nm
Ti:Sapphire	600–1,100 nm	Cytochrome aa3 Green/Blue/Black Tattoo ink	600 nm 694, 755, 1064 nm
Diode	670–1,550 nm	Green/Blue/Black Tattoo ink	694, 755, 1064 nm
Alexandrite	720–800 nm	Green/Blue/Black Tattoo ink	694, 755, 1064 nm
Nd:YAG	1,064 nm	Non-specific	—
Th:YAG	2,010 nm	Water	≥1,400 nm
Ho:YAG	2,140 nm	Water	≥1,400 nm
Er:YAG	2,940 nm	Water	Maximum at 2,940 nm
CO_2	10,600 nm	Water	≥1,400 nm

From: Rosenshein JS, Ph.D. *Physics of Surgical Lasers* Oral and Maxillofacial Clinics of North America, 1996.

Glossary

Laser light occupies several different positions within the electromagnetic spectrum. The infrared emitters are arranged in the near infrared (IR) [neodymium:yttrium-aluminum-garnet (Nd:YAG) 1064 nm, HO:YSGG/2080 nm, holmium (Ho):YAG/2100, erbium (Er):YAG/2920 nm], mid-IR (CO_2: 10,600 nm); the visible light group encompasses all colors (KTP/yellow, argon/green, helium-neon/red, tunable flash pump-dye/many colors, and the ultraviolet group mainly to 193 nm). All forms of laser light are properly characterized by the terms listed below.

Absorption length (Extinction coefficient) Absorption of the first 63% of the delivered energy (rather than 90% as for extinction coefficient). This 63% absorption is measured from the histologic specimen correlating with the vaporized region of the target specimen. There are approximately 2.3 absorption lengths in each extinction length.

Duty cycle Duty cycle refers to the percentage of time the laser is on per second when used in a repeat-pulse mode. It is the product of pulse width and repetition rate multiplied by 100.

Energy Energy is the capacity to do work or, in laser terms, to vaporize tissue. It is measured in joules (J) and can be looked upon as a measurement of dose. An important concept to remember is that a finite amount of energy will vaporize a finite volume of tissue. Studies have shown that it takes 2.4 J of energy to vaporize 1 mm^3 of soft tissue at a fluence of approximately 4 J/cm^2. Laser energy is a product of power (watt) and time of application (sec):

$$\text{Energy (J)} = \text{Power (W)} \times \text{Time}$$
$$10\text{ J} = 1\text{ W} \times 10\text{ sec}$$
$$10\text{ J} = 10\text{ W} \times \text{sec}$$

(The same amount of tissue is removed)

Extinction length Distance from the tissue surface at which the incident beam has been reduced to 10% of its initial intensity.

Fluence (ED) Fluence, or energy density, is the total amount of energy delivered per unit area of the applied laser beam. It is the product of irradiance (W/cm^2) and time of laser application, expressed in J/cm^2. This time of laser exposure also determines the amount of heat conduction to cells immediately adjacent to the target tissue, referred to as lateral thermal heat transfer.

Irradiance (PD) Irradiance, or power density, is the rate of energy delivery per unit area of target tissue. Practically speaking, it is a measure of how intensely the beam is concentrated over a given surface area (W/cm^2). The higher the irradiance, the faster a given volume of tissue is vaporized.

Laser pulse and pulse width (PW) Depending on the laser medium, the laser light emitted may be continuous or pulsed. A continuous wave laser beam (e.g., CO_2) emits an uninterrupted beam at the output power set for as long as the switch is turned on. It can also be chopped or gated to form a train of pulses. If the on-off duty cycle is controlled by repeated direct current cycling or by radio-frequency control, rapid superpulsed output pulses of brief duration occur. The superpulse beam has a peak power that far exceeds that set on the console power. Usual energy is 50 to 200 mJ/pulse at peak powers up to 1200 W per pulse. Ultrapulsed lasers maintain higher energy/pulse and produce pulses of 200 mJ/pulse. The laser exposure time, called pulse width or pulse duration, refers to the duration of an individual pulse during which energy is delivered. It has been estimated that a pulse width as long as 650 μs is short enough to prevent significant heat diffusion from the target tissue to adjacent tissue, thereby preventing significant unwanted thermal damage.

Power Power is the rate of energy delivery, or how fast energy flows. It can be thought of as an instant measure of energy output. The unit of measurement is the watt (W), which is defined as one joule per second. The line power output of a laser is the power of the laser beam at its exit point from the laser.

Pulse repetition rate (PRR) Repetition rate is the number of laser pulses per second, measured in Hertz (Hz).

Spot size Spot size refers to the diameter of the laser beam as measured by creating a laser impact of 0.1 sec at 10 W on a moistened wooden tongue blade. It varies with the distance of the incident beam from the laser handpiece to the target tissue (see Fig. 3–7). The energy distribution within the beam spot is not uniform. Rather, it follows a Gaussian curve, being highest in the center and tapering off toward the periphery, creating a laser crater as the beam hits the target tissue (see Fig. 3–4). Approximately 86% of this beam is available to create the vaporization crater. When the beam is in focus, the power density is at its highest for any given output power. Because the area of a circular spot changes with the square of its radius, a doubling of the spot size, when the beam is defocused, will result in a fourfold decrease in power density. Therefore, when the laser is used in the defocused mode, the beam geometry is flattened out, which permits controlled ablation of tissue to occur.

Thermal relaxation time The process by which heat diffuses through tissue by conduction is referred to as thermal relaxation. Thermal relaxation is the time required for tissue to dissipate 50% of the heat absorbed from the laser pulse by diffusion.

Zone of coagulation necrosis Lethally damaged tissue secondary to lateral thermal damage (heat conduction) adjacent to the vaporization crater. May also be a carbonized region.

Zone of sublethal injury Peripheral area injured by lateral heat conduction that has the capacity to recover.

Zone of vaporization Volume occupied by the vaporization crater. This is the tissue actually removed by the explosive vaporization of the laser pulse.

Index